NST

Spinal Integration

• OSTEOPATHY FOR THE NEW MILLENNIUM •

Michael Nixon-Livy

NST
Spinal Integration

• OSTEOPATHY FOR THE NEW MILLENNIUM •

edi·ermes

NST SPINAL INTEGRATION • Osteopathy for the New Millennium •
by Michael Nixon-Livy • www.nsthealth.com • e-mail: info@nsthealth.com

ISBN 978-88-7051-719-4 - Paper edition

ISBN 978-88-7051-720-0 - Digital edition

External relations - Edi.Ermes srl - Viale Enrico Forlanini, 65 - 20134 Milan (Italy)
Phone +39.02.70.21.121 - Fax +39.02.70.21.12.83
e-mail: editorial@ediermes.com

Drawings: Dr. Michael Nixon-Livy – Dr. Levent Efe/MedicalArts
Marco Fanuli, Andrea Rossi Raccagni and Raffaella Stilo/Edi.Ermes Archive

Paper edition printed in January 2021 by Aziende Grafiche Printing, Peschiera Borromeo (MI), Italy
for Edi.Ermes - viale Enrico Forlanini, 65 - 20134 Milan (Italy)
http://www.ediermes.com - Phone +39.02.70.21.121 - Fax +39.02.70.21.12.83

Preface

It is often said that there are two things in life that are always a certainty – death and taxes! Benjamin Franklin, 1789.

But birth is not mentioned in the same context, yet without it, death is not possible. Birth is therefore at least, equally as much an unavoidable certainty, as death and perhaps taxes are.

Consequently, what is also guaranteed for all of us is the temporary nature of life itself and barring accidents, life can be either more temporary or less temporary, but it's temporary! I am convinced that how our "life" is managed from birth and beyond will ultimately have a powerful determination on when and how death takes place.

Working with many thousands of patients, students and colleagues over a clinical career spanning thirty years, or more in one form or another, what has become blatantly obvious to me is that the single most precious commodity, holding apart the points of birth and death, making the process of life "less temporary" is a robust state of health.

And there is no question that millions of people around the world lack the ability to create this most precious yet fundamental commodity for themselves.

They engage in lifestyle practices that deplete their "vital life force" at such a rate that becomes unsustainable as they reach their 60's, 70's and 80's, and the points of birth and death draw ever closer together, courtesy of one type of disease, malady or health crisis or the other; then finally the organism can no longer act as a viable receptacle, and a life is cut short all too soon.

Yet science tells us that our human genetic potential is such that we can live to 120-140 years of age which is almost twice the average age that most people actually live to.

So where are we going wrong and how and what can we change?

Ultimately, the answer is multifactorial but some basic concepts and principles that are fundamental and perennial are worth considering, as they relate to spinal therapy and its underpinning philosophy.

First and foremost, I am a spinal therapist, and like many other spinal therapists share the belief that if we can ensure that everything from the cranium to the coccyx is in its right place then physiology will flourish, disease will diminish and health will abound.

And there's no doubt, that to a large extent "Structure Governs Function" is my philosophical and daily working mantra that I live by in clinical practice.

But the truth is it would be wonderful if it were only that simple!

In fact, I can adjust the spine, every day of a person's life, yet it won't make them healthy!

They might feel better for a while, but the issue(s) that provoked their malady in the first place, if not attended to, will serve to pull the spine and the organism with it, out of balance again and again.

In other words, if we could sit around all day eating hamburgers, drinking booze and smoking cigars, and it extended our life span and the quality of our life span, then *count me in*, as I'd be the first to do it, simply because like most stimulating experiences, it feels great when you are doing it!

But sadly the reality is that it's the opposite and practices such as these shorten our lives.

Sure, everybody knows somebody who lived to 90 or 100 years of age and smoked like George Burns (1896-1996) but it's not the norm, and I bet you that walking briskly up a flight of stairs would not have been possible for George!

So there's age and "quality of life" that both need to be considered in what determines a healthy life, and our spinal adjustments, indeed if they are going to be of use at all, need to be considered in that broader context.

This book is written with the professional therapist in mind whether he or she are at the beginning of their clinical career or further advanced.

It is primarily designed to provide an insight into the Neurostructural Integration Technique – NST – and its workings, plus the wonderful process of natural self-adjustment (autoregulation) that the human organism is capable of and readily moves into when stimulated with this unusually effective and dependable therapeutic approach.

Throughout the book I will make some important distinctions between being pain-free and being healthy as they are very different realities in many respects.

I will present NST as unique spinal integration method that can quickly be learned by professional practitioners and applied with exceptional effect to help the countless individuals who suffer daily from back pain, neck pain and any other pain to be quickly free of their maladies. And hopefully throughout the process learn that they are the ultimate drivers of their unique process of life.

In this context it's fair to say that NST can not only become wonderful pain removal technique, but a profoundly effective starting point from where good health and a better way of life may be attained, so that this wonderful but temporary process of life becomes somewhat less temporary and somewhat more energized, enjoyable, fulfilling and therefore meaningful.

Ultimately, NST will have tremendous appeal for a broad variety of professional therapists including physiotherapists, osteopaths, neurologists, chiropractors, craniosacral therapists, sports medicine therapists, postural and musculoskeletal therapists, who want to quickly and efficiently incorporate a world class therapeutic approach into their clinical practice, that will not only quickly and dependably help their patients on a daily basis, but will also rapidly build reputation and career success.

However, this book is far from scientific in that it will encourage you to buy into working more so with the "art of therapy" as opposed to the "science of therapy" which I seriously doubt exists to any great extent, in any case.

I am very favorably disposed to research and regard it highly for the insights and wisdom it can deliver, in helping to propel us forward as a species equipped with better knowhow.

It's my experience, that observing how the human organism is responding to a sequence of procedures, as opposed to trying to direct it into a predictable or premeditated response, can be the difference between a powerful and sustainable therapeutic outcome, or the opposite.

I will however provide you with logical ideas, concepts and models upon which NST was designed, and via which it can be best understood and operated, and to this extent I trust, that the content will have an appeal for the more scientifically minded, while striking a chord of common sense at the same time.

It is also my firm belief that the "context" in which therapy takes place is almost as important as the applied therapy itself, and that "context" can be influenced and created as much by what the therapist says, as what they do.

To be clear, NST of course is not a placebo-based approach, nevertheless we would do well as practitioners to recognize that "therapeutic momentum" is real, and is something that every client who chooses to come for therapy naturally brings with them to a greater or lesser extent.

That it can facilitate the process of therapeutic outcomes and healing is not in question.

Ultimately, the simple formula of enhancing therapeutic momentum, applying NST, observing what the organism does in response, and making further adjustments either in the clinic or in the lifestyle, will elicit extremely satisfying clinical outcomes for patient and practitioner alike.

Acknowledgements

My deep appreciation goes to the four men who had the most direct impact on the creation of NST and whose shoulders I firmly stood on to get NST up and running. They are Tom Bowen, Dr. Charles Krebs, Dr. Major Bertrand DeJarnette, and Dr. Trevor Creed.

Many thanks also go to a group of individuals who believed in NST and myself in the very early years, making it possible for NST to take flight in Europe and beyond. They are Alfred Schatz – IAK Institute Freiburg, Germany; Dr. Jean Claude Pigout and Dr. Jean Paul Romano – CFK Institute Marseille, France; Dr. Dominique Monette – IBK Institute, Brussels, Belgium; Dr. Riccardo Scognamiglio – Instituto di Psicosomatica Integrata, Milan, Italy; and Dr. Joe Mercola – Mercola Enterprises, Chicago, USA.

My heartfelt thanks also go to Burkhard Behm ND, Dr. Alessandro Aloisi, Dr. Eddy Milet, David Johnson MA, Gordon Dickson ND, and Olivier Ruppen ND, for their wonderful friendships and for the help, support, expertise and encouragement they unselfishly provided me, to find new ways forward in growing NST, whenever I needed it.

And to the other great organizers and sponsors who came after them, and who similarly believed in NST and myself, and continue to support the growth and proliferation of NST including, Dr. Geert Drenth and Dr. Jan Berx – Profon, Belgium; Dr. Emanuela Martinoli – Edi.Ermes – Milan, Italy; Anke Schilling ND – Gotha, Germany; Dmitriy Merkulov – Meridian – Saint Petersburg, Russia.

My thanks go also to the many wonderful NST Teachers who have come on board for a short while or longer, and through whose eyes I got to see the world of teaching NST from a completely other perspective.

Finally, to my beautiful wife Joanna, who was my sole sounding board throughout the writing of the book. Her unwavering patience, encouragement and expertise in all matters NST, physiotherapy, osteopathy and naturopathy, made the task of writing the book a lot of fun.

And to our beautiful and strong-willed little daughters, Kalina (3.5 years) and Viktoria (8 months) who always had so many clever strategies, for getting me away from my work station to be with them. Although I admit to sometimes being frustrated, I came to grasp the sheer wisdom in their demands, as they helped to make me relax and laugh countless times every day, ultimately keeping me sane.

Special Thanks

I would also like to extend a very special thank you to Raffaele Grandi and Emanuela Martinoli, directors of Edi.Ermes, for their generous invitation and encouragement to write this book, which has been sitting on the back burner for too many years.

After many years of prodding from other potential publishers, and never really getting close to a starting point, it took a single invitation from Raffaele and Emanuela for me to know that they were the right people to work with. The stars aligned perfectly because of whom they are, and their honesty, fairness and clarity throughout impressed me enormously. I thank them both sincerely for making the publishing of the NST book a reality.

To my amazing wife Joanna,
and our two beautiful little daughters Kalina and Viktoria.

The combination of your wonderful support, encouragement,
patience, capacity for distracting me a hundred times a day,
and endless love, all somehow fused beautifully,
to add so much enjoyment and merriment to writing the book.

With three such vibrant characters having my back,
there's nothing better I could have asked for.

Thank you all so much for everything – you mean the world to me.

Contents

Introduction

FROM PHENOMENA TO DAILY OCCURRENCE

Since the late 1980s when I first started using a very rudimentary version, of what would later become integrated NST, I was astounded by the sheer regularity with which many patients suffering from physical pain and mental stress would remarkably be free of their symptoms, and return to a state of balance, after just a handful sessions.

I had come from a background of chiropractic, manual therapy and kinesiology where I had also seen magical results taking place with some patients, but never in the same way or with the same regularity that I saw this work achieve it.

So little effort for such big improvements in such a short space of time. Surely, I must be dreaming, I used to think back then, because I was literally witnessing the beginnings of a phenomena occurring in my own clinic on a daily basis.

Never before had I worked so easily and experienced such outstanding results.

Long standing pain would dissolve, energy increased, spirits were lifted and my patients became happier and more hopeful about life without me even suggesting that that's what they needed to do; medications were reduced or discontinued and many surgeries completed avoided.

Now after almost thirty years of using NST and many thousands of patients later, I still see the same phenomena day after day. Perhaps the novelty of it all has diminished to some extent, but not the immense satisfaction I receive when a patient has finally discovered a solution to their health problems, and decided to make adjustments to how they plan to move forward on their life's journey from this point onwards.

And it's undoubtedly a double benefit for them, to be free from their symptoms, while discovering how not to create them again in the future.

My hope and wish is to share this phenomenal therapeutic intervention called NST with as many other professional clinicians around the world, so the reality that I and my patients have been experiencing for so long also becomes a reality for them and their patients.

Indeed, since May 1996 I have been teaching NST to groups of professional clinicians around the world, and today in 2020 the NST community of practitioners numbers approximately six thousand, who on a yearly basis consult approximately 8 million patients around the world.

I am delighted by what has happened over the last 24 years via this steady pace of growth, but I am not at all satisfied that the job is complete, and my wish and passion is to continue the teaching of NST at a postgraduate level well into the future.

I am also delighted and deeply grateful to have had the expert help of some excellent teachers over the journey, who have shared my passion, and contributed significantly to the growth and population of the NST practitioner community.

HISTORY

The genesis of NST as integrated and teachable system, unbeknownst to me at the time, began in 1993 when I joined the clinical practice of Dr. Charles Krebs in Melbourne, Australia, at his invitation, to help him with a burgeoning client load, that was most exclusively comprised of children suffering from Dyslexia, ADHD, Autism and a variety of other behavioral and "brain-related" conditions.

Charles, who had also been my main teacher in Kinesiology some years earlier, had developed his own system for correcting or improving the above conditions, and he'd called it LEAP (Learning Enhancement Advanced Program) and I had been one of his most avid supporters and practitioners for some years.

Exacerbating his client overload situation was the fact that Charles spent long periods out of Australia and therefore his clinic, teaching LEAP in Europe, where it had started to make a name for itself at many of the big Institutes there.

LEAP was fast becoming a revolution in the field of Kinesiology, and there was no mistaking why, as it literally worked wonders for children suffering in particular from Dyslexia and ADHD conditions. The positive benefits this had for the families of affected children were significant as well.

Up until 1993 I had run and operated no less than five of my own very successful clinics in and around Melbourne, namely in Maldon, Box Hill, Doncaster, Caulfield and Kew, establishing a solid reputation for resolving spinal, musculoskeletal, learning and emotional conditions, and I was passionate about everything I had become well known for.

But the opportunity to join Charles and deal almost exclusively with LEAP patients was also appealing and had many advantages, amongst which was the fact that his clinic was attached to a Kinesiology school that was a well-known hub for research in the field, but also a center for other highly capable and successful practitioners, who had their clinics under the same roof.

Indeed, once I joined the clinic it was an exciting time, but I quickly became afflicted with the same client overload issues as Charles had, and was booked in advance for up to three months at a time.

Part of the issue was that LEAP was exceedingly thorough, and required patients to come in for a two-hour session once a week for 8-12 consecutive weeks, depending on the severity of their condition and their rate of response.

One of the important parts of all LEAP treatment programs was to clear the patient of "neuro-energetic switching" perhaps better described as confusion within the body's meridians, energy systems and spinal reflexes.

This part of the LEAP program had to be done at both a superficial level and a deep level, and one of the frustrating issues was, that from week to week with certain children, the deep level corrections needed to be redone as they were not holding.

I wanted to find a solution to this and naturally defaulted to using my spinal work, which was my own blend of some of Tom Bowen's (Australian) osteopathic work, DeJarnette's (USA) chiropractic work mixed with a bit of classical osteopathy.

Having studied all three some years earlier I nevertheless regarded Bowen's work as the most efficient of all.

To my surprise at the time, I discovered that the spinal corrections not only corrected superficial and deep level switching, but the children's conditions stabilized much more quickly. I also discovered that access to deeper areas of the brain to do with visual and auditory memory, the limbic system generally, and the hypothalamus, became much easier, as did the LEAP corrections for them as well.

Undoubtedly to me this was a revelation, as I was able to reduce by 50% in most cases the time I needed to spend with each child to take them through the LEAP system.

Twelve two-hour sessions suddenly turned into 6 two-hour sessions and so on.

There were suddenly positives on all levels, in that the children could enjoy the benefits much sooner, I could see more children and the cost to parents was halved, resulting in a win on all levels.

My waiting list went from 3 months to about 5 weeks and never deviated from that.

The only issue I had was that Charles might not be so thrilled with me having dabbled with his system, and frankly at the time I did not know how to tell him, until one day after one of his overseas trips he dropped into the office and asked an obvious question: "How are you getting through the cases so quickly and effectively"?

I must admit to feeling uncomfortable about explaining it all to him at the time, but in true collegiate style, Charles simply celebrated the news, and said let's look into why this is happening.

Charles was a scientist and researcher at heart, and nothing delighted him more than setting up protocols and tests to garner the essence of some particular system, be it physiological or energetic.

Delving into why the spinal work accelerated and stabilized the LEAP correction so efficiently, became the starting point for building NST into a system although this was not the intention at the time.

After about twelve months of testing at the Carlton clinic, we were both convinced that my spinal work and kinesiology belonged together, and Charles could not have been happier or prouder that it had happened in his own workplace.

It was now October 1995 and he was heading off for another European tour, this time starting with a first stop at Lake Garda in Italy, to attend a large Kinesiology symposium with hundreds of attending delegates from around the world.

As I met him in the corridor one day a few weeks prior his departure, I enthusiastically implored him that he must share our discoveries with his colleagues over there. He said nothing for a few seconds and then with a steely gaze that I will always remember, retorted - "I'm not going to tell them anything, you come and tell them the story yourself".

I nervously laughed off the idea, saying that it would be far better him telling them about it all, as he had the credibility with LEAP and more, but again he insisted I come. I quickly started to realize that he was not joking at all, but indeed very serious.

"What about the clinic? Who would manage the patients?", I said. "Don't worry they will still be here when you get back", he quipped.

His plan suddenly started to take shape in my mind more and more, as he offered to connect me with all of the right people at the symposium, with the idea that I might be able to travel and teach at some level in the future as well.

Speaking appointments at the symposium were already filled, but having direct access to the principles of Europe's largest colleges in Kinesiology, really appealed to me.

Within days I had my ticket and hotel booked and was on my way not long after.

At the conference I got to meet principles from colleges in Belgium, France, Germany, Italy and Spain and gave many demonstrations.

To my great surprise, the overwhelming sentiment was that they were not so much interested in how my spinal work might interface with any current kinesiology programs, rather they wanted to see the work packaged into an integrated and teachable format, some even guaranteeing me, that if I could deliver a manual by March of 1996, that I would fit into their next cycle of seminars in 1996 and then 1997 and beyond.

I was really in a quandary now, as I had thought that my future was well mapped out in Melbourne, Australia, for at least the next decade.

I came back to Australia after that trip with more confusion than clarity, but family and loved ones, all solidly backed the idea and encouraged me to think about tackling it full on.

But even if I bought into the idea, how was I going to put my spinal collection of strategies of Bowen and DeJarnette's work into a system that made sense and could be taught?

As providence would have it, one of the visiting practitioners to our clinic in Melbourne was Dr. Trevor Creed, an accomplished SOT® Methods Chiropractor, who had designed and developed his own system of spinal work that involved somewhat unbelievably, correcting a patient's etheric template.

As challenging as it may sound to be able to adjust the spine, sacrum and cranium by not touching the body, this work was for real and he called it Chiron.

Trevor was no light-weight in respected professional therapy circles either, and had previously held the position as President for the Association of SOT® Methods Doctors in Australasia. He knew his SOT® Methods like no other, and had studied with DeJarnette personally.

When he adjusted the spine from 20-30 cm above the body you could literally "feel" every correction, and the results were identical to a high velocity thrust. However, the whole subject of Chiron is a story for another day, but suffice it to say that I was speaking with the right person when it came to building teachable systems around unknown concepts.

As Trevor knew that I had studied some SOT® Methods, he initially simply challenged me with the concept of exploring the relationships between Bowen's work and DeJarnette's work as a single integrated system, claiming that they must be very similar. He provided me with many stimulating suggestions to point me in the right direction.

As it turns out, the research and testing that Charles and I had previously undertaken, to integrate the spinal work with LEAP, would serve as a template for investigating the corollaries between Bowen's work and DeJarnette's work more precisely.

From that point onwards, I undertook months of intensive evaluation of the two systems, and built the various works of Bowen that I knew, around the operating system that was the core of DeJarnette's work - namely the Secondary Respiratory Mechanism.

By February 1996, the body of work that would become known as NST had finally taken shape, and had been trialed on some hundreds of patients with great effect already.

Both in my heart and gut I knew that something very special had taken place with the whole story of NST, but I was yet to trial it on professional practitioners in a seminar setting who were paying good money to attend.

The first manual became a reality by April 1996, and by May 1996 I was presenting NST to a group of thirty Osteopaths and Physiotherapists at the CFK College in Marseille France.

The seminar was a great success, and NST had taken root at the highest level, in one of Europe's most demanding and critical osteopathic and physiotherapeutic landscapes of France.

Since that time, I have personally taught over 450 multi-day seminars, in various countries around the globe, while an additional 200 more multi-day seminars have been taught by my band of wonderful teachers.

NST is now a very well-established and respected spinal integration system, throughout Europe, United Kingdom, Switzerland, Russia, USA, Canada and Australia.

This book I trust, will help to convey the NST message and know how, with more depth and clarity, for both the already experienced practitioner, and those interested in learning NST.

About NST 1

OVERVIEW

Let's look at a black and white objective definition of what NST is, and how it is applied, so that we have a general framework within which we can add more detail moving forward.

NST is a uniquely designed and remarkably effective soft tissue Osteopathic method, developed in Australia in the early 1990s by myself with valuable input from a variety of colleagues along at the time. NST's construction and underpinning philosophy were significantly influenced by the Osteopathic work of Thomas Bowen, Australia, and the Chiropractic work of Dr. Major Bertrand DeJarnette, USA.

NST or "Neurostructural Integration Technique" refers to the manner in which the technique is applied and points to some of its underpinning philosophy. Said in reverse (technique integration neurostructural), NST is a technique for the integration of the structure via stimulation of the neurological and neuromuscular systems.

NST utilizes absolutely zero mechanical adjustments to the bones themselves, as in classical Osteopathy or Chiropractic, preferring instead to adjust the spine, pelvic girdle and cranium directly through applied sequences of specialized rolling movements called Pri-moves (proprioceptive rolling impulse movements), and remarkably the results achieved would make any Osteopath, Chiropractor, Physiotherapist and others, feel extremely gratified.

The Pri-move is unique to NST and has three fundamental steps to it.

1. Firstly, there is a stretch over a designated muscle, tendon, ligament or nerve.
2. Once the stretch is performed, contact is made to the same underlying structure, and in many cases, the patient is advised to inhale and exhale.
3. On exhalation, the same underlying structure is crossed in the reverse direction to which the initial stretch was performed (Fig. 1.1).

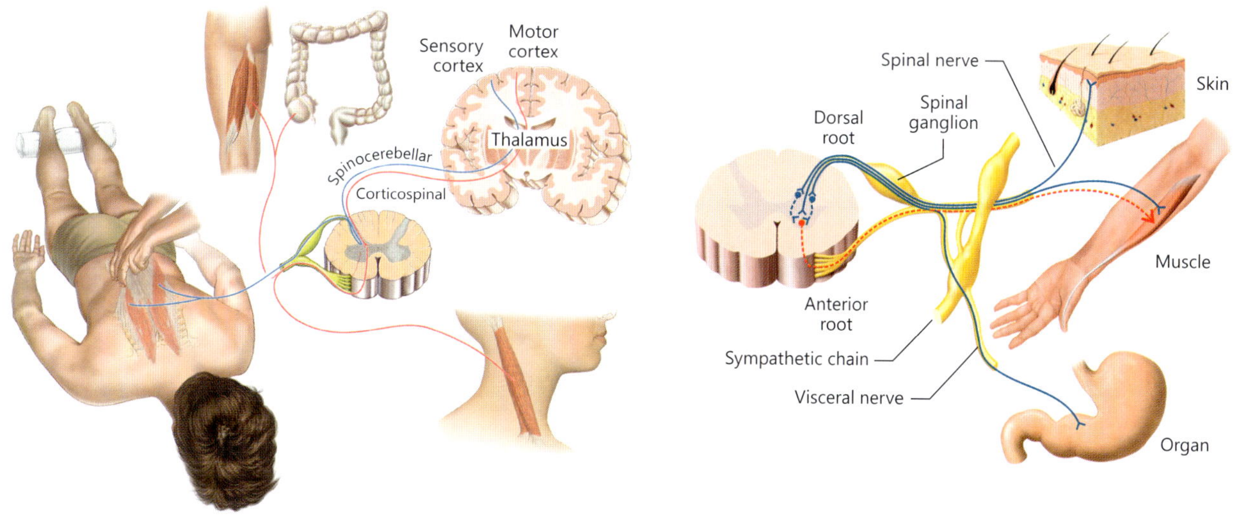

Figure 1.1 The Pri-move is performed using a "stretch-contact-move" formula. A Pri-move may simultaneously affect muscles, organs, fascia and nerves depending on where it is performed. The basic physiologic model of the Pri-move is akin to the functionality of a spinal segmental reflex, where stimulating one structure within the reflex arc may cause all parts to integrate.

The basic physiologic model of the Pri-move is akin to that of the spinal segmental reflex response, where I can stimulate the skin with an acupuncture needle and create a response in an organ or muscle innervated by the same neural pathways. Or I can stimulate an organ and affect the surface tension of the skin and subcutaneous connective tissue and muscle. Or I can stimulate a muscle with a Pri-move and affect the skin, subcutaneous connective tissue and organ as well as the muscle.

Pri-moves applied to the spinal column musculature will create a multi-level response, including local sedation and pain removal, while, at the same time, a similar response in muscles of the upper and lower body, remote to the site that has been treated, may be experienced.

As an example, the first Pri-move applied to start an NST session is at the level of L3-L4 lumbar vertebrae, and will cause a general sedation of the lumbar spine, a relaxation of the hamstring muscles and general relaxation of various neck muscles.

Whereas Pri-moves applied to the upper and lower extremities (arms - legs) tend to be more local in their effect, arguably mediated via more direct muscle spindle and Golgi tendon reflex responses.

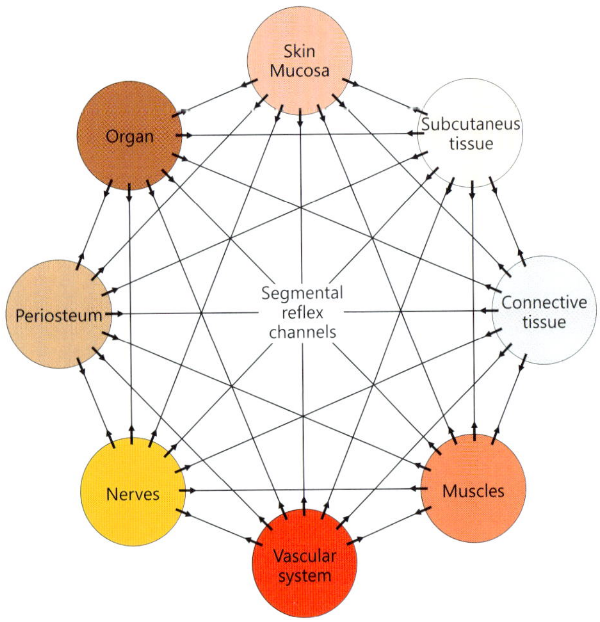

Figure 1.2 Interpreting the outcome of every Pri-move is not possible or useful to the therapeutic outcome of NST. Pri-moves appear to have a chaotic "Random Reflex Response", the sum total of which serve to induce the organism back to homeostasis.

The combination of the both spinal and extremities Pri-move stimulation creates an unmistakable total body integrative outcome.

Interpreting and tracing the effect of every Pri-move is considered to be both irrelevant and unrealistic, as the degree and intensity of response of every Pri-move is highly subjective.

Rather, the practitioner looks for changes in muscle tension and tone compared bilaterally, and at the same time, evaluates the status of the iliolumbar ligaments. Leg length is also considered to be a very helpful guide, as to the effectiveness that the sequences of Pri-moves has achieved and TMJ likewise, are yet another valuable barometer.

The level of integration that exists in the human organism via muscular, fascial, nervous, endocrine and energetic systems is far too complex I believe, to even warrant attempted interpretation. I can stimulate a muscle with a Pri-move on one person and an organ may function better, whereas the same Pri-move in the next person will cause a leg muscle to twitch or perhaps a subtle movement in the scalp.

The sheer breadth and level of complexity that the human organism has within its own reflex systems, and therefore at its disposal for self-adjustment, it almost limitless.

Indeed, it appears as though the body knows how best to adjust itself, when stimulated in a systematic manner such as with NST.

It is for this reason that, after observing thousands of patients go through their own unique journey back to balance, I like to think of the Pri-move sequences as causing a "Random Reflex Response" where the stimulation of a strategic NST point or points, can cause relaxation or release in "seemingly" unrelated and unpredictable structures elsewhere in the body. If there is any magic in NST, then it is the "Random Reflex Response" phenomena, that creates the sleight of hand (Fig. 1.2).

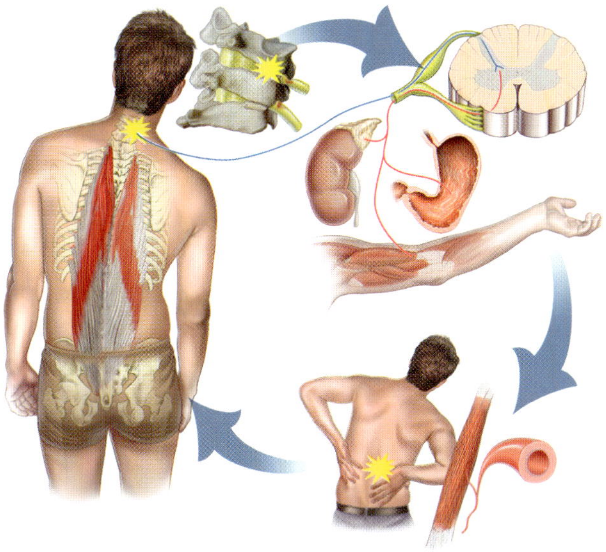

Figure 1.3 Poor lifestyle and postural habits may lead to muscular tensions that become cumulative and progressive, causing pain, dysfunctional physiological conditions and stress.

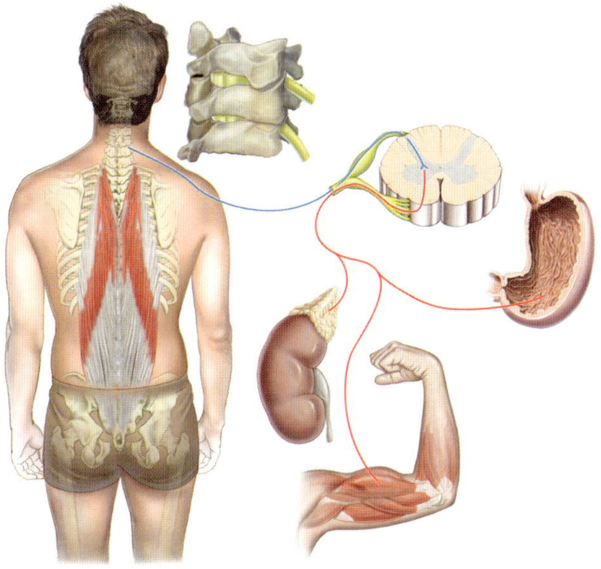

Figure 1.4 Balanced bilateral tensions in the Micro (cranial-neck) and Macro (below the neck) systems are the goals of NST to ensure optimal physiological function between nerves, muscles and bones.

If there is one important lesson that I have learned in applying NST, it is to "observe" what a person's body does after the stimulation, as the results, although similar in many cases, are also highly subjective and definitely not always predictable. Curiosity and ignorance can help to create a potent context in the therapeutic setting.

AIM

The main aim of applying NST is to remove pain, correct dysfunctional physiological conditions and psychosomatic stresses, by eliminating irregular muscular tensional patterns that have manifested in the body, due to poor postural habits, injury, and poor lifestyle habits (Fig. 1.3).

To this extent, correcting the tensional relationships between nerves, muscles and bones is paramount, and indeed, one of the main guiding principles surrounding NST's application.

Adhering to the basic principle that muscles move bones primarily, and not the other way around, emphasis therefore is placed squarely on ensuring that the muscular system is balanced bilaterally, both at Macro and Micro levels.

However, the ultimate goal of any NST session is to restore the systematic and involuntary function of the sacro-spino-cranial system, including the autonomic nervous system, via the restoration of balanced muscular tensions and consequently "tensegrity" throughout the body (Figs. 1.4 and 1.5).

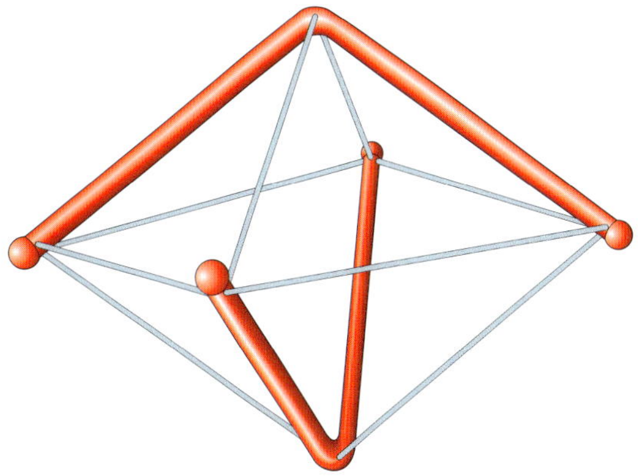

Figure 1.5 This tensegrity model helps explain the tensional relationships existing between the bones of the body (red tubes) and the collective soft tissues (gray cables) that act on the bones. When tensions are balanced the bones are ideally positioned to permit proper nerve transmission and optimal function of the sacro-spino-cranial system.

APPLICATION

NST's application is firmly rooted in the philosophy that "symptoms" are manifestations of the "system" having lost its integration at one level or the other.

Consequently, regardless of the symptoms that patients might present with (for example, back pain, neck pain, autoimmune issues, menstrual disorders, digestive disorders, headaches, etc.), the whole system is evaluated and adjusted as an integrated system.

At the very minimum, each and every patient receives a core spinal balance consisting of lumbar, thoracic and cervical spine adjustments that form the platform for any further corrections that may be necessary.

Most typically, however, an integrated session will include the core spinal balance plus some releases for the upper and lower extremi-

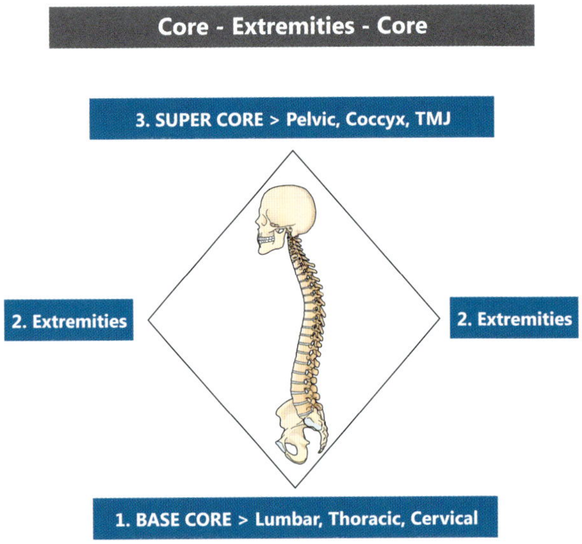

Figure 1.6 Following a structured Core-Extremities-Core template, patient assessment and subsequent choice of appropriate procedures, becomes a simple and organic process. Clinical process is simplified while powerful autoregulating responses are guaranteed.

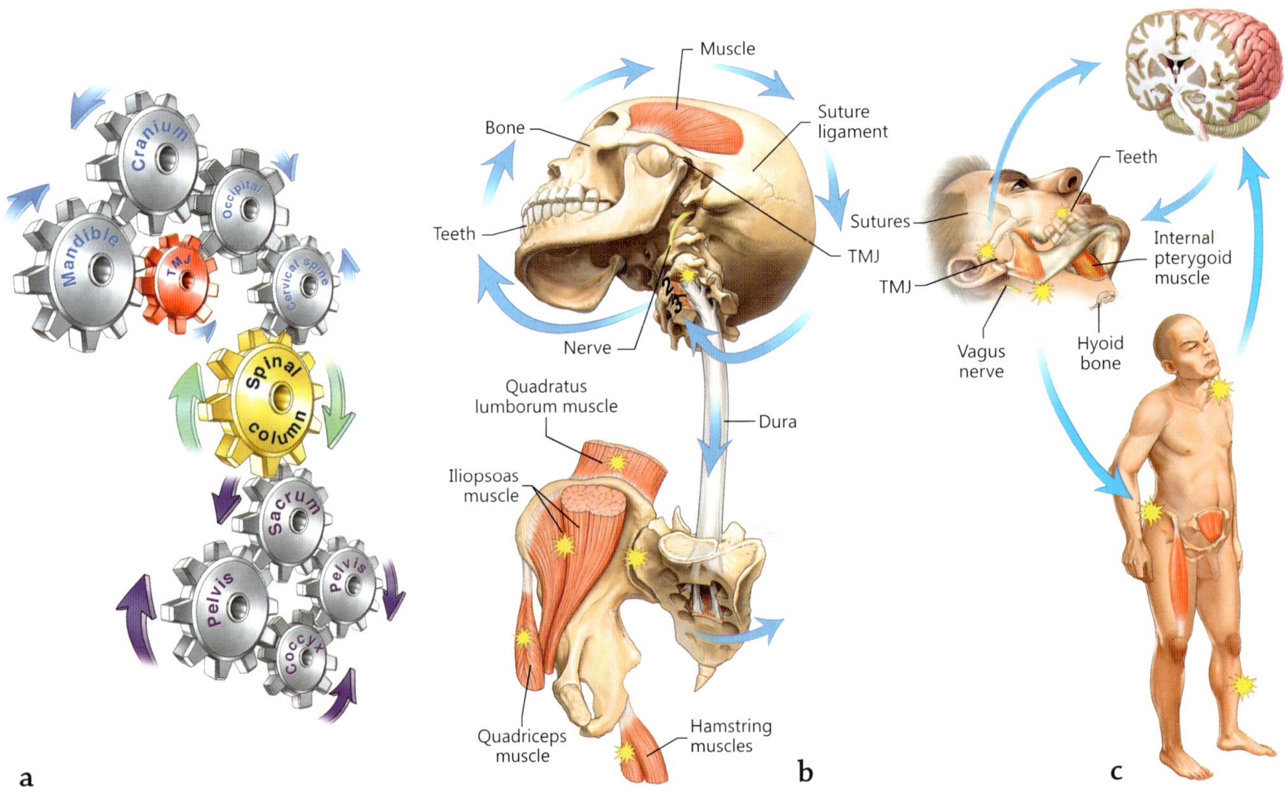

Figure 1.7 Micro-Macro system concepts. (**a**) Interlocking gears with TMJ highlighted illustrating its connectivity to all body parts. (**b**) Image illustrating that all components of the cranium (Micro system) need to be integrated for the spine and rest of the body to be integrated. (**c**) Image illustrating when Micro-Macro system integration is lost that the body enters a perpetual imbalance cycle that is frequently evident in chronic and/or degenerative conditions.

ties and most likely further adjustments for the diaphragm, sacrum, pelvis and TMJ.

Importantly, working in this Core-Extremities-Core fashion clearly "alerts" the innate autoregulating capacity of the body to get to work, thereby providing much of the unique and powerful unlocking and integration, that takes place within the human organism after an NST session (Fig. 1.6).

The practitioner quickly experiences and realizes that what they have at their fingertips is a powerful and dependable Osteopathic system, that is quickly and simply applied with dramatic and convincing outcomes for a high percentage of patients.

Significantly, a great deal of importance is attached to the temporomandibular joints (TMJ) and their ability to affect almost anything and everything in the body, which is a hallmark of NST system.

The relationship of the TMJ to the rest of the body is viewed in a Micro-Macro sense, where the TMJ, along with the teeth, tongue and chewing muscles belong to the Micro system, that exerts a hierarchical influence over the Macro system represented generally by the vertebral spinal column, pelvic girdle and the rest of the body (Fig. 1.7).

RESULTS

Using a "System before Symptom" approach means that there is no health issue that cannot be safely and effectively addressed with NST. In fact, NST is suitable for all acute and chronic conditions and for all age groups, from newborn babies to the elderly.

However, as history would have it, NST is renowned around the world as a "wonder technique" for correcting back and neck pain but, in reality, this is a very small percentage of the vast array of maladies and conditions that respond quickly and profoundly to the application of a few NST sessions (Fig. 1.8).

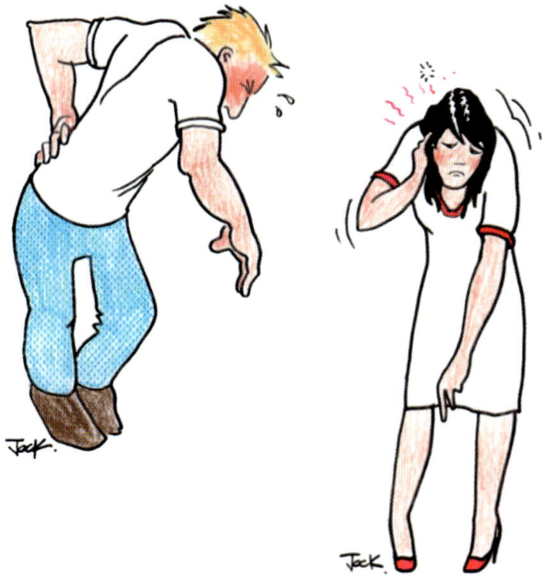

Figure 1.8 Acute and chronic back and neck pain conditions are routinely resolved in just 2-4 sessions using NST and with a high degree of sustainability in the corrections.

International NST statistics confirm that in general clinical practice, where patients are presenting with conditions from back pain to autoimmune disorders, over 85% of patients will require just 2-4 sessions of NST to achieve total resolution of their presenting condition. If the condition is not fully resolved, it will be significantly and noticeably improved for the better.

Of the 15% of patients who do not experience total resolution after 2-4 sessions, 10% will require between 5-8 sessions to achieve total resolution while 5% will require ongoing sessions at approximately one visit per every 7-14 days, depending on individual symptoms.

As an example, a patient suffering with Parkinson's disease may require ongoing sessions at the rate of one every 10 days to remain symptom free.

And results also appear in stages that I call Stage 1, Stage 2 and Stage 3.

Stage 1. Results are those that are most obvious and apparent directly after a session, and in the first 24 hours. These are typically rapid reduction in pain, increased range of motion and better energy levels.

Stage 2. Results are those that become apparent over the ensuing two to five days, and are more gradual and progressive. Often a patient may feel pain free directly after a session only to find themselves either back in discomfort or dealing with a new symptom 36 hours after their session. This will typically be followed by a partial or full return to balance within 72 hours after the session. This is testimony to the process of autoregulation at work, that NST initiates.

Stage 3. Results are those that tend to trickle in seven to ten days after the session, whereby the organism is continuing to adjust and heal itself. This may involve the reduction of chronic inflammations through improvement in blood and lymph flows. These results tend to be progressively more and more settled and permanent.

IN THE CLINIC

NST has been designed with the modern practitioner in mind, and is both user-friendly and does not require heavy physical effort on the part of the practitioner. In fact, many practitioners switch to NST for this reason alone!

An NST session may last 15 minutes or 45 minutes depending on presenting symptoms.

Yet another unique feature of NST in application, is that symptom patterns unlock more effectively by giving the patient a pause on the treatment table for around 5-10 minutes, at strategic points in the session.

For many practitioners, this creates the practical opportunity to start working with another patient and likewise leave the patient rest for a while as well.

Although the resting periods are not mandatory, they are most often appreciated by patients, and do allow the practitioner to treat around 3 patients per hour on average.

On the other hand, some practitioners prefer to use a more holistic approach, where they spend extra time with each patient by giving lifestyle recommendations after the session, and NST lends itself very well to this style of clinical application as well.

CONCLUSION

NST is a modern day soft tissue Osteospinal (Osteopathic) system that is easy to learn and reproduce instantly in the clinic, for outstanding results, that greatly satisfy patient's requirements, whilst building reputation and success for the practitioner.

Bowen and DeJarnette 2

THOMAS AMBROSE BOWEN

Thomas Ambrose Bowen (1916-1982), who called himself an Osteopath but never formally qualified as one, enjoyed a tremendously successful clinical career that spanned 30 years, and had the unrivaled status of treating some 13,000 patients per year with a success rate of 88% in just 1-3 sessions (Fig. 2.1).

They are staggering statistics and certainly caught the attention of many other doctors and professors back in the 1950s, 60s and 70s who wanted to know how he did it. They simply wanted to know how his system worked.

Frustratingly, for one and all of his interrogators, was his simple response that "explanations are not important when people are getting well".

Whether he knew and understood the mechanisms behind what he had created or not remains unknown to this day, but what we do know about him is that he had a freakish ability to feel nerve and energy flows in the body, and based his therapeutic interventions to a large extent, on this alone.

However, coupled with this uncanny knack was his ability to feel changes in tissue tension, both gross and subtle, and also used this as a mandatory rule to achieving a successful therapeutic outcome.

He observed patterns of muscular imbalance in the body that could run from a hamstring muscle then contralaterally via the sacrum through the erector spinae muscle group and up into the cervical spine.

According to the five students he taught throughout almost 30 years and who learned largely by observing him, his penchant for rules also went further, in that he insisted that the "cycle of the body" needed to be balanced to ensure that the therapeutic goal had been achieved for the patient.

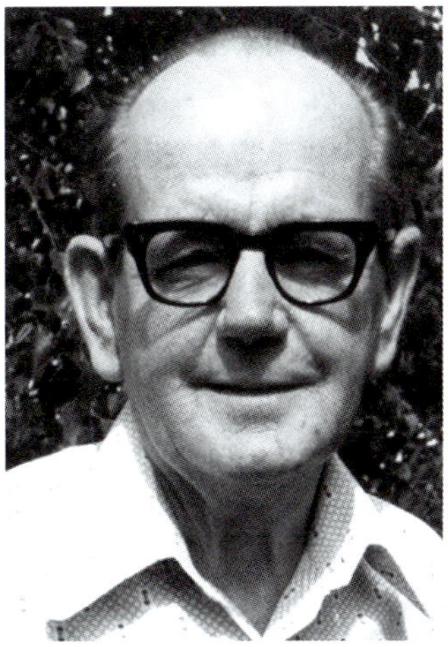

Figure 2.1 Thomas Ambrose Bowen (1916-1982). A great humanitarian and gifted genius in the field of Osteopathy, whose ideas and methodology inspired the development of NST, that continues to help millions of individuals annually to loose their pain and enjoy better health.

He paid special attention to the coccyx and TMJ, in particular citing that if the coccyx was left unbalanced, the "cycle of the body" would not come back into balance either. And the TMJ he considered to be the "black box" or "radar control" of the body.

MAJOR BERTRAND DEJARNETTE

Major Bertrand DeJarnette (1899-1992), on the other hand, was a qualified Osteopath and Chiropractor and famously developed SOT® Methods (Sacro Occipital Technic™). He was far more detailed and scientific in the way he approached the body and evaluated its connec-

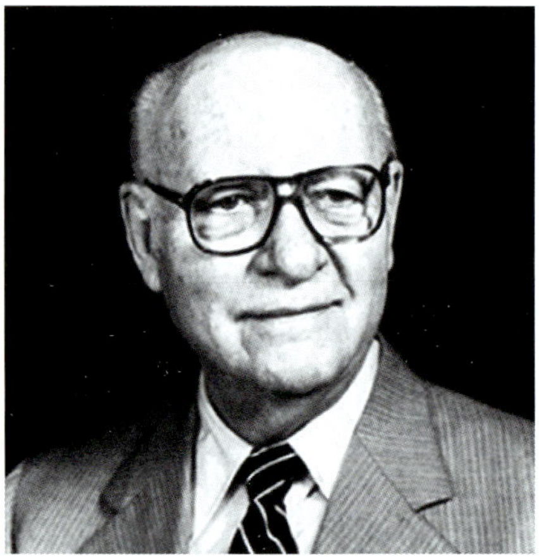

Figure 2.2 Major Bertrand DeJarnette (1899-1992). A deep scientific thinker and humanitarian who developed SOT® Methods, and whose ideas and methodology helped inspire the development of NST, that continues to help millions of individuals annually to loose their pain and enjoy better health.

tions and unravelings. His clinical career lasted 60 years and he continually researched and perfected his techniques (Fig. 2.2).

It cannot be said perhaps, that he treated the same number of patients with the same degree of success as did Bowen, but he certainly taught many more than five students, and made massive contributions to the world of health generally, and like Bowen, has a rich progeny who continue to flourish and help millions around the world to find pain relief and better health to this day.

DeJarnette observed patterns of whole body muscular imbalances that ultimately manifested in localized fixations. He identified three distinct categories simply called Category I, Category II and Category III, and used them as a way to help the physician diagnose and treat the patient accurately and appropriately.

Briefly, Category l faults had to do with disturbance of the Primary Respiratory Motion (discussed later), disturbing the relationship between sacrum and occiput, cranial meninges, cerebrospinal fluid flows and vasomotor function.

Category ll faults are specifically related to mechanical dysfunction between the sacrum and ilium, hence pelvic girdle. When the sacroiliac weight-bearing capacity is affected, symptoms may manifest as whole body pattern proprioceptive and muscular imbalances, with faults in the spinal column, cranial sutures, TMJ and extremities.

Category lll faults manifest as an ongoing instability at the sacroiliac joints causing S1-L5 and L5-L4 upward pressure on intervertebral discs, resulting in disc herniation and nerve root compression at those levels. Psoas and piriformis muscles were considered in this category along with sciatic nerve irritation and/or compression.

Leg length is also considered a valid assessment, as are sacral ligaments.

SOT® Methods use strategically placed cushioned wedges between the patients anterior-superior thigh to help the pelvis and sacrum come back into balance, after which a variety of additional hands-on adjusting techniques may be used to complement the affect that blocking has had.

POINTS IN COMMON

Although terminologies, ways of looking at patterns of imbalance and corrections may differ, SOT® Methods and Bowen's work nevertheless have a lot in common.

The fundamental principle that patterns of muscular imbalance pull the bony skeletal system out of place causing pressure on nerves and intervertebral discs, resulting in stagnation of the vascular, visceral, endocrine, energy and fluid systems of the body, creating further consequential muscular imbalance with more chronic and degenerative outcomes, is ultimately identical in both systems (Fig. 2.3).

In my working with both systems, I have come to respect both men enormously for being creative geniuses and masters of their respective systems.

DeJarnette's ability to provide elegant descriptions of the complexity of imbalance in the human organism, and ultimately categorize it, is second to none. Bowen's ability to see the patterns of imbalance from his own unique per-

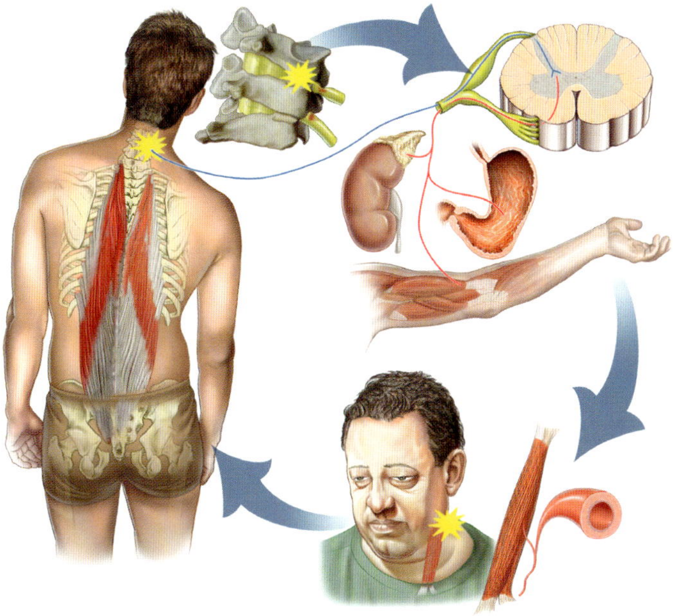

Figure 2.3 Patterns of muscular imbalance pull the bony skeleton out of place, resulting in bones coming into contact with nerves, leading to a host of consequences for the body's systems and physiology, ultimately resulting in further muscular compensations and pain.

spective and adjust them with so much simplicity, yet elegance, is both astonishing and inspiring (Fig. 2.4).

It is my opinion that the essence of both men's work remains with them, as it is only they who saw it, and they who knew it, the way they did. That so many others have been able to use their work in one form or another, and even more people benefit from it as patients, is a testimony to the insatiable passion that both men had to find solutions to help their fellow man.

In the creation of NST, I was obviously inspired by SOT® Methods and Bowen's work, and wanted to deliver to the global therapeutic community a technique that embraced the essence and spirit of both men's work, but fashioned it in such a way that both assessment and application became simple and straightforward to learn and use.

I believe that you could teach the basic mechanics of NST to a child and they would get great results, but beyond that point there is still so much more scope for learning the subtleties of the work that, once learned, render even the most difficult of cases resolvable.

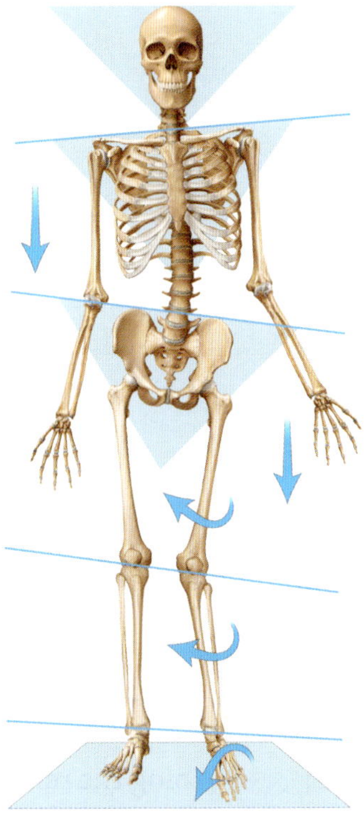

Figure 2.4 Both DeJarnette's and Bowen's approaches identified complex patterns of musculoskeletal conditions within the body and both systems were capable of unraveling them in a systematic fashion with excellent clinical outcomes.

NST Operating Systems 3

The first principle of NST is that the human body is highly integrated organism capable of self-adjustment or autoregulation. Indeed, the human body's vigilant and unrelenting ability to continue to adjust and adjust itself until it can do so no longer (and life itself expires) is a testimony to perhaps its most defining feature of all – "adaptation".

To understand why and how the human body has this level of integration and consequently ability to adjust itself, we need to go back to the point when we all started biological life as a fertilized egg.

SPINAL DEVELOPMENT

In the process of embryogenesis an embryo forms and develops. And from the moment fertilization of an egg or ovum takes place by fusion with a sperm, a myriad of chemical and electrical changes commence, intelligently conspiring to ensure that embryological development unfolds with both the right timing and precision to ensure life continues.

The ovum is typically asymmetrical in shape and has an "animal pole" that later becomes the ectoderm and mesoderm, and a "vegetal pole" that later becomes the endoderm. The fertilized ovum is called a zygote (Fig. 3.1).

At every step of the way new associations are made, resulting in the formation of new cells, tissues and systems. At every step of the way "integration" is the guiding mantra of the living cell, and it achieves this both profoundly and thoroughly at all levels, of the organism it is building.

Scientists studying embryogenesis have

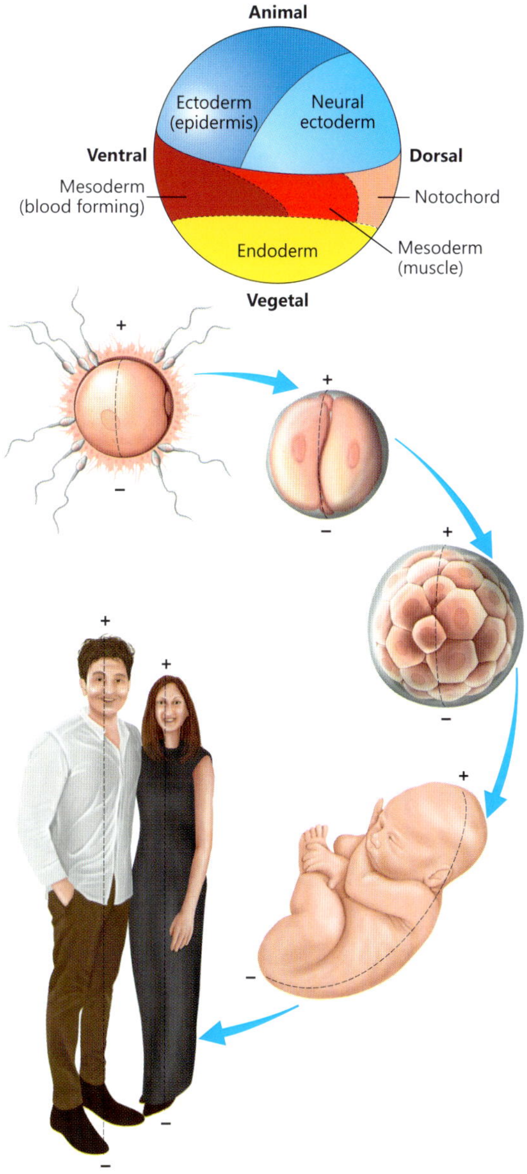

Figure 3.1 From the single fertilized ovum up to the fully developed fetus, integration is the guiding mantra of the unfolding embryo as it is swept throughout its development along the migrating layers of ectoderm, mesoderm and endoderm, coerced by the steady rhythmic flux of the cells electrical system.

known for decades now, that at the moment fertilization takes place, a measurable electrical impulse is established across the fertilized egg that has a positive and negative aspect to it. In other words, an electrical polarity. And this electrical polarity communicates along a very specific axis that effectively divides the egg into two equal halves.

Significantly, this electrical polarity guides the process of embryological development through to fetal development and then full gestation, finally manifesting as the craniosacral flows that can be detected by holding certain points on the head and base of the spine (Fig. 3.1).

Interestingly, if we follow the migration of the cells clustered around the positive and negative poles in the single fertilized egg, into when it becomes a more recognizable miniature human at approximately 12 weeks, we discover that the cells adjacent to the positive pole in the single fertilized egg migrate to form the cranium and the brain while the cells adjacent to the negative pole migrate to form the tip of the vertebral spinal column, namely the coccyx (Fig. 3.2).

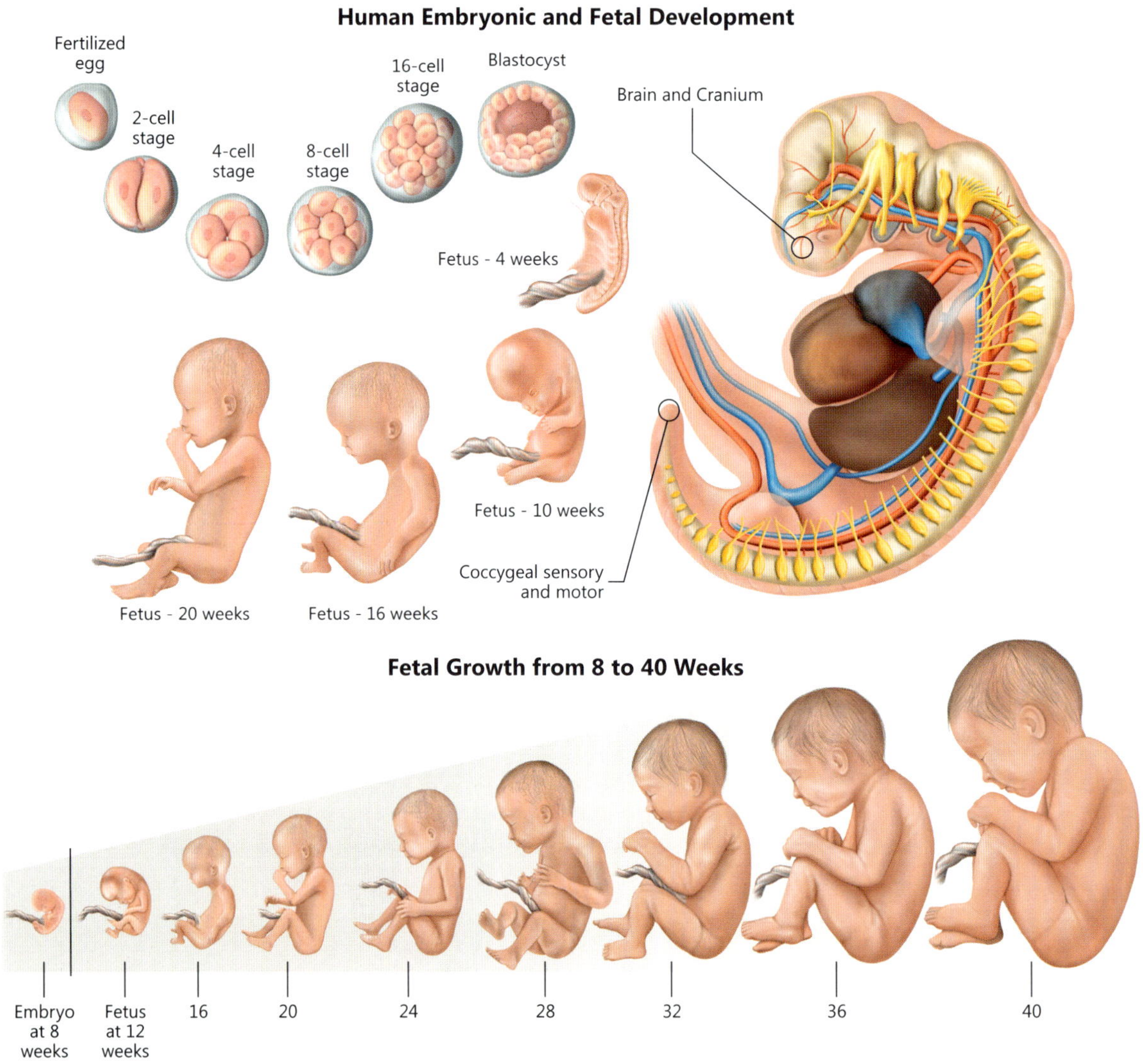

Figure 3.2 The integration that exists in the single fertilized ovum is perpetuated throughout embryological and fetal development with predictable results in the formation of the human body. The opposing poles of the single fertilized egg migrate away from each other to form the cranium and coccyx both major regulating centers of the craniosacral system and hence physiology.

The specific axis, that once formed the pathway for communication in the single fertilized egg, unfolds into the neurological spinal cord and its membranes plus the vertebral spinal column and its ligaments and muscles.

That such specific integration exists in the human organism is not a fluke, but an evolutionary phenomenon, without which there would be no organism, let alone the ability for it to be able to regulate and sustain itself throughout a lifetime.

And indeed, when we reflect on the musculoskeletal system itself, through which NST seeks to adjust the whole organism, we should not be surprised on reflection, that its function is entirely dependent on and interdependent with all other systems in the body.

Each and every movement we could logically argue belongs to the muscular system, but to the extent that these muscular movements are dependent on the cooperation of the circulatory, respiratory, nervous, lymphatic, excretory, digestive, skeletal, integumentary, endocrine and immune systems cannot be overlooked or underestimated.

Indeed, without the active cooperation of all systems the body cannot create movement, far less maintain it for any length of time.

And when we understand these simply facts as we approach the human body with therapeutic intervention, such as NST, any response therefore must be considered as a change to the whole organism. An attempt therefore by the organism to better organize and regulate itself in its ongoing pursuit of preserving life.

OPERATING SYSTEMS

The three important functional and autonomous systems that are observed and manipulated in using an NST approach are: the Secondary Respiratory Mechanism, the Stomatognathic System and the Primary Respiratory Mechanism.

I have intentionally referred to them in that order, as this is how they are prioritized and attended to in every NST session. And following this hierarchy of application not only creates the best unlocking of the sacro-spino-occipital system, but it creates the most sustainable results.

Irrespectively, all three systems are more or less interactive and interdependent, and responses may be generated by working on any one or two, or all three in any given session.

We owe much of our understanding regarding the existence of these systems, their function, and relevance to health, to highly celebrated pioneers in the industry of Osteopathy, Craniopathy and Applied Kinesiology such as Sutherland, Upledger, Walther, DeJarnette and Bowen.

The following I present are my own explanations of how I see these systems at work, and are conceptual descriptions, that provide practical insights to enable the practitioner to assess, and use them with NST procedures and protocols.

As we can see in Spinal Development above, the human organism is designed to function as an integrated self-regulating somewhat phenomenal "whole" from the moment fertilization of an egg takes place.

SECONDARY RESPIRATORY MECHANISM

When a baby takes its first breath, the diaphragm muscle moves, and in doing so a myriad of life sustaining activities commence, from gas exchange in the lungs, oxygenation of the blood and cellular metabolism.

The diaphragm also plays a vital role in mobilizing all of the organs in a rhythmic fashion, from which the body arguably takes many queues in organizing itself in a postural and locomotive sense, while at the same time, helping to stabilize the spinal column itself.

Remarkably, when the diaphragm muscle ceases to function, so too does the human organism and life itself ceases.

Indeed, it is not only that the diaphragm permits the lungs to breathe, as a consequence of its involuntary movement, but the whole

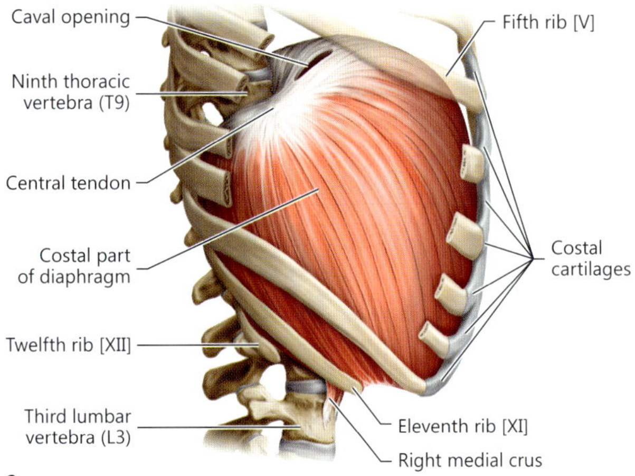

a

Figure 3.3 The diaphragm separates the thoracic and abdominal cavities. The muscle itself has two parts consisting of a fibrous central tendon, to which certain organs attach, and an external active muscular section that surrounds the central tendon. The main muscular motor nerve input is via two phrenic nerves emerging from C3-C5 segments in the cervical spine. The central tendon is also supplied with two phrenic nerves for sensory nerve output. Further sensory nerve output from the external muscle fibers is supplied from T7-T10 segments of the thoracic spine.

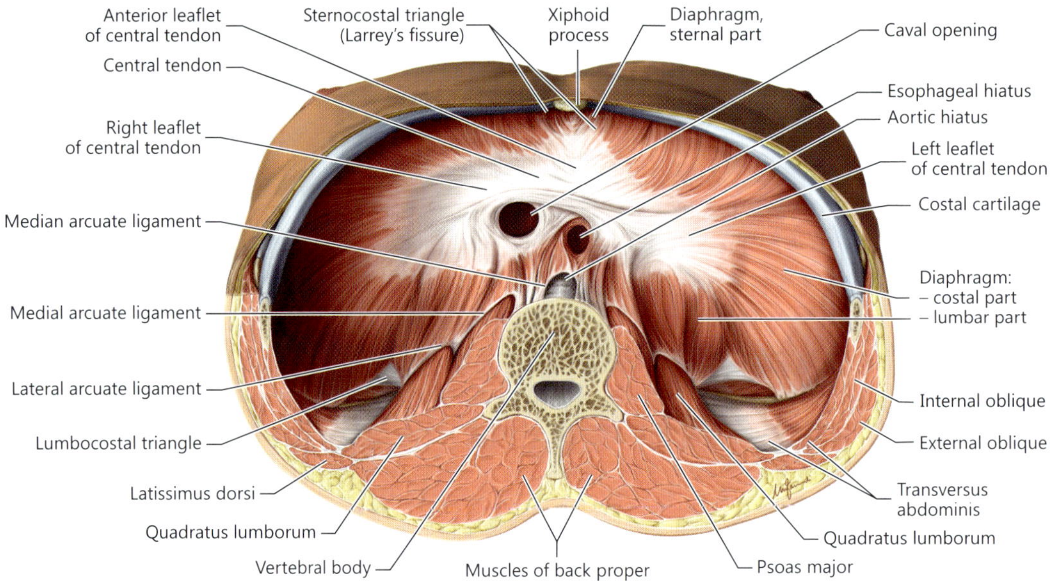

b

body itself expands and contacts from the level of the deepest cells to the most superficial level skin itself.

In so many respects the diaphragm is the muscle of life! (Fig. 3.3).

Andrew Still, the original father of Osteopathy, had the following to say about the diaphragm muscle: "Through you, we live, and through you we die" – Still's biography.

It will come as no surprise therefore, to know that once inhalation takes place and the diaphragm muscle distends, a series of other predictable and life sustaining activities take place that ensure indeed another breath will take place and life itself perpetuate.

These activities are conveniently summarized in the Secondary Respiratory Mechanism – SRM model, popularized in osteopathic and chiropractic circles, by Major Bertrand DeJarnette D.O., D.C., SOT® Methods (Sacro Occipital Technic™).

There are a few variations on the components that make up the SRM, and a few variations on how the model works, but in general, most models carry the same message of an autonomous system that has three interactive diaphragms namely the Thoracoabdominal diaphragm, the Pelvic diaphragm and the Cranial diaphragm, that work in a synchronistic fashion as an integrated unit.

SRM FUNCTION

As inhalation takes place, the inferior movement of the central tendon of the diaphragm muscle pressurizes the abdominal organs in a downward and outward movement, at the same time causing pressure on the abdominal muscles and pelvic floor muscles.

This causes the pelvic ilia to flare in an anterolateral direction, creating an obligatory reciprocal movement of the sacrum, whereby it moves forward at its distal apex, whilst the coccyx moves backwards into the perineal cavity. This sequence of movements then reverses on exhalation.

These movements are to some extent supported by the iliopsoas muscle, which also pulls the lumbar spine into flexion. And along with the diaphragm muscle, the scalene muscles also become involved in this initial stage of respiration, helping to cause an elevation of the thoracic rib cage, and a reciprocal extension of the cervical spine.

To extend things a little further, once the diaphragm distends, the pelvic girdle flares and the sacrum and coccyx both move; the non-elastic dura mater also exerts its own influence on the cranium via "dural" pull, firstly assisting the scalene muscles, in creating the extension of the cervical spine, and secondly, initiating a cranial flare similar to the pelvic flare. This is a sacro-occipital influence.

However, we must also consider the reverse, in that when inhalation takes place, the sphenobasilar junction flexes, also tightening the dura mater, which in turn pulls on the second sacral segment rotating the sacral apex in an anterior direction. This is a craniosacral influence.

Another of the unique outcomes of the cranial flare on inhalation and the subsequent cranial bone repositioning, that takes place on exhalation, is that mechanoreceptors embedded in the cranial sutures are compressed, and "fire".

This micro flexion and extension at the sutures causes nerve impulses to arise in the cervical plexus, that transmit into the phrenic nerves, thereby ensuring that the diaphragm distends once again, and both respiration and therefore life continue.

Yet another unique outcome, is that there is a mimicking of movements between the pelvic girdle and the cranium, whereby the pelvic flare is copied by a flare of the temporal bones, while sacral bone movement appears to be copied by the movement of the base of the cranium, as it flexes and extends at the sphenobasilar junction, and finally the sphenoid bone itself appears to copy the movement of the coccyx.

However, it's important to remember that, despite all of its unique characteristics and sophisticated micro integration, fundamentally the general autonomous behavior of the SRM is

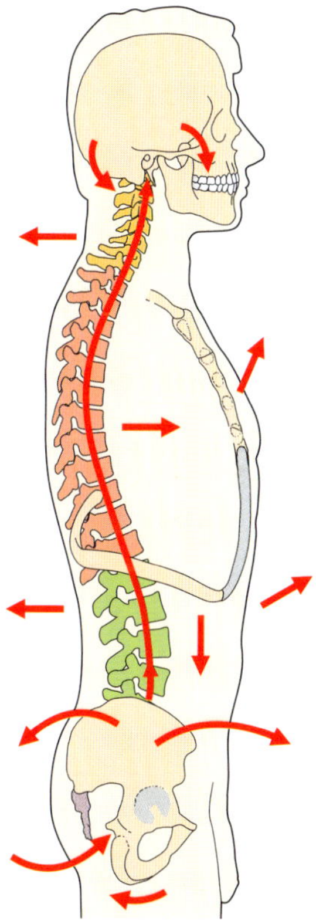

Figure 3.4 The autonomous Secondary Respiratory Mechanism maintains synchronous rhythmic relationships between the diaphragm, pelvic girdle and cranium. Its proper unimpeded function is dependent on the level of balance, integration and function at those three levels. If any level is compromised, the whole system is compromised with far reaching effects for the musculoskeletal system, deeper structural aspects of the organism and therefore physiology itself.

very much governed by the general state of balance within its major components – the diaphragm, pelvic girdle and cranium.

And it is expressly for this reason that much of the core work of NST is designed around ensuring that these important components of the SRM are in balance and communicating with one another, prior to delving deeper and correcting more specific faults within the organism.

In the final analysis of the situation, it's more likely that the system breathes and moves as one, and both ends exert an influence on each other and therefore the system as a whole (Fig. 3.4).

DURA MATER

Importantly, we also have to factor in some of the unique characteristics of the dura mater and the role it plays, to better understand the

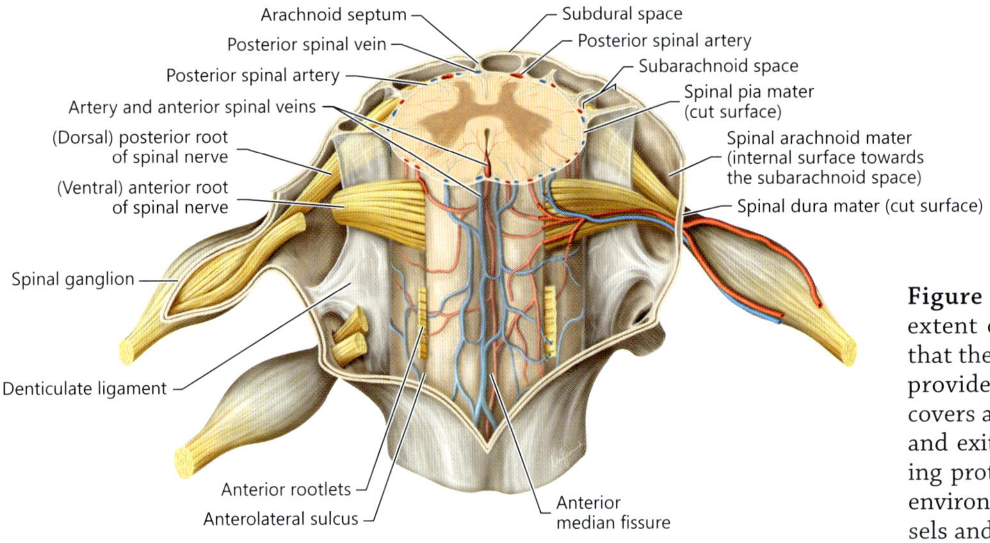

Figure 3.5 Image showing the extent of the enveloping coverage, that the 95% non-elastic dura mater provides. Note how it thoroughly covers all surfaces of the spinal cord and exiting nerves, thereby providing protection and a self-contained environment for nerves, blood vessels and cerebrospinal fluid.

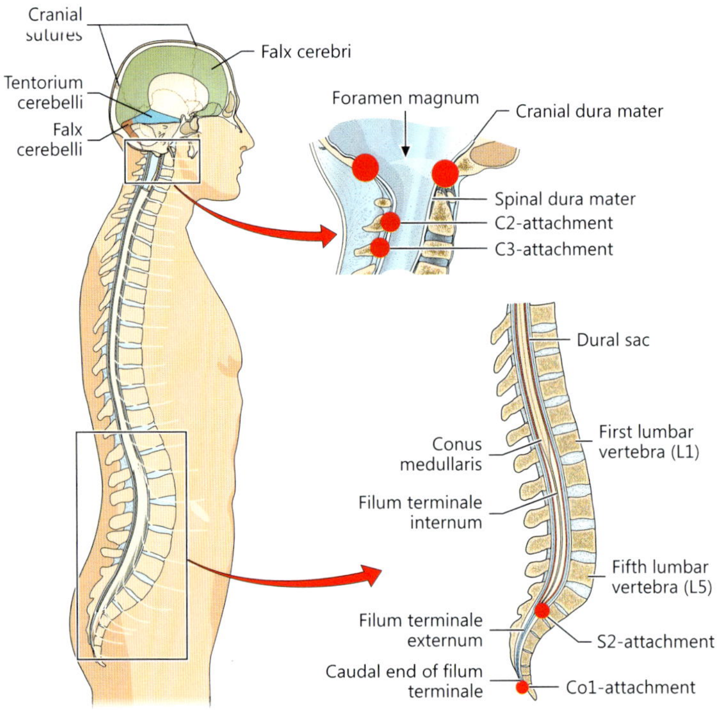

Figure 3.6 Image highlighting the important points of attachment of the dura mater. Note the significant attachments at the Co1, S2, C3, C2, foramen magnum, cranial vault and its sutures. Collectively they share an intimate bond that renders the system into one highly integrated mechanical unit. The right bottom image shows the dural sac in a cross-section view, anchoring to S2 of the sacrum and its ultimate attachment to Co1 of the coccyx. Note the relationship of the conus medullaris of the spinal cord to the dural sac, spinal column, and both the filum terminale internum and externum.

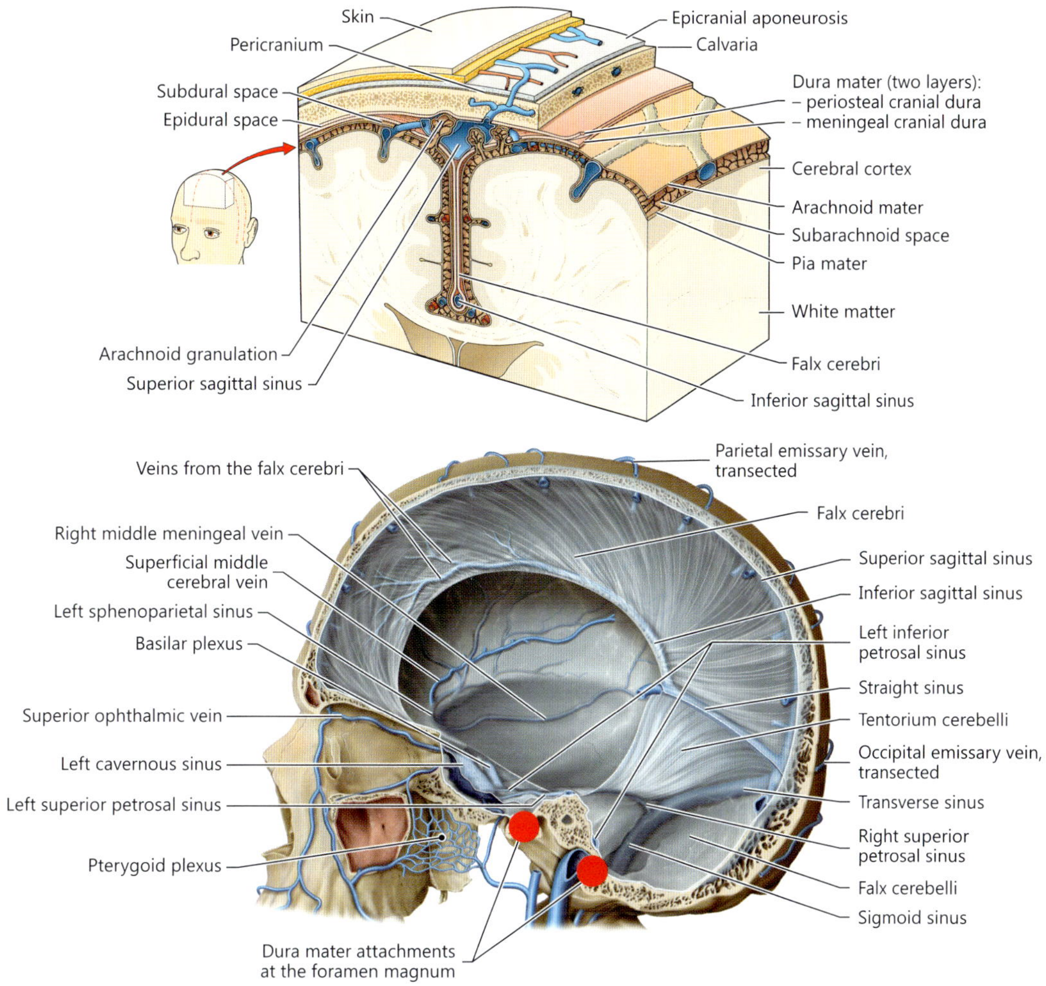

Figure 3.7 Top image shows the extremely intimate relationship (continuity) that the dura mater shares with blood vessels, calvaria (skull), pericranial layer and skin. The bottom image highlights the dura mater attaching to the foramen magnum, then lining the cranial vault and blending with the falx cerebri, falx cerebelli and the tentorium cerebelli.

deeper implications this has for, not only our structure and nervous system, but also our ongoing health (Fig. 3.5).

The dura mater (tough mother) is a 95% non-elastic membrane that runs continuously from Co1 of the coccyx to S2 of the sacral body via the filum terminale; it firmly attaches to S2 of the sacrum (anterior aspect) but then runs comparatively loosely inside the cranial canal, until it re-attaches strongly to the internal circumferences (posterior aspects) of the third and second cervical vertebrae. It then jumps over the atlas and re-attaches firmly to the foramen magnum and cranial base, from where it securely adheres to, and runs continuously with the inside of the cranial vault, blending with its internal membranes (falx cerebri, falx cerebelli and the tentorium cerebelli) (Fig 3.6).

The endosteal layer of the dura is continuous through the cranial sutures (amalgamating with nerve endings) and foramina with the pericranium, and through the superior orbital fissure and optic canal with the periorbita (Fig. 3.7).

As the non-elastic "dural" membrane system is also a closed envelope filled with cerebrospinal fluid under pressure (ultimately rendering it a non-elastic, fluid filled, reciprocal tension system), mechanical faults such as an angulated coccyx may have far reaching effects in other parts of the system via "dural drag" leading to a

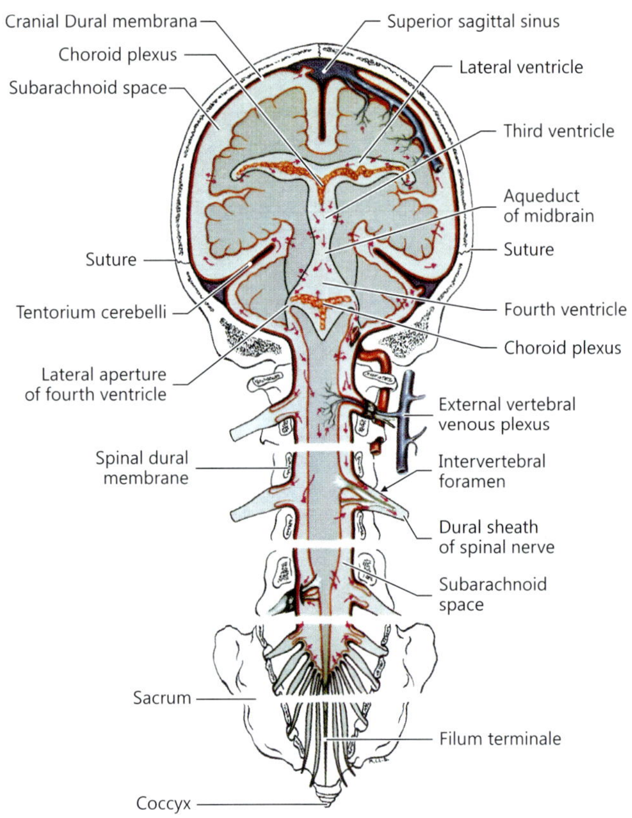

Figure 3.8 The image shows the extent of the pressurized dural envelope or sac from cranium to coccyx. Note the ventricles through which cerebrospinal fluid flows.

myriad of symptoms remote to the mechanical fault itself (Fig 3.8).

Consequently, a coccyx fault may cause "dural drag" resulting in neck pain or headaches. Conversely cranial suture faults may cause "dural drag" leading to lumbo-sacro-coccygeal symptoms, such as back pain and urogenital conditions.

And either of those outcomes will most certainly interfere with the autonomous function of the SRM, and indeed another of the organism's important operating systems, known as the Stomatognathic System.

In the section on the Stomatognathic System that follows just after the completion of this section on the SRM, we will add further clarity to the overall situation, by considering the micro and macro relationships that exist between the cranium and its many intricate structures and the pelvic girdle.

What is clear is, that from sperm and egg to fully unfolded sacro-spino-occipital system, nature has decreed that integration and autoregulation are the main operating codes that underpin the function of the body at all levels.

SRM: A BLUEPRINT FOR NST

The significance of the autonomous Secondary Respiratory Mechanism to NST is that it was the "blueprint" around which much of NST is built.

In fact, the core NST balance referred to as the Dynamic Body Balance – DBB alone, is designed to integrate the components of the SRM as a starting point for correcting all conditions.

The DBB contains corrections for the lumbar, thoracic and cervical spines, and is designed to be applied as a complete and integrated body balance. Importantly, DBB also targets elements of the pelvic girdle, spinal column, diaphragm and cranium that provoke autoregulation and integration of the SRM (Fig. 3.9).

Although the DBB is very powerful, it represents the least amount of work that an NST practitioner would do at any given session, and in fact more often than not, additional procedures are added that increase specificity, unlocking and sustainability of corrections.

As an example, more specific adjustments may be added to the DBB such as releases for the legs, arms, diaphragm muscle, pelvis, sacrum, coccyx and TMJ.

This means a more rapid reduction in pain, greater range of motion throughout the body and noticeably improved energy levels all in shorter time frames.

STOMATOGNATHIC SYSTEM

While using NST's Dynamic Body Balance – DBB correction for the lumbar, thoracic and cervical spines, will bring the SRM back into balance for the vast majority of individuals, and

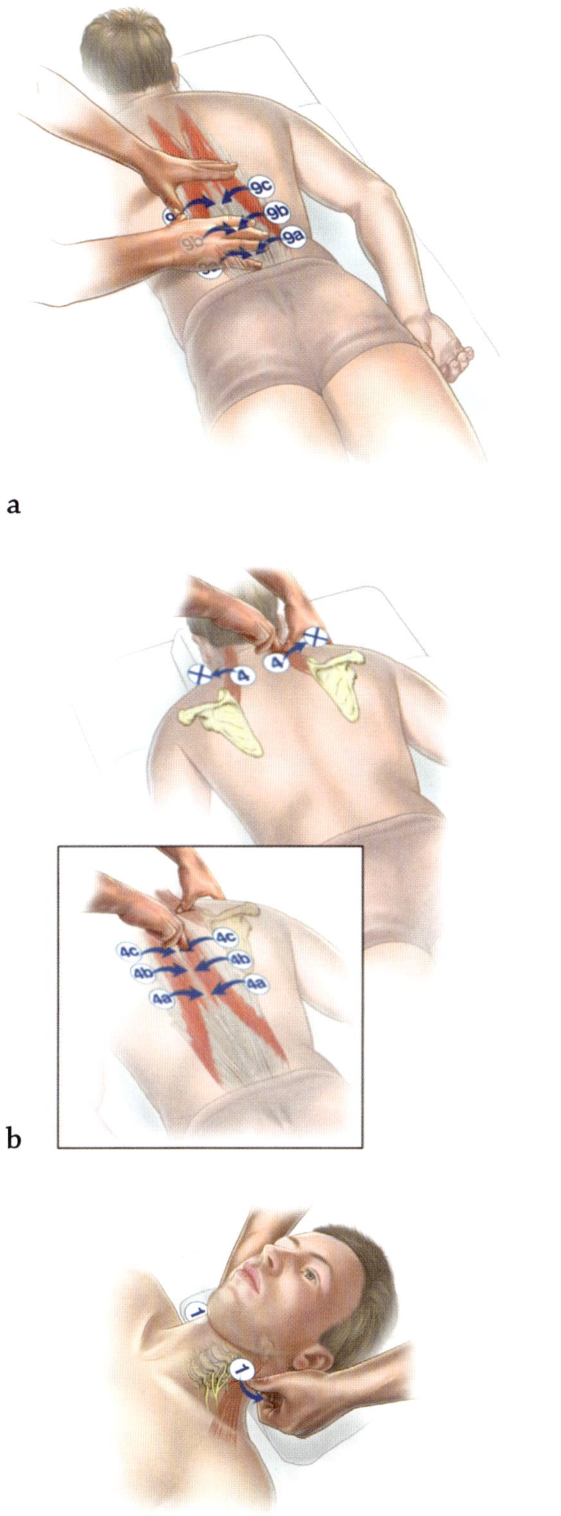

Figure 3.9 NST – Dynamic Body Balance (DBB). The DBB is designed to integrate the components of the Secondary Respiratory Mechanism. Examples of typical points from the DBB. (**a**) DBB1 – lumbar section; (**b**) DBB2 – thoracic section; (**c**) DBB3 – cervical section.

correct thereby, a myriad of structural, pain and health conditions; the corrections achieved will not hold for long if there are more chronic or degenerative imbalances, in particular at the level of the cranium and cervical spine, sabotaging the SRM's ability to maintain integration.

Structural faults or imbalances at the level of the temporomandibular joints (TMJ), cranial sutures, crainal and hyoid muscles, cranial nerves and the teeth themselves, serve to keep the body in a state of perpetual imbalance, where the SRM seeks balance, but that balance is constantly sabotaged by these more insidious faults, that need detection and correction if indeed the body is to remained balanced.

As nature would have it, the body is regulated very much in a hierarchical sense, and although the SRM is a major regulating system of the body, its influence is to some extent trumped by another very precise regulating system call the Stomatognathic System – SGS.

"Stomato" meaning of the face and mouth and "gnathic" meaning to gnaw or chew, the SGS controls the functions of chewing biting and swallowing and to some extent speech as well.

The hard components of the SGS in the upper body include all of the teeth, all bones of the cranium including the mandible, the hyoid bone, the seven cervical vertebrae, the first three thoracic vertebrae, the first two sets of ribs, both scapulae, both clavicles and the sternum.

In the lower part of the body the hard components are the pelvic bones, sacrum and coccyx.

Further soft components include both TMJ, the dura mater and all of the associated muscles, fasciae, nerves and blood vessels that make the system a fully functional system.

The fundamental operational characteristic of the SGS is, that every time we chew, bite, swallow or speak, the system moves as an integrated whole at one level or the other, be it osseous, muscular, fascial or nervous.

At a glance it is easy to observe that some of

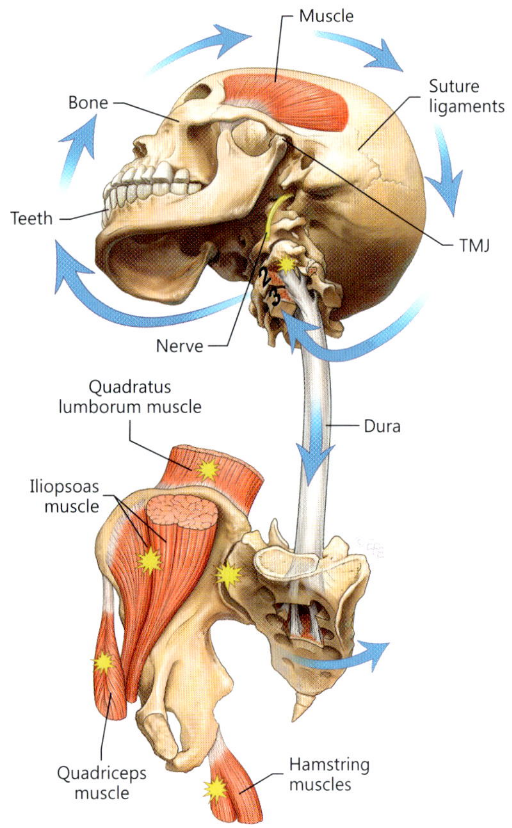

Figure 3.10 Stomatognathic system (SGS) - highlighting the relationship between Micro and Macro sections of the SGS. The components of the Micro section (TMJ, teeth, muscles, sutures, nerves and ligaments) must remain dynamically balanced to assure an appropriate relationship between the cranium and cervical spine. If this relationship is compromised by any one of the components of the Micro section, then via "dural drag" the sacrum will be affected resulting in a number of predictable postural muscle faults (hamstring, psoas, quadratus lumborum and erector spinae muscles).

the components of the SGS such as the pelvis, sacrum and coccyx bones are identical to the SRM as indeed they are.

And given that the cervical vertebrae, some thoracic vertebrae, upper ribs, scapulae, clavicles and sternum are also involved, it quickly tells us that the SGS can very directly influence the rise and fall of the thoracic cage and therefore affect respiration itself.

In reality, if the SGS is imbalanced it can quickly and negatively affect the SRM's operation, by creating muscular compensations at the level of the cervical spine and thoracic cage or at the level of the pelvic girdle or both.

An unbalanced SGS if you will, in layman's terms, "puts the brakes on" the SRM's function, not only impacting respiration but everything dependent on it, including locomotion.

A simple way to think of the SGS itself, and indeed its relationship to the SRM, is to view things in Micro and Macro systems terms, where the Micro system controls the Macro system (Fig. 3.10).

The "main" components of the SGS Micro system, that if imbalanced, will quickly apply torsion to the upper cervical vertebrae (to which the dura mater attaches, and hence affect the whole SRM), are the teeth, the TMJ, the cranial sutures, the cranial nerves and the cranial muscles (including cranial, facial, hyoid, tongue, chewing and swallowing muscles).

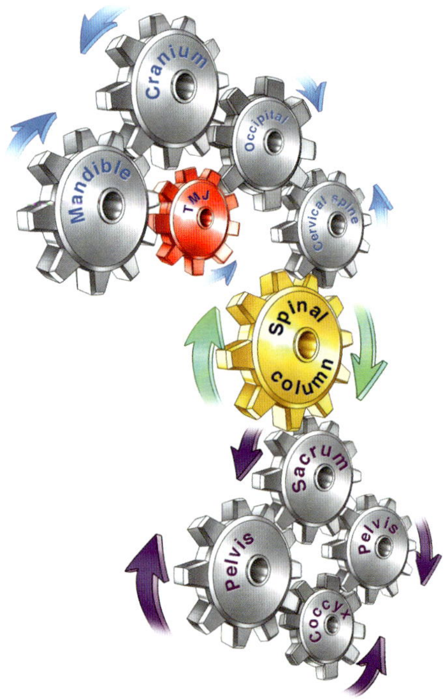

Figure 3.11 Interlocking gears with TMJ highlighted illustrating its connectivity to all body parts. A dysfunctional TMJ may cause symptoms locally in the Micro section of the SGS, but its influence may affect the Macro section of the SGS just as easily. See also Chapters 7 and 9 for further information on the TMJ and SGS.

In other words, if any one of these components is imbalanced, resultant muscular torsions will appear in the rectus capitis posterior major and minor, obliquus capitis superior and inferior (all posterior neck muscles) and longus capitis (anterior neck muscle) muscles, that connect the upper cervical vertebrae to the cranium, and this quickly transfers into distortions in the dural membrane system and SRM generally. This is characterized by predictable postural muscular imbalances in the hamstring, psoas, quadratus lumborum and erector spinae muscles.

In SGS thinking, the Micro system clearly exerts a hierarchical structural influence over the Macro system (Fig. 3.10).

Correcting the Macro system via SRM integration may not guarantee a correction of the Micro system, but correcting both the Macro and Micro system together, when necessary as determined by assessment, will ensure total body integration and sustainability of structural corrections.

Of the Micro system components, the TMJ are the most frequently imbalanced and this may or may not be associated with reciprocal issues of the teeth. When imbalanced, or in a state of deterioration, the TMJ disturb the function of the SGS and the SRM, causing both local and remote symptoms (Fig. 3.11).

A more thorough discussion on the TMJ is presented in Chapters 7 and 9.

One of the other defining characteristics of the SGS, when it is imbalanced, is the fact that the body is no longer able to sustain proper afferent input to the brain from the Micro or Macro systems and, as a consequence, efferent output to both Micro and Macro system muscles is compromised, to the extent that more poor afferent input leads to more poor efferent output, creating what can only be described a perpetual imbalance cycle.

Treating back pain and neck pain locally with individuals suffering from this condition will not bring about sustainable outcomes. Rather the whole system needs to be balanced, with the practitioners two eyes firmly fixed on the status and integration of the Stomatognathic System (Fig. 3.12).

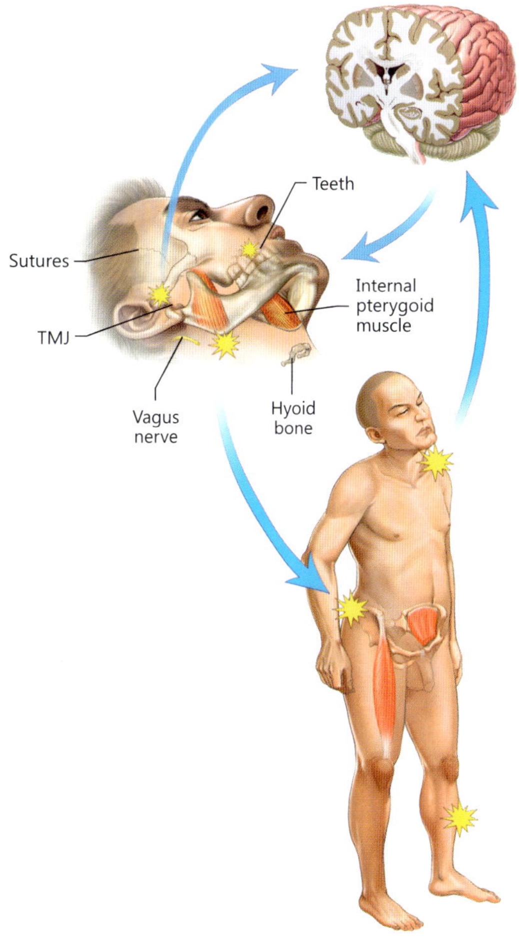

Figure 3.12 Relentless compromised afferent input to the somatosensory cortex of the brain will result in compromised efferent output via the somatomotor cortex to the muscles of the Micro and Macro systems of the SGS. When this occurs over time, a perpetual imbalance cycle is established in the human organism, frequently evident in cases of chronic pain and illness.

PRIMARY RESPIRATORY MECHANISM

The final and least directly utilized operating system in NST is the Primary Respiratory Mechanism – PRM.

It is referred to as the PRM because it is the "primary" rhythm of the body, "respiratory" because it controls cellular respiration of the body and "mechanism" because it is capable of regulating other aspects of the human organism such as the SRM and SGS (Fig. 3.13).

If we refer back to the beginning of this chapter, in the section on Spinal Development, we will realize just how significant the PRM ebb and flow or craniosacral flows are to the body's development and ongoing health.

The PRM in reality is just another term for the body's craniosacral rhythm and system.

Referred to by DeJarnette as the PRM and by Bowen as the "Cycle of the Body", its correction is mainly used in NST as a final balancing strategy, after the main work of integration has been achieved via correcting the SRM and the SGS.

The PRM generally comes back into balance automatically once the SRM and SGS have been balanced.

However, a craniosacral therapist or craniopath might use it exclusively as their only correction strategy for any presenting condition. It is my observation that this is a slower and more time consuming way to approach things.

The PRM is described variously by different experts in the osteopathic, chiropractic, craniopathic and craniosacral fields, but the following summary as proposed by Sutherland (1873-1954) is generally well accepted.

The PRM is a combination of subtle movements that take place at the body's core and consist of:

- The inherent motility of the brain and spinal cord.
- Fluctuation of the cerebrospinal fluid.
- Mobility of the intracranial and intraspinal membranes.
- Articular mobility of the cranial bones.
- The involuntary mobility of the sacrum between the ilia (sacroiliac joints).

At a glance, and in particular if one has never considered such subtle movements, let alone tried to distinguish them from one another, you could be forgiven for wanting to place this whole subject quickly into the "too hard to do" basket.

Nevertheless, a skilled practitioner is able to distinguish between all of these movements in much the same way a practitioner using Traditional Chinese Medicine (TCM) may distinguish between the various qualities and attributes of the energy pulse found at the wrist.

However, I have found it to be much more efficient to correct the SRM and SGS before correcting the PRM, and it is for this reason that the PRM is our final NST operating system.

Ironically, in reality the PRM is perhaps the easiest of all three operating systems to work with, providing the SRM and SGS have been firstly corrected, as the practitioner need only

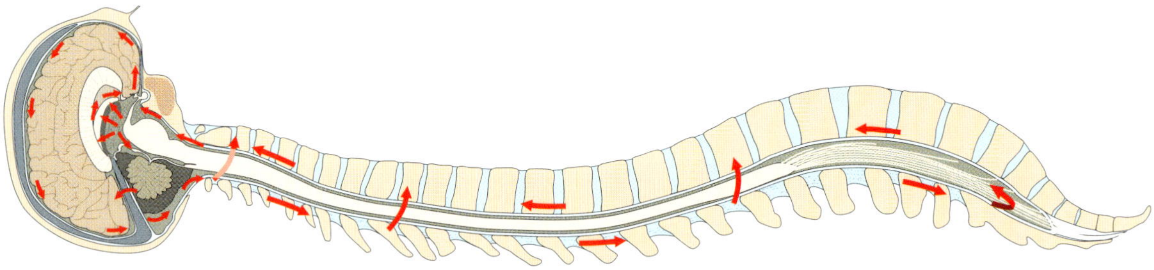

Figure 3.13 The Primary Respiratory Mechanism (PRM) may regulate the SRM and SGS. It is evident as an energetic "pulse" in the single fertilized ovum but then develops into a system with more recognizable characteristics such as the inherent motility of the brain and spinal cord, fluctuation of the cerebrospinal fluid, mobility of the intracranial and intraspinal membranes, articular mobility of the cranial bones and the involuntary mobility of the sacrum between the ilia (sacroiliac joints).

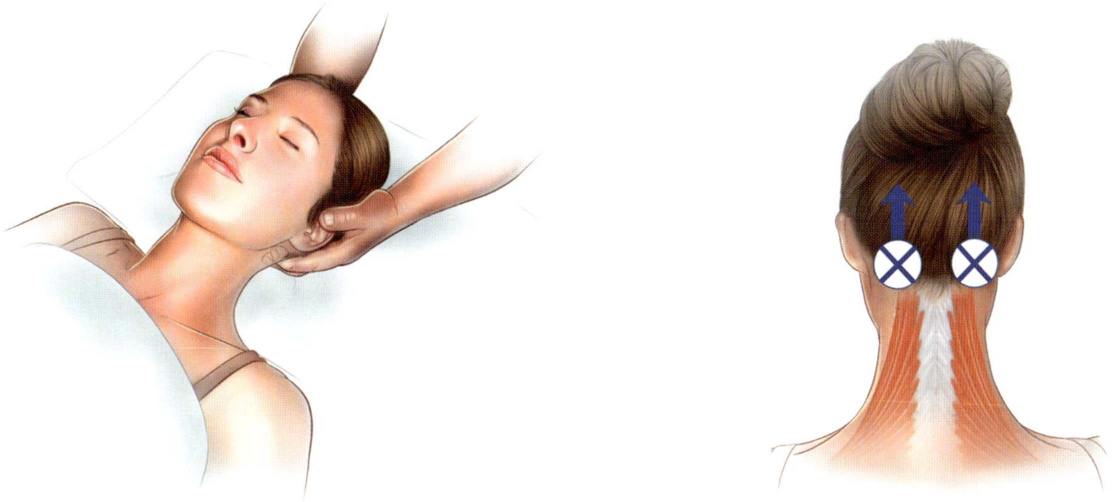

Figure 3.14 The PRM rhythm may be detected and corrected at the bilateral insertions (cranial origins of descending part) of the upper trapezius muscle. In NST the correction of the PRM is typically performed after integration of the SRM and the SGS have firstly been achieved. Doing things in this order makes for a much quicker correction of the PRM.

sit at the patient's head and wait to feel for the rhythm.

With the index and middle fingers conjoined from both hands, the insertions of the upper trapezius muscle are contacted with soft pressure. The practitioner simply needs to wait, when using the simplest version of all (Fig. 3.14).

Without trying to distinguish between motility, mobility and cerebrospinal fluid flows, the various other pulses that may be detected in beats per minute (bpm) are the vascular at 60-70 bpm, the pulmonary respiration rate at around 40 bpm and the primary respiratory pulse which can be as slow as 2 bpm up to 18 bpm. Most practitioners feel it at around 5-12 bpm.

In my own clinical practice, I use a technique called the CRIT (cranial respiratory impulse technique) for inducing the PRM at the end of the session, and I typically spend no more than 5 minutes applying it, as the primary rhythm appears and settles very quickly after the NST bodywork is complete.

Exceptions to this rule however, for using the PRM correction as a singular intervention strategy, may be for when certain individuals cannot tolerate touch, and/or the reflex responses generated by the NST Pri-moves. Patients presenting with fibromyalgia, some aged and frail patients or even babies are good examples. So a singular correction strategy using the PRM definitely has its place in NST, albeit typically not a first choice option. But as a finishing strategy - every day of the week.

Further Operating Principles 4

TENSION – PRESSURE – ENERGY

In the mid 1980s, my passion in medicine was the chiropractic approach, and I was both an ardent patient and practitioner alike.

My simple philosophy was that if all vertebral bodies of the spinal column were in their right place, there would be no nerve impingement and muscles and organs would function optimally.

Underpinning my belief was the notion that bones in the spinal column were stacked on top of each other and needed to be in the right place. All true enough to some extent, but I was never taught to consider muscles let alone fascia as viable systems of adjustments for the bones.

I was not alone in my thinking either, and had some highly talented Australian peers such as Dr. Gerry Baenisch D.O., Dr David Warry D.C., and Dr. David Lovett D.C., collectively from whom I learned so much about spinal and articular adjustments, and from whom I received many hundreds of sessions of old school chiropractic and osteopathic adjustments.

The "crack" (high velocity thrust – HVT) was in fashion, and the more the merrier. If someone was out of balance the motto was to "crack them back" to balance!

I had also learned to combine chiropractic adjustments with yoga as an after care system, and it was pretty effective for the most part, except that a chiropractic adjustment was still necessary at least once a week to keep patients balanced.

As a patient and student, I had also followed this thinking faithfully and over a number of years, and had received as many as 3 chiropractic session per week for lower back and neck problems, however things had progressively become worse, to the point that I had become hypermobile in both lumbar and cervical spines, and I was in constant pain.

Yoga was not helping either and, by the late 1980s, I felt I was destined for the human scrap heap.

My chiropractor at the time Dr. Mark Brown D.C., had also struggled to help me with his softer approach and in frustration sent me to a Bowen therapy practitioner.

My first session of Bowen therapy was a revelation for several reasons, as it immediately and significantly improved my condition and completely flipped my thinking about the spinal column 180 degrees.

I was suddenly confronted with the philosophy that, it is muscles that move bones and not the other way around, and if this philosophical shift produced these types of results, I was sold.

I had not received one HVT adjustment at all, just a series of comfortable rolling motions over strategic muscles along my back, neck and legs and the result was astounding!

The source of all strains of Bowen Therapy was Mr. Tom Bowen, who passed away in 1982, and as much as I would have loved to have meet him, I had the good fortune of meeting, working with or being treated by several people who were very close to him, including three of his direct students, who only numbered six in total.

If my own experiences with Bowen Therapy were not enough, the collective influence of Oswald Rentsch, Romney Smeeton and Kevin Ryan decisively moved me away from using HVT adjustments, into a new world of therapy.

Bowen's work had few rules but much common sense to it.

His main rules were to "balance muscle tensions equally on both sides of the body" to ensure that the "cycle of the body" came back into balance. As simple as those two rules might sound they contain mountains of solid wisdom and technical knowhow.

TENSEGRITY AND HYDROSTATIC PRESSURE

One look at the human skeleton will quickly confirm, that it was not designed by a stone mason or carpenter.

If a stone mason fashions building blocks, they have flat surfaces that are designed to be stacked on top of each other, in an interlocking style to build walls, structures and buildings that stand upright because of the enormous compressive strength they possess.

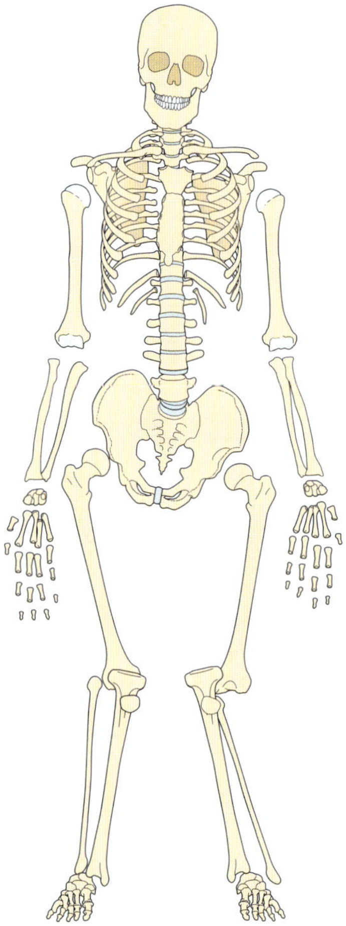

Figure 4.1 The bony skeleton in and of itself has no structural integrity. Without the support of the muscles, various soft tissues and hydrostatic pressure, it would crumble into a stack of bones on the ground.

Not only can they support their own massive weight, they will not move or crumble when other weights are added to them.

Carpenters use the same principle that applies to the construction of chairs, tables, furniture and almost anything else that is designed to sit in one place and support weight.

This is compressive strength at work, however the human skeleton in and of itself, possesses zero compressive strength as a structure.

If the human skeleton was not supported by and held together with fasciae, ligaments, tendons and muscles, it would crumble in a stack of scattered bones on the ground (Fig. 4.1).

In and of itself it is not capable of standing upright, yet it apparently does so as humans clearly stand vertically and of course move about as well.

A closer examination of the human skeleton reveals that there is not one flat surface anywhere; rather it is made up of bones that are bent, twisted or curved and have odd looking lumps and protrusions on them as well. The cranial bones, clavicles, scapulae, ribs, femurs and metatarsals are just a few quick examples.

However, once we consider the simple fact that the skeleton is a highly sophisticated system of levers and spacers, designed to permit locomotion by muscles pushing and pulling against it, we can start to appreciate its elegance and beauty from a much more functional point of view.

Although the bones of the human skeleton are very strong, they are nevertheless not responsible for bearing much of the weight of the human body at all.

So, the question arises, can muscles bracing against the skeleton make it stand upright?

Not entirely, but they can certainly help, when we combine them with one of the body's other unique structural attributes of hydrostatic pressure, which it has in abundance.

Hydrostatic Pressure

An oft-made joke about the human body is that it's nothing more than a big bag of water that moves about; which is not entirely untrue, given that our bodies are indeed comprised of and 65-70% water.

From an evolutionary perspective, our species originally emerged from the oceans and seas. And as necessity dictated, that we eventually become terrestrial land dwelling creatures, in our very earliest migrations, therefore, we took with us the necessary life sustaining vital elements of our embryonic womb, in sea water. By necessity, the sea water needed encapsulation for transportation onto land, and hence the first membrane was formed.

As various species evolved, and amongst many other evolutionary marvels and miracles, the tendency to encapsulate fluids in membranes became part and parcel of how organisms are built.

Indeed, every living cell in the human body is a marvelous liquid filled microcosm encapsulated by an equally marvelous membrane.

As essential to life as the internal functions of every cell is, the hydrostatic pressure is possesses helps it not only maintain its own structure, but the structure of is closest neighbours. And when we consider alone that the human body has some 37.2 trillion cells, we start to appreciate how much naturally occurring hydrostatic pressure we have.

But the creation of hydrostatic pressure is not made by cells alone. Our tough connective tissue matrix, a "metamembrane" of astounding intricacy, that literally binds specific cells into tissues, tissues into organs, organs into systems, cements muscles to bones, coats every bone, ties bones into joints, wraps every nerve and every vessel, laces all internal structures firmly into place and envelops the body as a whole, also helps to create significant hydrostatic pressure as well.

In fact, the connective tissue matrix is so pervasive that, if every other tissue and liquid were removed from the body and only empty compartments of connective tissue remained, the form it would create, would be that of our complete three-dimensional physical body in extremely fine detail.

It has many different properties from diffuse and watery to tough mesh like with tensile qualities superior to steel wire. But in reality it is one continuous metamembrane from the scalp on our head to the soles of our feet, and from the exterior of our skin to the interior of our bone marrow (Fig. 4.2).

Apart from being inextricably woven with our bones in the form of tough flexible ligaments and tendons that help hold our frame together supporting our posture, it compartmentalizes all structures and fluids of the body trussing them into cylindrical shapes and pressurizing their liquid contents creating structural rigidity, thereby massively adding to our weight-bearing capacity.

Joint capsules, intervertebral discs, bursae and all compartments in the body that contain lymph, blood, synovium or water, contribute to the hydrostatic pressure in the body as well.

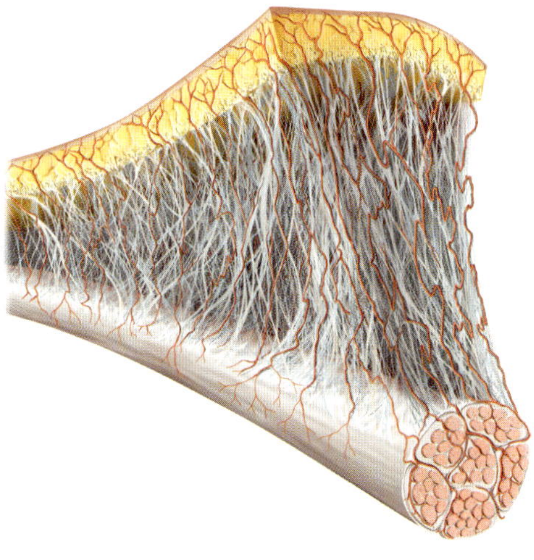

Figure 4.2 Our body's system of fascia or "metamembrane" is one continuous network from the scalp on our head to the soles of our feet and from the exterior of our skin to the interior of our bone marrow. It serves many purposes in the human body one of which is to compartmentalize structures and fluids thereby adding to our weight-bearing capacity and essentially assisting the body to remain upright.

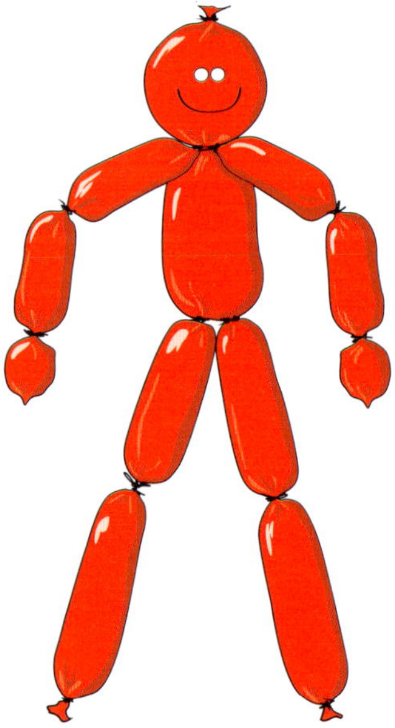

Figure 4.3 The collective hydrostatic pressure derived from the compartmentalization of lymph, blood, synovium and water in the human body lends greatly to the body's ability to remain upright, prior to considering the role of the skeleton.

Indeed, there is enough hydrostatic pressure in the body to keep it upright without a skeleton, but add a skeleton for pushing and pulling against, and we start to form a clearer picture as to how we stand upright and the true relationship between muscles and bones, that in fact, permits this compartmentalized bag of water to move around, and indeed, interact with its environment (Fig. 4.3).

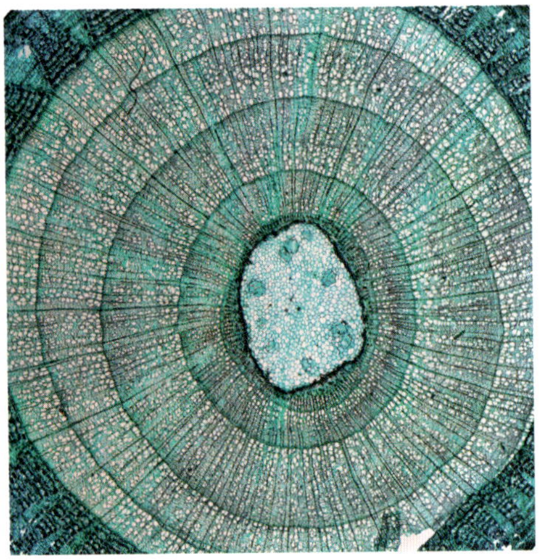

Figure 4.4 The principle of compartmentalization of fluids in a membrane to create rigidity and structure is not unique to humans and animals, as nature also utilizes the same principle in the plant kingdom, to keep a flower upright, albeit using cellulose in place of fascia.

And it's worth sparing a thought for the fact that connective tissue left unattended tends to loose its tensile strength, and along with it, the quality of the body's hydrostatic pressure.

Add insufficient intake of water, and we can quickly start to see just how important it is to exercise and hydrate to keep our skeletons, joints and bodies in top shape.

Hydrostatic pressure is not unique to humans either, as nature uses it throughout the plant kingdom as well, where it performs such tasks, as keeping a flower upright, albeit with a cellulose membrane instead of the collagen one, that we have in the human body. But the principle of compartmentalization of fluids in a membrane to contribute to structure is the same! (Fig. 4.4).

In humans, however, the reality is that we need to move around and therefore our compartmentalized water bag has been invested with a skeleton, and consequently, we are much closer to the truth of the matter when we acknowledge, that in fact, it is the combination of strong hydrostatic pressure and balanced muscular tensional forces acting on the skeleton that permit us to stay upright and indeed move around.

As we delve further into our ability to stand upright and move about, understanding the relationships between the various parts and systems can go a long way to helping us appreciate not only how and why NST was built, and how to use it as a structural realignment technique, but indeed how to keep ourselves and our patients stronger and healthier for the journey ahead.

Tensegrity

The term tensegrity was coined by the celebrated architect and inventor Buckminster Fuller in the 1960s to refer to the tensional integrity of structures both animate and inanimate.

In structural medicine it refers to the concept of musculoskeletal relationships that exist between the forces of tension provided by muscles, tendons, ligaments and fasciae interacting with bones and joints that help keep the body stable and efficient, in both mass and movement.

Tensegrity was exactly the principle that Tom Bowen was referring to back in the 1950s when he said that if the muscles and tissues of the body are balanced bilaterally, the "cycle of the body" would come back into balance, pain would diminish, and energy levels improve. History has now vindicated how correct he was.

One of the characteristics of tensegrity in building is that it is a highly efficient methodology that uses a minimum amount of building materials to create a maximum amount of strength. Buildings covering large areas can be built using cables and rods as the main skeleton of the building which sits in place because of its "tensional" and not "compressive" qualities.

Stone masons and builders stack things on top of one another, to build structures and frames that stand upright, because of the compressive qualities they possess.

The human body applies and exemplifies the usage tensegrity at many levels, but it is most on display when we consider the relationships between muscles and bones in particular.

In Figure 4.5, the red poles represent the bones of the body, and the cables attached to the poles keeping them in their unique positions represent the muscles, tendons, ligaments and fasciae. The cable anchoring fixtures represent the articulations.

The critical message in this model is that the better balanced the cables are, the better the load-bearing qualities of the structure will be.

Importantly, if all cables are balanced, heavy load may be applied to the apex of the tensegrity structure and it will not collapse. In fact an open structure such as this can easily support

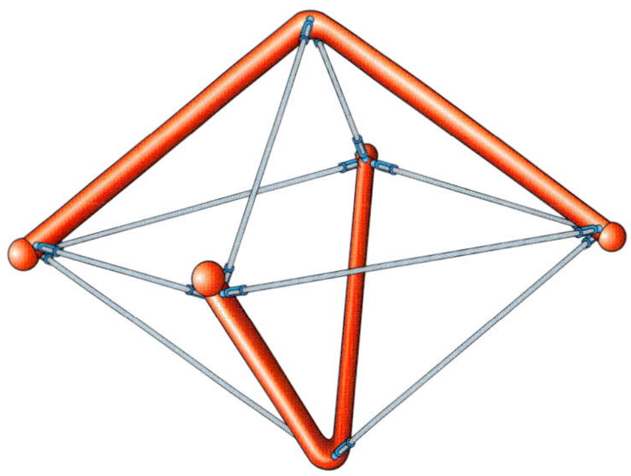

Figure 4.5 This tensegrity model helps explain the tensional relationships existing between the bones of the body (red tubes) and the collective soft tissues (gray cables) that act on the bones. When tensions are balanced the bones are ideally positioned to permit proper nerve transmission and optimal function of the sacro-spino-cranial system. Importantly the load is taken up by the tensional members and not the bones themselves. Our skeleton therefore is not a direct load-bearing system – this places enormous significance on ensuring that the collective tensions in our soft tissue system are optimal.

the same or more weight as a structure built from solid materials of equivalent weight.

Significantly it's the "tensional integrity" of the cables or soft tissues that will take up the load as the hard members spread under load, and not the bars or hard tissues themselves (Fig. 4.6).

Conversely, if any one or more of the cables looses its optimal integrity, the whole structure will move, and in moving it will loose some of its load-bearing capacity.

Of course, this is exactly what happens in the human body when in particular muscle tensions are imbalanced.

When tensegrity is compromised or lost tensional forces acting on bones literally pulls them onto or against nerves preventing nerves from firing correctly, in turn, causing other muscles, organs and glands to experience lack of supply, ultimately leading to stagnation of lymph and blood supply finally causing pain (Fig. 4.7).

And this description is an over simplified account of what really happens, as muscles al-

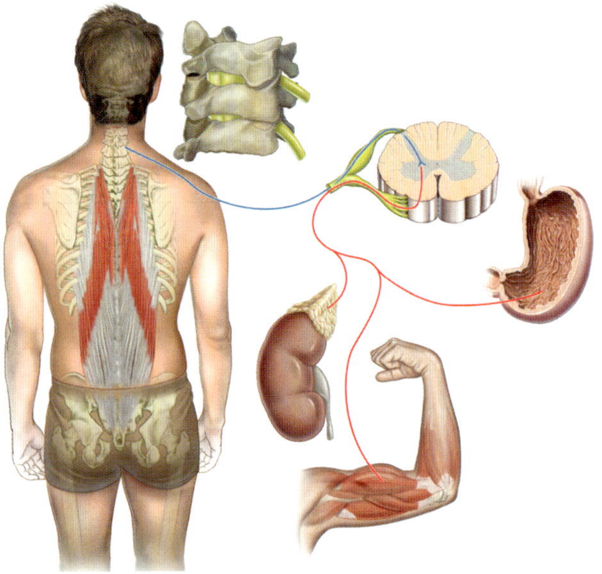

Figure 4.6 Optimal tensegrity leads to flexibility of movement, strength, conservation of energy, a robust physiology, vitality and health.

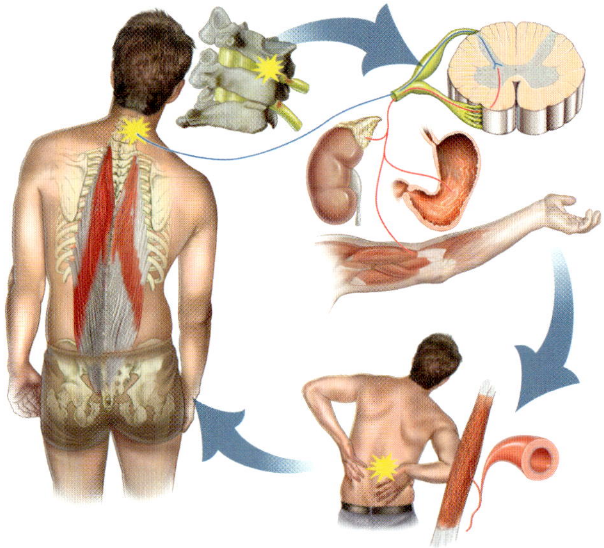

Figure 4.7 Compromised tensegrity leads to restriction of movement, less strength, over consumption of energy, sluggish physiology, lack of vitality, pain and poor health.

so directly affect nerve function with pressure. Nerves need appropriate amounts of pressure to fire both electrically and hydraulically, and when muscles become too tight or too laxed, nerves fail to transmit effectively with yet further consequences.

This principle can be applied to any muscle pair anywhere in the body, and the consequences are always the same with unbalanced tensions leading to either excessive bone or muscle pressure, or both, on nerves with compromised muscle function elsewhere, leading to circulatory problems, inflammation and pain (Fig. 4.8).

Again, there is some over simplification and convenience of description in this story as well, and we need to keep in mind that muscles do not operate in isolation. Although muscles have individual names, locations, shapes, and other characteristics that oblige us to refer to them singularly, they do not however have functional singularity. Rather they operate in patterned groups depending the task being performed.

When the body is in a state of compensation with muscular contractions, it is always a pattern of imbalance and not just a single muscle that is affected.

As an example, a patient may have a tight hamstring on the left side, a tight gluteal muscle on the left but then the pattern will often switch to the right side of the body where portions of the erector spinae musculature will be involved. Ultimately, the patient might be presenting with neck pain on the left hand side, and perhaps headaches as well.

Furthermore, these patterns do not always conform to classical muscle train patterns either. Actually, when we consider the fact that the connective tissue that binds, connects, penetrates, wraps around and indeed forms the mold for each and every one of our 640 odd muscles, is completely continuous, is it any wonder that disturbing one muscles function may have consequences far and wide.

So we will be closer to the complex truth in our conceptulization of muscular activity, if we regard the body as having one muscle, whose millions of fiber-like cells are distributed throughout the fascial network and are orient-

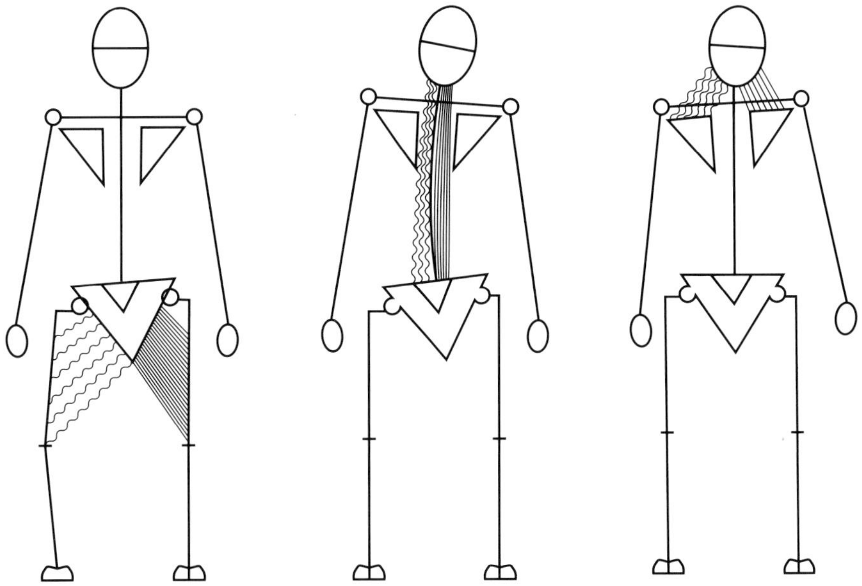

Figure 4.8 Compromised tensegrity can be found throughout the body from the feet to the cranium, and in all cases, the resulting consequence is that bones are pulled onto nerves impeding their function. Bones may also apply pressure to ligaments causing their mechanoreceptors to fire inappropriately. In both cases further tension, compromised function, inflammation and pain are the consequences.

ed in innumerable directions, creating innumerable lines of pull.

Throughout his career Bowen had identified irregular muscle patterns as being the main indicator that the body as a whole was out of balance, and therefore, unsurprisingly, in discomfort and pain.

It is also worth pondering the fact that smooth muscles that make up our organs, has its own influence on skeletal muscle, either through direct pull or via organ-muscle reflex effect. Indeed, a visceral organ struggling to function optimally may have very rapid and painful affect for the muscles it is reflexively connected to.

The heart, lungs, liver, gallbladder, stomach, pancreas and spleen are common culprits in neck and shoulder pain conditions, whereas kidneys, intestines and urinary bladder are often involved in lower back, pelvic and leg conditions.

It has also been my experience in observing some thousands of patients over 20 years or more for "muscle pattern imbalances" that the patterns can be very random and often very mild in terms of the numbers of contracted fibers involved in any one muscle compartment.

But when the body is balanced systematically the pattern clears as a whole.

Of course, when we reflect on the body's operating systems SRM, SGS and PRM discussed in Chapter 3, we start to appreciate how muscle compensations can not only create local symptoms but indeed that they can compromise the whole body with mechanical, neurological and hormonal consequences.

Simply put, any point of imbalance, particularly chronic patterned muscular imbalance, introduced into an integrated operating system will have systematic consequences, and those outcomes can manifest in any part of the system.

It should come as no surprise to discover that the improvement of the body's general tensegrity by systematically correcting these patterns of wasteful muscular contractions, and thereby the systems they effect, has an immediate and positive impact on pain level reduction, energy level increase and even mood improvement.

WASTEFUL MUSCULAR CONTRACTIONS

To have a somewhat deeper appreciation about the consequences for our health, and indeed our life span, that chronic wasteful muscular contractions can have, we need to consider the blood.

The average heart beats about 70 times a minute and with each beat pumps 60 to 90 milliliters of blood out of the heart. At rest, the blood travels around the body and back to the heart in roughly one minute. It can therefore move 5 to 7 liters of blood in about one minute which translates into 7,000 to 10,000 liters per day – at rest!

But since most people are not always resting the figure in reality is potentially much higher.

Astonishingly the distance the blood travels daily is around 20,000 km which is about half way around planet earth.

Briefly, the blood is built from the food we eat, the liquids we drink and the air we breathe. And the quality of our blood depends on the quality of the fuel we invite into our bodies for processing and breakdown.

The foods, liquids and air we ingest are broken down into micro nutrients such as glucose, fatty acids and amino acids that are eventually converted into ATP (adenosine triphosphate), one of the most abundant molecules in all of the cells of the body, that muscles desperately need to function.

Importantly, therefore, the blood carries nutrition and oxygen to its trillions of cells, amongst other things, providing us with energy to move around using our musculoskeletal systems. Not surprisingly, muscles, and therefore muscular effort, consumes more of our nutrition and oxygen supplies (energy) than any other tissue in the body, for the simple reason, that muscles comprise about 70% of the tissue bulk of the body and are, as noted, the "principle system" we use to move around (Fig. 4.9).

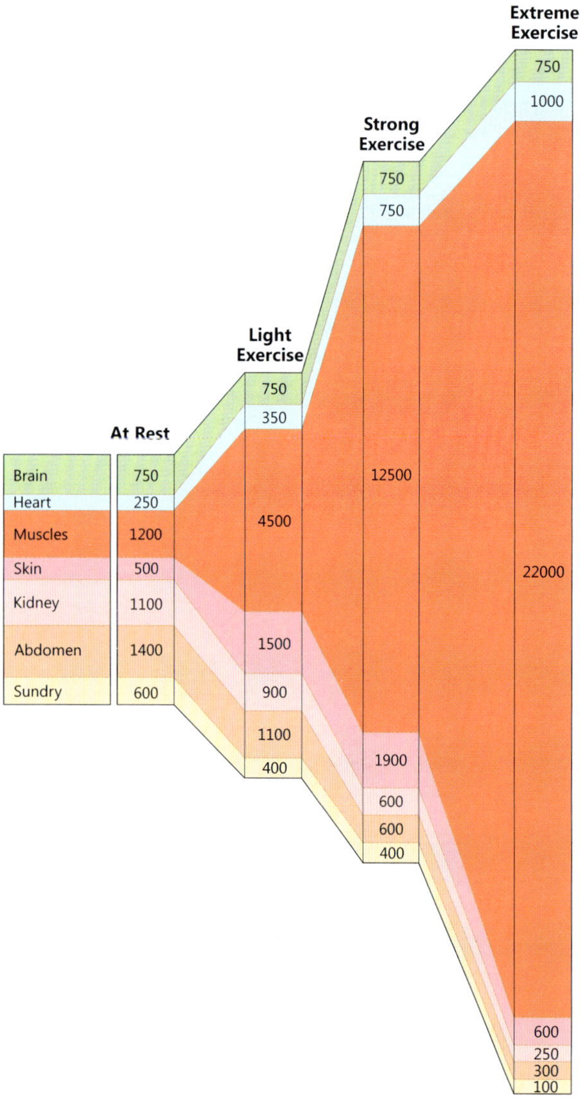

Figure 4.9 The chart shows the varying levels of energy consumption (metabolic support) in milliliters of blood flow per minute, that the indicated body parts require throughout rest, light exercise, strong exercise and extreme exercise. Apart from at rest, when digestion demands slightly more metabolic support than muscles, all other phases of movement (muscle activity) from light, to strong, up to extreme, dictate that the muscles demand for blood supply and hence metabolic support, progressively and exponentially outweighs any other part of the body. It is for this reason that chronically restricted muscular patterns left unattended, are a drain on the organism, thereby predisposing it to other more serious diseases over time, if not corrected.

However, nor is it just the skeletal muscles that we use to move around that demand so much of our energy supplies.

Every swallow of food, every breath of air, the distribution of every drop of blood, every exploration, every defense, even reproduction of the species – all are muscle activities. And the degree to which the muscular system is compromised, the entire organism is weakened, limited.

It is really not going too far to regard the musculature as the primary organ of the body, the dominant tissue of animal life.

In this context then, it is our vital organs that are the servants to the higher demands of the muscles and not the other way around!

THE FENN EFFECT

In 1922 Wallace O. Fenn ran a series of experiments to determine and compare how much energy was utilized and liberated in isotonic muscle contractions when passively contracting versus contracting during work performance. His experiments also involved looking at isometric muscle contractions and energy consumption.

Although some of the accuracy concerning the outcomes he laid claim to have been disputed over the years, and in the modern age in particular, as myothermal measuring equipment has evolved, nonetheless the basic principles that contracting and relaxing muscles consume and release heat and energy in differing amounts holds true.

Fenn's fundamental premise that is relevant, is simply that a muscle that is actively working whilst contracting, demands far more nutrition, oxygen and metabolic support than does a muscle that is simply contracting without doing any work.

And a chronically restricted muscle is working very hard because it is typically pulling against fixed resistance like a joint, bone or other muscle or muscle pattern, thereby increasing demands for energy whilst not producing any useful active work (Fig. 4.10).

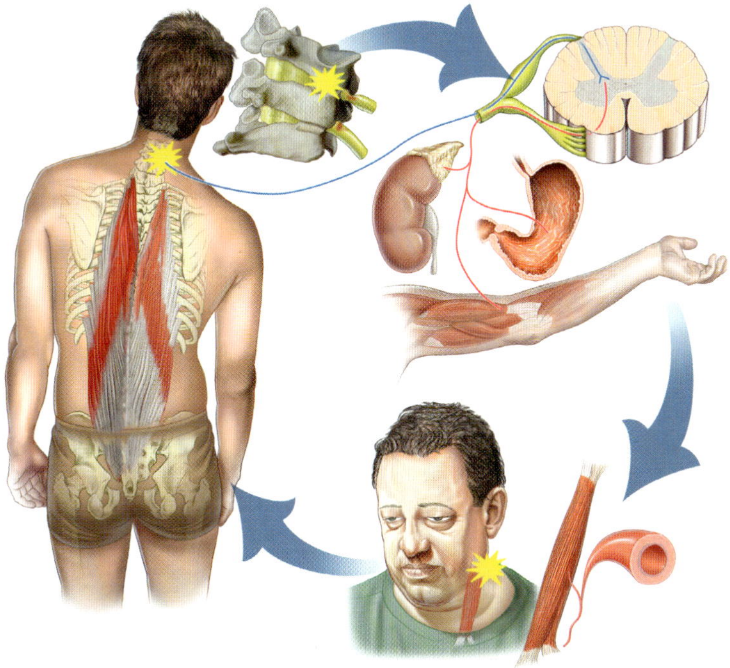

Figure 4.10 Whilst a chronically restricted muscle may eventuate in movement and pain symptoms, what is not obvious is the amount of unnecessary energy it is using without producing any output benefit. When groups of muscles are restricted in a patterned fashion, the drain on the organism over time can be significant.

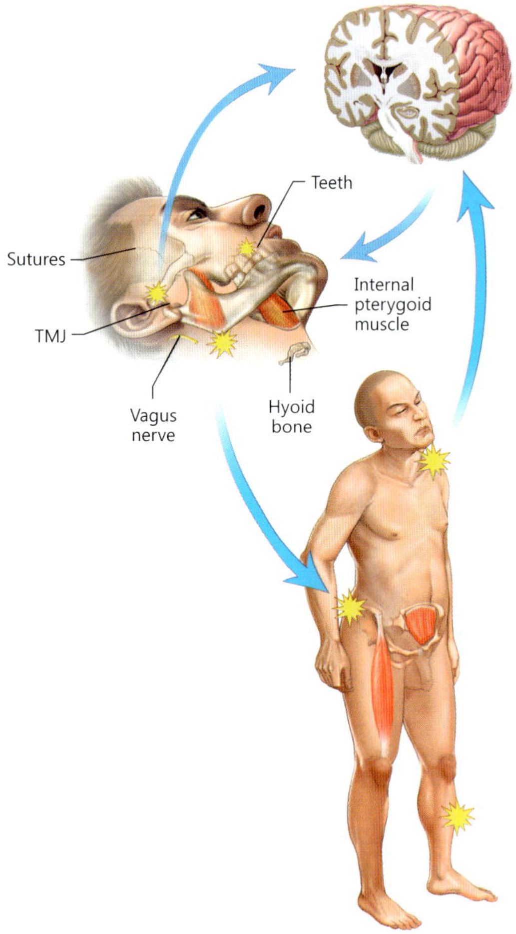

Collateral side effects occur when we consider that the tissue around the contracted muscle(s) site will be impeding circulation and nerve operation thereby starting a vicious cycle that can only lead to further pain and discomfort.

A "perpetual imbalance cycle" is an apt description for the state that many patients present to a clinic for help with, and when the practitioner can offer a solution such as NST to comprehensively unlock the troublesome muscular holding patterns, it is not only a gift for the moment but "potentially" one for a lifetime! (Fig. 4.11).

Figure 4.11 Wasteful patterns of chronic muscular imbalance frequently lead to the human organism entering a "perpetual imbalance cycle", where further pain generates further tension and further tension further symptoms and so on. Over time a greater predisposition to disease is unavoidable.

What Causes Muscles to Go out of Balance 5

STRUCTURE GOVERNS FUNCTION

As remarkable as results are with NST, it must be firmly understood that any therapeutic endeavor including NST is just that, an intervention. However, results become more sustainable and lead to a greater state of health and wellbeing for the individual, if the role of NST is considered in the broader context of the patient's lifestyle behaviors, patterns and choices.

Performing NST or any other therapeutic intervention every day of someone's life will not make them healthy, and it's clearly a mistake to think that it will.

When patients make this critical distinction and realize that, in fact, their previous lifestyle choices have lead them to a state of compromised health, then they are in clear position to adopt different choices, that will yield a whole new reality.

It's at this point that patients can "choose" to adopt the practitioners' recommendations to embrace such changes as inclusion of exercise and appropriate movement behaviors, detoxification programs, dietary changes including suitable supplementation or not.

As noted earlier in the preface of this book, Structure Governs Function is the motto I work by in daily clinical practice, but at the same time, I have a very focused eye on lifestyle and how or what my patient is doing to contribute to their current state, and also what they might be likely to do once they leave the clinic.

But the "choice" always rests with the patient, and bringing a patient to a point where they can make an "informed choice" is, in my opinion, the best and indeed most empowering outcome a practitioner can assist their patient to arrive at.

And the reality is that some patients just want their pain removed and others want more, and both are achievable.

The following is how I see it: assuming that our main philosophical tenant, that Structure Governs Function or physiology is indeed correct, then we make a further conclusion and believe that physiology, especially a robust physiology, if sustained will deliver health. And we can therefore logically conclude that Function Governs Health.

Taking it yet another step further we can logically conclude that, if we can maintain constant health, we will experience a better "quality of life" that will invariably lead to a long life span.

So packaging everything into a nice tidy formula we may logically conclude that Structure Governs Function, Function Governs Health and Health Governs "Quality of Life" and Life span.

To help prove this logic is correct, you can challenge any patient about why they want to loose their pain, they will tell you in one form or another, that they want to feel better, with more energy and have better mental capacity or, in other words, they want a better "quality of life". And if you push the point somewhat and question further, the answer will be that they want a better "quality of life" as they believe this will lead to a ripe old age.

But to make the story more complete, as practitioners we need to ask ourselves a defining question about structure itself. How and why does structure loose its balance so chron-

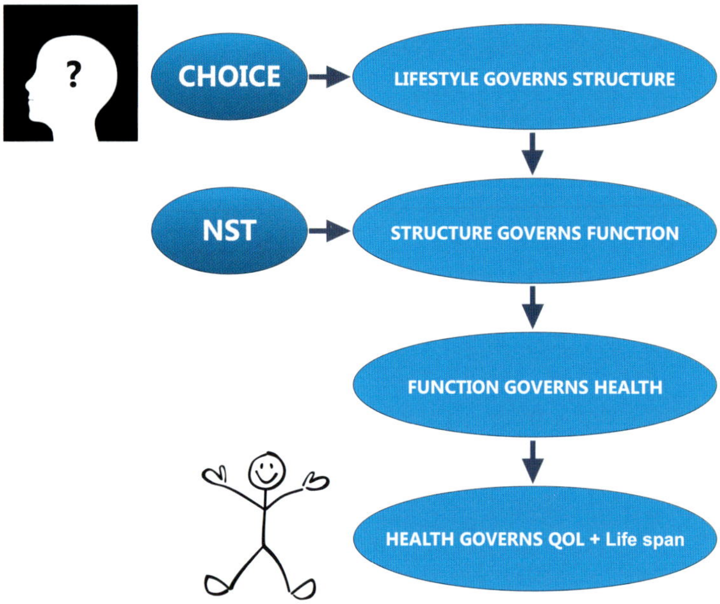

Figure 5.1 Our patients ongoing lifestyle choices – informed or uninformed – around exercise, nutrition, detoxification, emotional well-being and recreation all have a cumulative effect – positive or negative – on the organism. Ultimately it is choice that governs the make up of our lifestyle, lifestyle that governs the status of structure, structure that governs physiology, physiology that governs health and health that governs the quality of our life and ultimately life span. In this context NST is a therapeutic intervention into structure enabling the organism to self-regulate itself back to balance. How long it stays there will largely be dependent on how efficiently the patient conducts their lifestyle.

ically, that it leads to poor health? Do we just wake up one day and discover that we are unhealthy, or is being unhealthy something that builds over time?

Barring perhaps congenital diseases or genetic diseases and unfortunate accidents, with serious consequences, I am convinced that the very vast majority of poor health, pain and suffering is created by the individual themselves, by having made poor lifestyle choices and decisions, that have become habitual and thereby started to have a negative impact on the organism itself. As an extension to this outcome, the choices and habits have become a confortable and seemingly normal part of their life. Frequently, they have no idea as to the intrinsic danger that accompanies these uninformed choices.

So choice whether informed or uninformed, is going to have a consequence that ultimately governs the "quality of life" we experience, and ultimately our life span itself (Fig. 5.1).

So NST is just an intervention into structure that typically causes a rapid reduction in pain, better range of motion and increased energy levels. But all of this does not mean that our patient is suddenly healthy.

The cultivation and maintenance of good health is a responsibility that nature decrees, must be attended to by each and every individual. We alone must "figure out" how best to manage our own unique set of choices and disciplines, built around the structural, nutritional and emotional requirements that our organism depends upon for health and longevity.

Building an Integrated NST Session 6

DYNAMIC BODY BALANCE – INTRODUCTION

There are many ways to build an integrated NST clinical session, with the simplicity or complexity of the session being determined, firstly, by applying fundamental principles and rules and, secondly, by tailoring the session around the patients presenting symptoms or physical indications.

And whilst the patient's symptoms may be known (e.g., back or neck pain) clarifying exactly which procedures may be the most relevant, additional specific indications must be considered.

Particular muscular tensions, ligament tightness, inflexibilities within certain articulations, clicking articulations, leg length discrepancies and the results of various specific tests carried out throughout every session, all carry their own significance, indicating which other procedures and protocols need to be added to deliver a session that is perfectly tailored for the individual.

In considering the foregoing, it may appear that designing and building an integrated NST session is complex, but in fact, the opposite is true as NST employs some basic rules and guidelines coupled with predetermined sequences, procedures and protocols that make it more like using a clever modular approach rather than having to design a new one every time (Fig. 6.1).

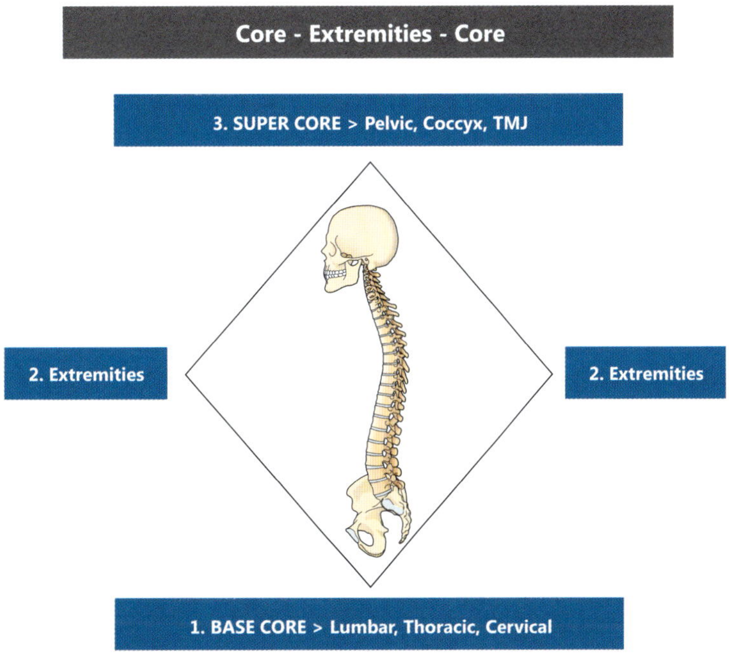

Figure 6.1 Following a structured Core-Extremities-Core template, patient assessment and subsequent choice of appropriate procedures, becomes a simple and organic process. Ensuring at the very minimum, that the "base core" is attended to, sets up a platform for any session, where the addition of other procedures is determined by presenting symptoms coupled with simple routine checks.

And building a session with the minimal amount of sequences, procedures and protocols, that will get the job done, is far a more desirable and elegant approach than just throwing the book at every patient using a scattergun approach.

If the minimum will do the job then the minimum will be used. If more detail is required more detail is added accordingly.

In Chapter 1, we learned that the flow of an NST session follows a Core – Extremities – Core approach starting with a Base Core, adding work for the extremities if necessary and then dealing with Super Core specifics as required, determined by applying specific tests throughout the session.

Following the Core – Extremities – Core approach, the minimum that any patient (excepting babies) would receive is Dynamic Body Balance (Parts 1, 2, 3), the highly dependable Core Balance for lumbar, thoracic and cervical spines.

Dynamic Body Balance is an integrated body balance designed to release and integrate imbalances in the lumbar, thoracic and cervical spines, and in doing so, bring the Secondary Respiratory Mechanism (SRM) back into dynamic balance.

NST is carried out using Pri-moves applied to muscles, tendons, ligaments and nerves that are well known structures in body work.

Apart from utilizing musculoskeletal considerations in its design, NST's makeup is also influenced by the basic principles of energy movement, especially PRM or craniosacral energy flows to unlock and integrate the body, and this unique design feature is on full display in the Dynamic Body Balance.

Importantly, much of Bowen's thinking in balancing the body was centered around balancing "Channel Energy flows" that he'd identified early in his career in the late 1950s. Specifically, he identified a bilateral channel running from sacrum to cranium, through and along which channel energies were manipulated by way of creating specific neuromuscular releases.

In other words, once the channel muscles were released, the channel energies came back into balance. Alternatively, if for example, a coccyx or TMJ fault was left undetected, the channels could be prevented from coming back into balance fully, thereby impacting the outcome.

Perhaps the closest concept to Bowen's channel theory would be that of the Bladder Meridian and its extremely significant Association Points in Traditional Chinese Medicine, that may be stimulated in a variety of ways including with needles or suction cups to name just two. The Central and Governing Vessel meridians may also be considered as good examples.

For structural therapists from the worlds of Physiotherapy, Osteopathy, Chiropractic and other manual therapies, the concept of energy alone can be challenging for many, let alone working with it. And there's no doubt working with something we cannot see, or perhaps even feel, is going to understandably pose a challenge to our way of thinking, and more particularly so, when we view things from an entirely scientific perspective.

However, even if one cannot "feel" energy movement it is not that important in terms of working with NST, as the sequences, procedures and protocols are already tried and proven, enabling the practitioner to just observe soft tissue responses and forget about what the energy is doing.

Nevertheless, it is worth noting that Quantum Physics has rapidly bridged the gap between pure science and energy concepts in the last two decades in particular, and it may not be long before energetic concepts become a commonplace inclusion in Western medicine, as they have been in Eastern medicine for several thousands of years already.

DYNAMIC BODY BALANCE – IN DETAIL

The Dynamic Body Balance (DBB) has three distinct sections – DBB 1, 2 and 3 – and is designed to integrate the lumbar, thoracic and cervical spines and thereby the Secondary Re-

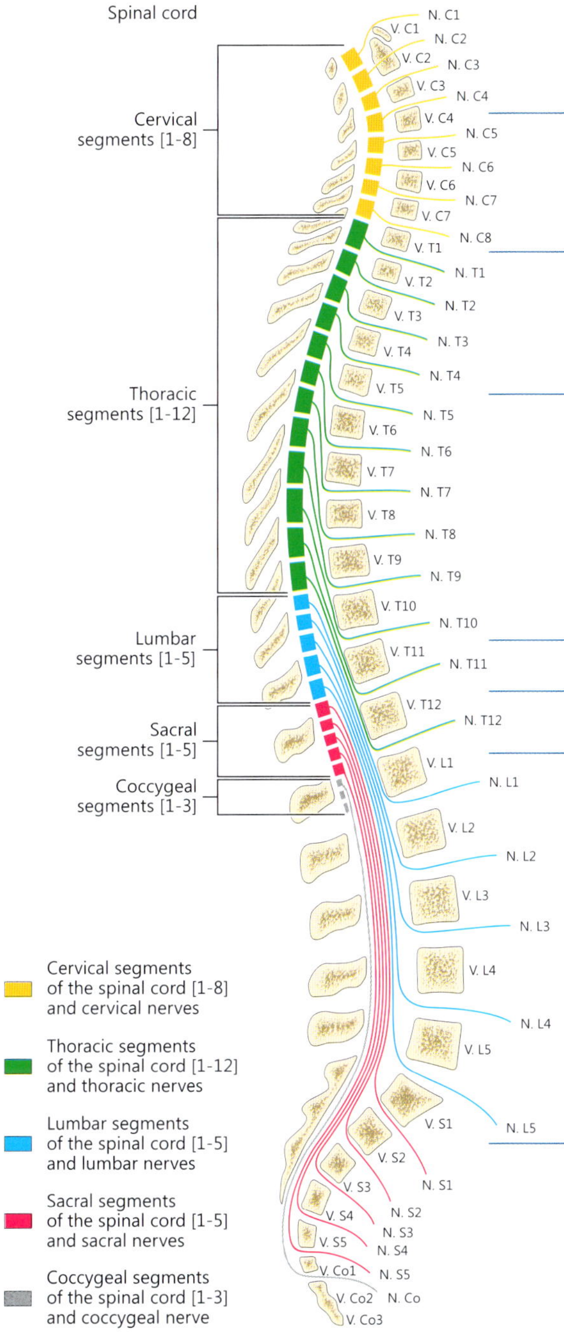

Innervation	Possible Symptoms
Intracranial Blood Vessels - Eyes - Lacrimal Gland - Parotid Gland - Scalp - Base of Skull - Neck Muscles - Diaphragm	Headaches - Migraine Headaches - Dizziness - Sinus Problems - Allergies - Head Colds - Fatigue - Vision Problems - Runny Nose - Sore Throat - Stiff Neck - Cough - Croup - Arm Pain - Hand and Finger Numbness or Tingling - Asthma - Heart Conditions - High Blood Pressure
Neck Muscles - Shoulders - Elbows - Arms - Wrists - Hands - Fingers - Esophagus - Heart - Lungs - Chest	
Arms - Esophagus - Heart - Lungs - Chest - Larynx - Trachea	Wrist, Hand and Finger Numbness or Pain - Middle Back Pain - Congestion - Difficulty Breathing - Asthma - High Blood Pressure - Heart Conditions - Bronchitis - Pneumonia - Gallbladder Conditions - Jaundice - Liver Conditions - Stomach Problems - Ulcers - Gastritis - Kidney Problems
Gallbladder - Liver - Diaphragm - Stomach - Pancreas - Spleen - Kidneys - Small Intestine - Vermiform Appendix - Adrenal Glands	
Small Intestines - Colon - Uterus	
Uterus - Colon - Buttocks	
Large Intestines - Buttocks - Groin - Reproductive Organs - Colon - Thighs - Knees - Legs - Feet	Constipation - Colitis - Diarrhea - Gas Pain - Irritable Bowel - Bladder Problems - Menstrual Problems - Low Back Pain - Pain or Numbness in Legs
Buttocks - Reproductive Organs - Bladder - Prostate Gland - Legs - Ankles - Feet - Toes	Constipation - Diarrhea - Bladder Problems - Menstrual Problems - Lower Back Pain - Pain or Numbness in Legs

Figure 6.2 The vertebral spinal column - nerve pathway map provides a reliable guide to help understand what symptoms may be affected by the three parts of the NST Dynamic Body Balance (DBB). DBB1 correlates to T7-L5, DBB2 correlates to T2-T6 and DBB3 correlates to C1-T1.

spiratory Mechanism as a whole, which it will do extremely effectively for the vast majority of individuals.

DBB is specifically indicated for individuals who do not have a lot of chronic muscular compensation in the body. Good examples of individuals who would fit this category are children and athletes.

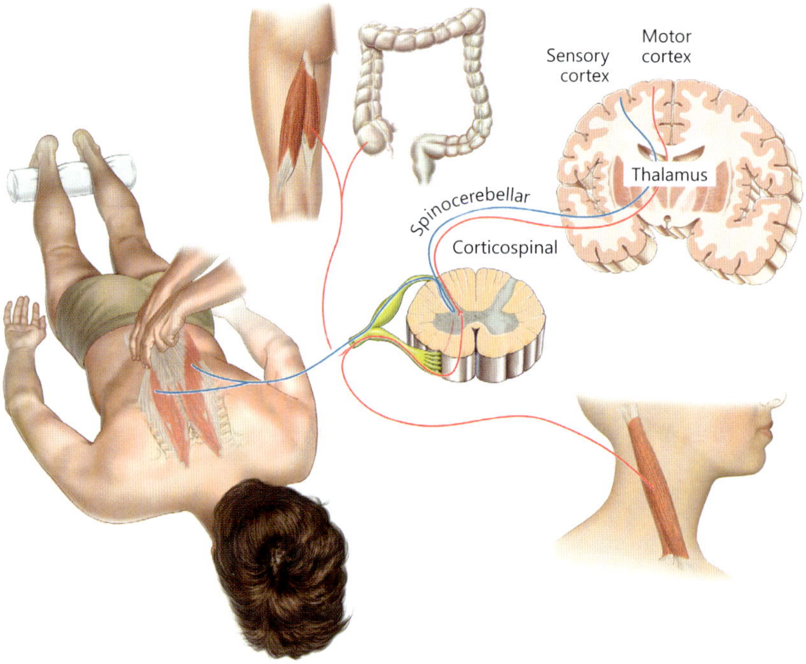

Figure 6.3 To execute every point throughout the DBB a Pri-move is performed, that employs a "stretch-contact-move" formula. A Pri-move may simultaneously affect muscles, organs, fascia and nerves depending on where it is performed. Sequences of Pri-moves typically create a neurological tipping point that initiates the process of autoregulation. Patient's responses are always subjective.

To be clear, this is not to say that individuals who do have a lot of muscular compensation, will not benefit from the DBB alone, as they generally will; however, achieving a complete resolution of associated presenting conditions for such individuals, will, as a rule, require more specific attention, such as the addition of further procedures and protocols as outlined after this section.

As a general guide to understanding which sections of the DBB will effect which part of the body, following the sensory and motor nerve pathways exiting the vertebral spinal column, is a reliable map (Fig. 6.2). Note: Energy pathways will often mimic neurological pathways but not always.

But first, let us deal with the DBB alone to get a clearer picture of just how the sequences of steps and Pri-moves are applied (Fig. 6.3).

Each step will be described by way of an "Action" with basic anatomical references and the "Resultant effect" being the typical outcome achieved based on clinical outcomes for approximately 5,000 patients and/or NST students since 1996.

An additional "Note" will be provided where necessary and refers to any further relevant information to do with the point itself, and its energetic significance according to Bowen's observations or, indeed, the principles of Traditional Chinese Medicine (TCM), both of which have many similarities theoretically and practically.

In particular, the notes relating to energy movement are just for informational purposes and are not essential to comprehend in order to ensure that the NST Pri-moves work effectively.

The DBB has three parts simple referred to DBB1, DBB2 and DBB3.

- DBB1 contains 9 steps.
- DBB2 contains 5 steps.
- DBB3 contains 6 steps.

Indications: Lumbar back pain, hip pain, leg pain, sciatica, knee pain, cramps, kidney and bladder problems, menstrual problems, large intestine problems, small intestine problems, adrenal problems, chronic fatigue and emotional depression.

Point 1

Action: Bilateral Pri-move applied to the lateral border of the iliocostalis lumborum muscle at the level of spinal vertebrae L3-L4 (Fig. 6.4).

Resultant effect: Sedation of the general lumbar spine musculature. Reduction in tonus of the general hamstring musculature. Reduction in tonus of the upper cervical spine musculature.

Note: In energetic terms, points 1 are referred to as a "block" and general sedation point, designed to temporarily slow the energy in the channel so that it can re-establish its proper flow and rhythm.

Relevant corollary points in TCM are governing vessel 4, bladder 23, 24 and 25.

Point 2

Action: Bilateral Pri-move applied to the common lateral border of the longissimus and semispinalis thoracis muscles at the level of spinal vertebrae T7-T9 (Fig. 6.5).

Resultant effect: Sedation of the thoracic spine musculature around T7-T9. Relaxation and improved function of the diaphragm muscle and respiration. Heart rate may slow and blood pressure may start to normalize.

Note: In energetic terms, points 2 are referred to as a "block" and general sedation point, designed to temporarily slow the energy in the channel so that it can re-establish its proper flow and rhythm.

Relevant corollary points in TCM are governing vessel 9 and 10, bladder 16, 17 and 18.

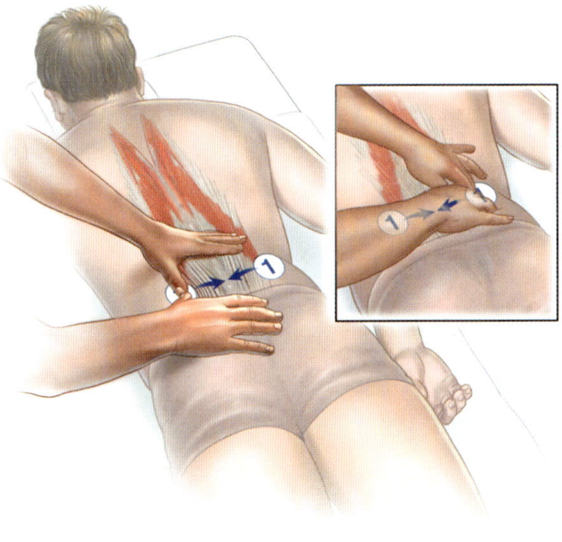

Figure 6.4 Medial bilateral Pri-move applied to L3-L4 level. In energetic terms, point 1 is a sedation block for the lumbar spine.

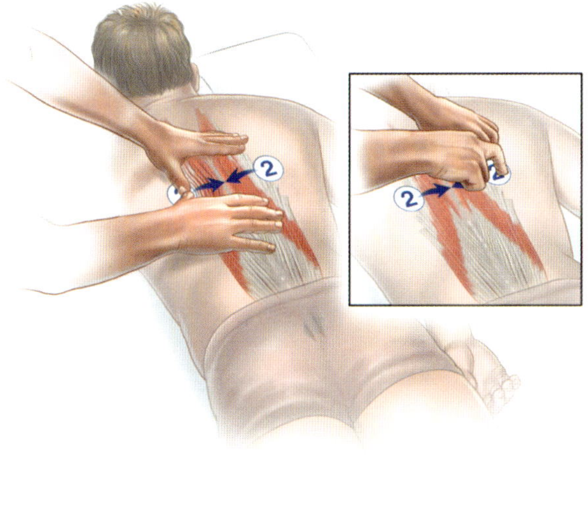

Figure 6.5 Medial bilateral Pri-move applied to T7-T9 level. In energetic terms, point 2 is a sedation block for the thoracic spine but a stimulus for the diaphragm.

Point 3

Action: Pri-move applied to the intersecting border of the gluteus maximus and gluteus medius muscles on a line consistent with the superior level of the gluteal crease. Action is bilateral (Fig. 6.6).

Resultant effect: Reduction in tonus of the general musculature of the buttock. Reduction in tissue tension over the sacral body.

Note: Helps prepare the sacrum for release by equalizing muscle tensions via gluteus maximus muscle. Helps with hip articulation because of its effect on both the gluteus maximus and gluteus medius muscles.

Relevant corollary points in TCM are bladder 48 and 49, gallbladder 30.

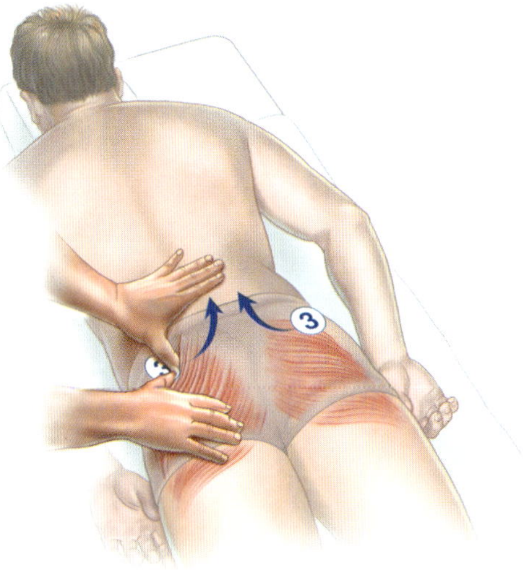

Figure 6.6 Medial bilateral Pri-move applied to the intersection of gluteus maximus and gluteus medius muscles. Helps improve function of the sacrum.

Point 4

Action: The sacral body is stabilized while manual lateral traction is applied to the sacrum and simultaneous flexion and torquing pressure of the lower extremity applied in a contralateral direction. Action is bilateral (Fig. 6.7).

Resultant effect: Additional reduction in tension over the sacral body and improved mobility of the sacrum with reduction in sacroiliac joint pain.

Note: In energetic terms agitates the sacral energy pool readying it for reintroduction into the channel with activation of point 8.

Relevant corollary points in TCM are governing vessel 2 and 3, bladder points 26-35.

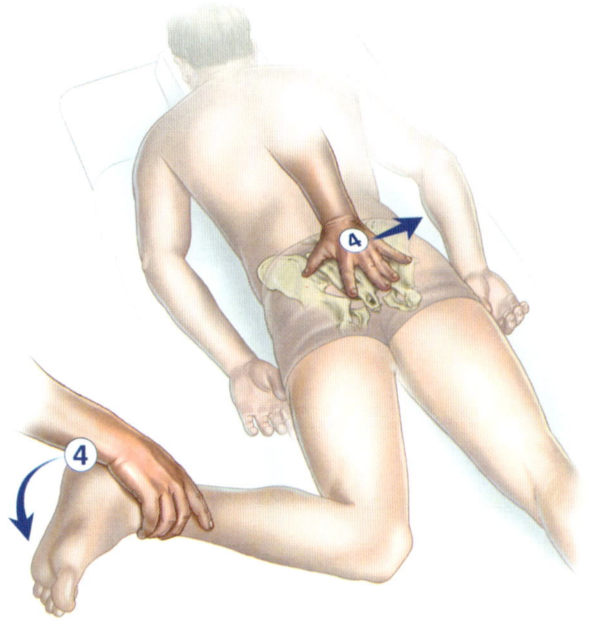

Figure 6.7 Bilateral mobilization applied to the sacral body and sacroiliac joints. Helps improve function of the sacrum.

Point 5

Action: Deep lateral Pri-move applied to the common tendon of the hamstring muscles immediately distal to the ischial tuberosity, followed by three posterior Pri-moves applied to the iliotibial tract in a distal to cranial direction. Action is bilateral (Fig. 6.8).

Resultant effect: Deep relaxation of the hamstring muscles and reduction in tension of the iliotibial band. Further improvement in mobility of the sacrum.

Note: Points 5 and 5a, 5b, 5c are often joined by point 5d which is simply an additional optional Pri-move applied over the belly of the tensor fascia latae muscle.

In clinical practice, the patient is given a strategic pause of between two to ten minutes duration after points 5 have been completed. The duration is determined according the severity of muscular compensation. The more compensation the longer the pause.

Fundamentally, the pause is given to allow the process of natural autoregulation (sacro-spino-cranial integration) to start and deepen, thereby providing a guarantee that a favorable result will be attained. Importantly, the mobility of the sacrum starts to resume its involuntary figure 8 "fish swim" motion.

When patients are not afforded a pause after points 5, the results are still quite satisfactory although typically more superficial. As a consequence, the patient may require four sessions rather than two to achieve total resolution of their presenting condition.

In energetic terms, points 5 further increase the energy potential (volume) in the sacral pool.

Relevant corollary points in TCM are bladder 35 and 50, gallbladder 30, 31, 32 and 33.

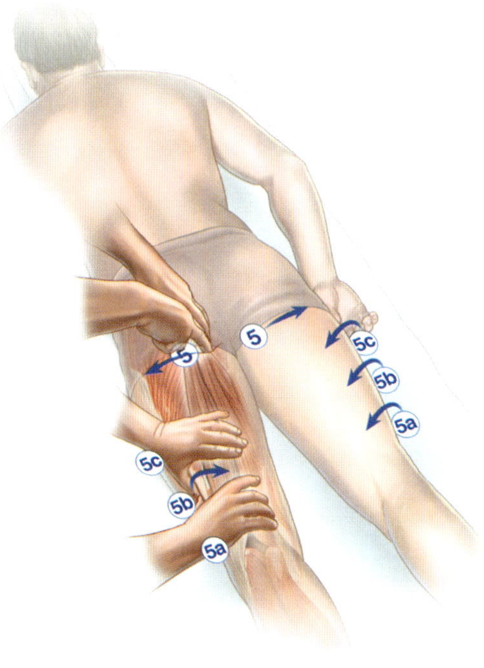

Figure 6.8 Lateral and medial Pri-moves applied to the common tendon of the hamstring muscles and the iliotibial band respectively. Firstly left leg and then right leg. Helps equalize tensions acting on the pelvic girdle, and in doing so improves function of the sacrum.

Point 6

Action: Bilateral Pri-move applied to the common lateral border of the longissimus and semispinalis thoracis muscles at the level of spinal vertebrae T7-T9 (Fig. 6.9).

Resultant effect: Maintains sedation of the thoracic spine musculature around T7-T9 plus relaxation and improved function of the diaphragm muscle and respiration. Maintains heart rate and blood pressure normalization.

Note: In energetic terms, points 6 are referred to as "re-blocking", and keep the channel energy flows between the sacrum and diaphragm constant.

Relevant corollary points in TCM are governing vessel 9 and 10, bladder 16, 17 and 18.

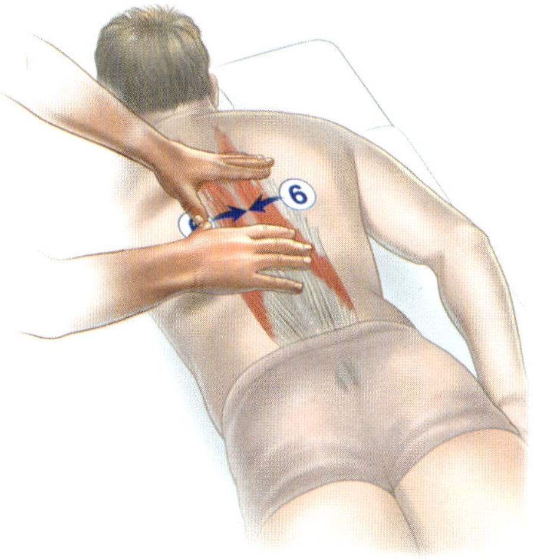

Figure 6.9 Medial bilateral Pri-move applied to T7-T9 level. Acts as a re-confirmation of point 2.

Point 7

Action: Three lateral Pri-moves applied to the longissimus thoracis muscle at the approximate levels of spinal vertebrae T10, T12 and L2, respectively. Action is bilateral (Fig. 6.10).

Resultant effect: Deep relaxation of the longissimus and spinalis thoracis muscles and deeper paraspinal muscles between T7 and L5 section of the spine.

Note: In energetic terms, points 7 are referred to as "opening the channel" and the action is designed to permit the flow of energy from sacrum to diaphragm.

Relevant corollary points in TCM are governing vessel points 4-8, bladder points 18-22 and also 42-45.

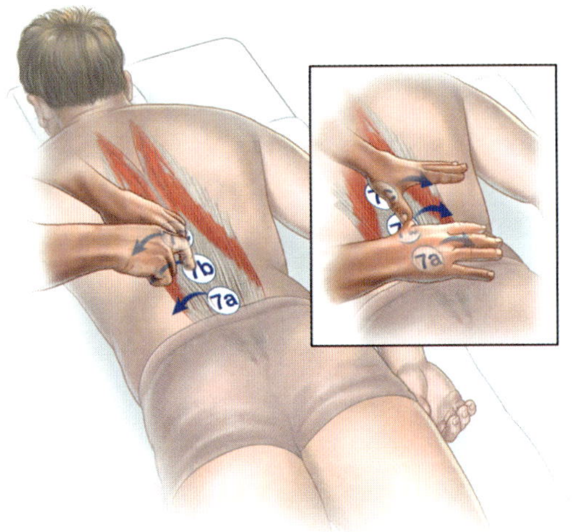

Figure 6.10 Lateral Pri-moves applied to T10, T12 and L2 levels. Firstly left side and then right side. Referred to as "opening the channel" these points also assist in relaxing musculature in and around the lower thoracic and lumbar spines.

Point 8

Action: A medial Pri-move is applied to the common intersection of the longissimus and semispinalis thoracis muscles at the level of spinal vertebra T8. At the same time moderate torquing pressure is applied to the fully flexed lower extremity in a lateral direction. The pressure is sufficient to create a gentle integrative line of force through the sacrum, hips, lumbar and lower thoracic spines, elevating the anterior or pelvic bone off the table by a few centimeters. Action is bilateral (Fig. 6.11).

Resultant effect: Increased flexibility and integration between T8 and the general pelvic girdle.

Note: In energetic terms, points 8 are referred to as "shooting" or propelling the energy through the open channel, from the sacrum to the diaphragm, thereby reinstating appropriate channel energy flows.

Relevant corollary points in TCM are governing vessel 9 and 10, bladder 16, 17 and 18 and, to some extent, all of the preceding TCM points mentioned in DBB1 (points 1-7) are involved in one way or the other, whether that be fully discharging and emptying out or replenishing.

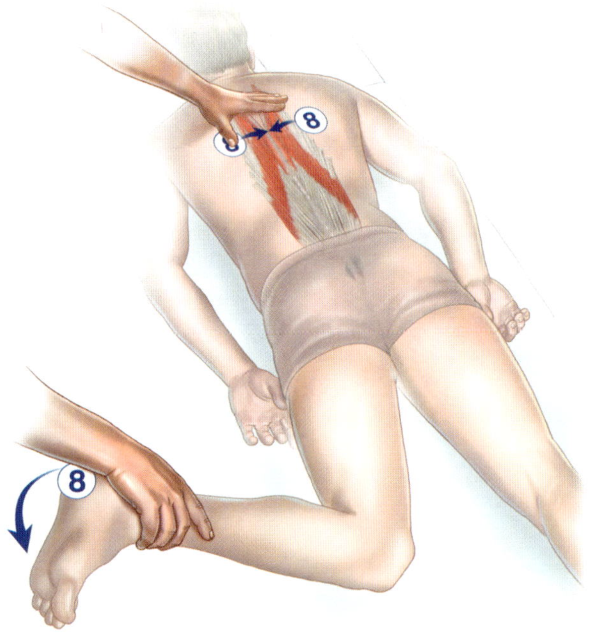

Figure 6.11 Medial bilateral, torque assisted Pri-move applied to T8 level. Assists in re-establishing integration between the hip, sacrum, lumbar and thoracic spines.

Point 9

Action: Three medial Pri-moves applied to the longissimus thoracis muscle in a medial direction at the approximate levels of spinal vertebrae T10, T12 and L2, respectively (Fig. 6.12).

Resultant effect: Ensures and maintains deep relaxation of the longissimus and spinalis thoracis muscles and deeper paraspinal muscles between T7 and L5 section of the spine.

Note: In energetic terms, points 9 are referred to as "closing the channel" and are designed to ensure the channel energies are maintained at appropriate flow rate.

Relevant corollary points in TCM are governing vessel points 4-8, bladder points 18-22 and also 42-45.

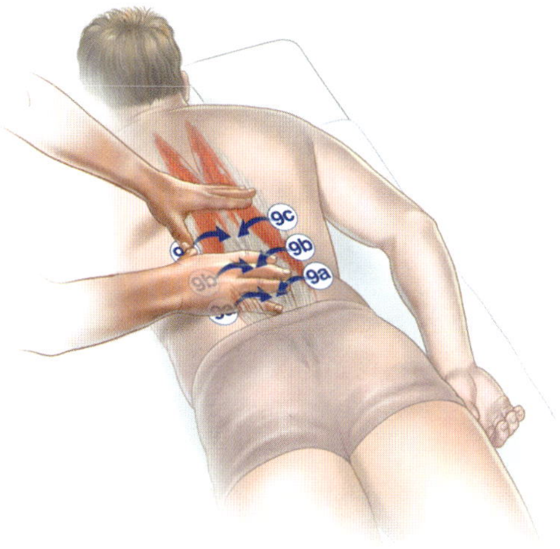

Figure 6.12 Medial Pri-moves applied to T10, T12 and L2 levels. Firstly left side and then right side. Referred to as "closing the channel" these points also assist in relaxing musculature in and around the lower thoracic and lumbar spines.

DBB2 – Prone position – 5 steps

Indications: Thoracic back pain, shoulder pain, neck pain, headaches, chest pain, breathing problems, adrenal gland problems, spleen problems, pancreas problems, stomach problems, liver problems, gallbladder problems, heart problems, chronic fatigue and emotional depression.

Point 1

Action: Bilateral Pri-move applied to the common lateral border of the longissimus and semispinalis thoracis muscles at the level of spinal vertebrae T7-T9 (Fig. 6.13).

Resultant effect: Sedation of the thoracic spine musculature around T7-T9. Relaxation and improved function of the diaphragm and respiration.

Note: In energetic terms, points 1 are referred to as a "block" but in fact are "re-blocking" having been performed three times in DBB1 already. They continue to provide a block in the lower channel and keep the channel energy flows between the sacrum and diaphragm constant.

Relevant corollary points in TCM are governing vessel 9 and 10, bladder 16, 17 and 18.

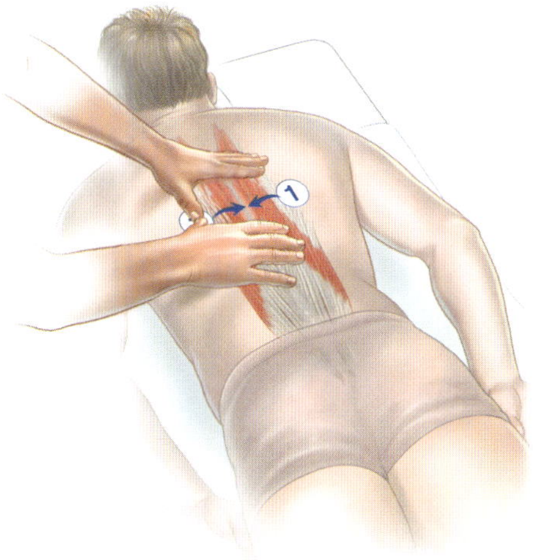

Figure 6.13 Medial bilateral Pri-move applied to T7-T9 level. Acts as a re-confirmation of point 2 in DBB1.

Point 2

Action: Three lateral Pri-moves applied to the medial border of the spinalis thoracis muscle at the approximate levels of spinal vertebrae T7, T5 and T3, respectively. Action is bilateral (Fig. 6.14).

Resultant effect: Deep relaxation of the upper thoracic spine musculature and the rhomboid muscles. Activation of these points also activates the thoracic origin of the upper trapezius muscle, and relaxation of the general trapezius muscle will also be noticeable. Improved range of motion in shoulder articulation.

Note: In energetic terms, points 7 are referred to as "opening the upper channel" and the action is designed to continue the flow of energy from sacrum to the cranium.

Relevant corollary points in TCM are governing vessel points 11-14, bladder points 11-16 and 36-40.

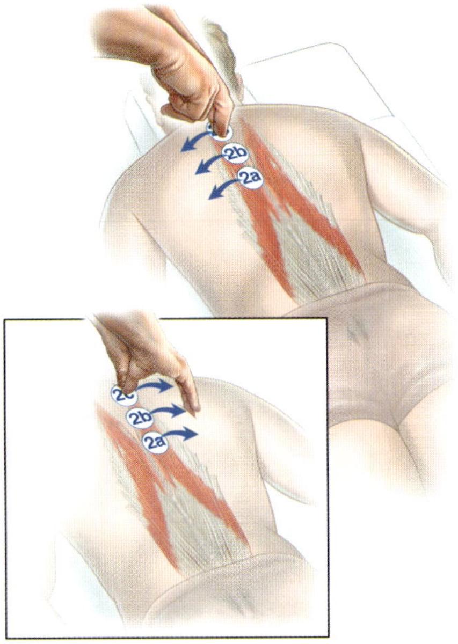

Figure 6.14 Lateral Pri-moves applied to T7, T5 and T3 levels. Firstly left side and then right side. Referred to as "opening the channel" these points also assist in relaxing musculature in and around the upper thoracic spine including rhomboids.

Point 3

Action: A medial Pri-move is applied to the common intersection of the longissimus and semispinalis thoracis muscles at the level of spinal vertebra T8. At the same time moderate torquing pressure is applied to the fully flexed lower extremity in a lateral direction. The pressure is sufficient to create a gentle integrative line of force through the sacrum, hips, lumbar and lower thoracic spine elevating the anterior pelvic bone off the table by a few centimeters. Action is bilateral (Fig. 6.15).

Resultant effect: Reinforces flexibility and integration between T8 and the general pelvic girdle.

Note: In energetic terms, points 3, like points 8 in DBB1, are referred to as "shooting" or propelling the energy through the open channel from the sacrum to the diaphragm, thereby reinstating appropriate channel energy flows. When done as part of DBB2, the lower channel energies are reactivated just prior to opening the gates at points 4 that permit the upper thoracic channel energies to flow into cranial channel. Relevant corollary points in TCM are governing vessel 9 and 10, bladder 16, 17 and 18.

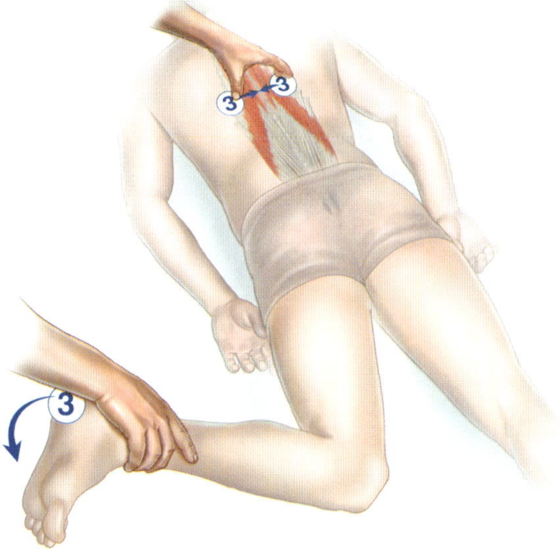

Figure 6.15 Medial bilateral, torque assisted Pri-move applied to T8 level. Acts as a re-confirmation of point 8 in DBB1.

Point 4

Action: Oblique Pri-move is applied to the levator scapulae muscle adjacent to its insertion into the scapula and at the approximate level of spinal vertebra T2. The levator scapulae muscle is retained in a rotated position, while three medial Pri-moves are applied to the lateral border of the spinalis thoracis muscle, at the approximate levels of spinal vertebrae T7, T5 and T3, respectively. Action is bilateral (Fig. 6.16).

Resultant effect: Reduction in tonus and relaxation of the levator scapulae muscle and upper thoracic spine musculature. Reduction in tonus of the upper trapezius muscles. Relaxation of the general deltoid muscles of the shoulder. Further reduction in tonus of the upper cervical spine musculature, initially achieved with points 1 - DBB1.

Respiration may noticeably deepen and coincide with overall general body relaxation.

Note: Point 4 is one of those seemingly insignificant points until activated when a "lot of change" follows. This may be because of the fact, that so much preparation has already been accomplished via DBB1 and the DBB2 channels being cleared, and the associated spinal musculature relaxation.

In energetic terms, points 4 open the "gates" permitting upper thoracic channel energies to flow into the cranial channels via the direct vertical spinal pathways and the secondary "small intestine" energy pathways that terminate at the TMJ. Relevant corollary points in TCM are bladder 11, governing vessel 14, small intestine 15 and 19.

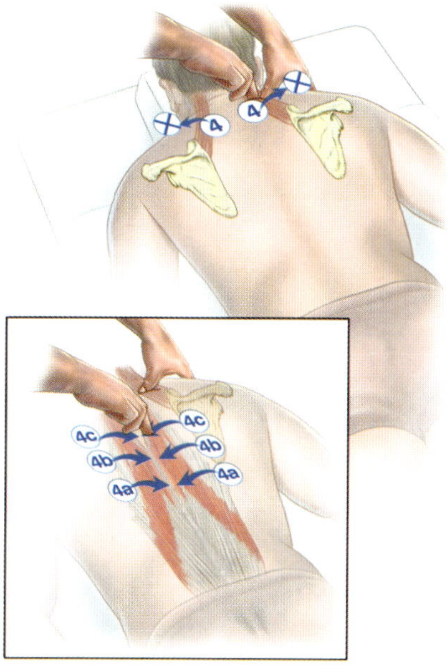

Figure 6.16 Oblique and medial Pri-moves applied to levator scapulae muscle and T7, T5 and T3 levels respectively. Firstly left side and then right side. These points assist in establishing a continuity of release between the upper thoracic spine and the cervical spine.

Point 5

Action: Circular Pri-moves applied to the common lateral border of the teres major and latissimus dorsi muscles and inferior angle of the scapula, respectively. Action is bilateral (Fig. 6.17).

Resultant effect: Reduction in tonus of the teres major and latissimus dorsi muscles. Enhanced range of motion of the shoulder articulation.

Note: In energetic terms, points 5 function as enhancement points for cranial channel flows to the TMJ.

Relevant corollary points in TCM are large intestine 15 and small intestine 10.

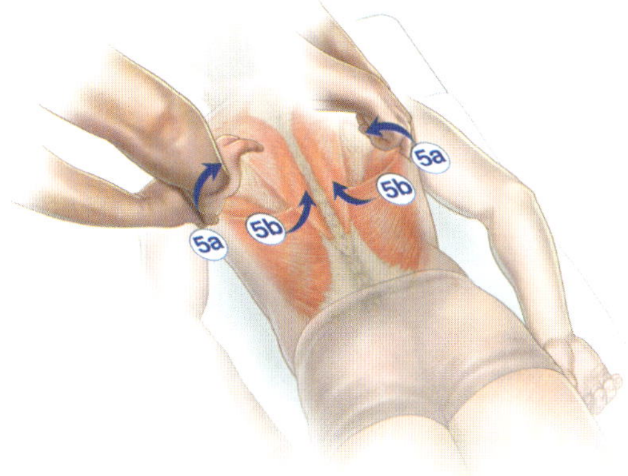

Figure 6.17 Circular Pri-moves applied to common border of the teres major and latissimus dorsi muscles and around the inferior angle of the scapula respectively. These points assist with enhanced range of motion of the shoulder articulation.

Indications: Neck pain, shoulder pain, headaches, throat problems, thyroid gland problems, facial pain, tooth pain, ear problems, eye problems, breathing problems, high blood pressure, dizziness, chronic fatigue and emotional depression.

Point 1

Action: Pri-move applied to the levator scapulae muscle immediately distal to its 4th point of origin at cervical vertebra C4 and crossing the cervical nerve plexus at the same level. Action is bilateral (Fig. 6.18).

Resultant effect: Further reduction in tonus and relaxation of the general neck musculature. Enhanced range of motion of the cervical spine generally. Enhanced respiration. Heart rate and blood pressure normalization.

Note: The phrenic nerves that innervate the diaphragm muscle originate largely from the cervical plexus but also receives some nerve supply from the brachial plexus.

In energetic terms, points 1 give impetus to the craniosacral energy flows.

Relevant corollary point in TCM is triple heater 16.

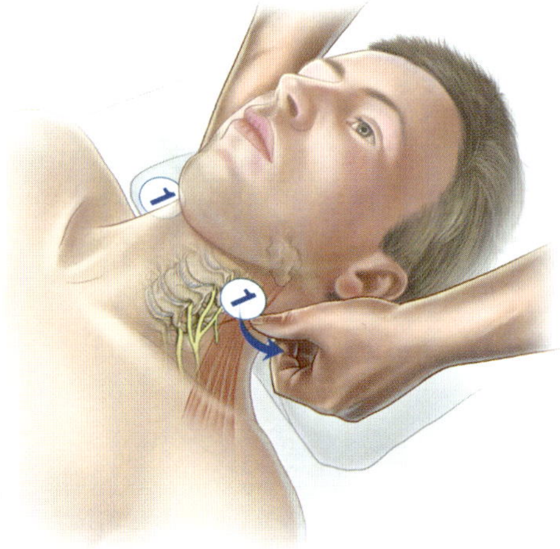

Figure 6.18 Posterior Pri-move applied to levator scapulae muscle at C4 level crossing the cervical nerve plexus. Firstly left side and then right side. Improvement in respiration can often be observed after the activation of point 1 due to the origin of the phrenic nerve at this point. Assists with enhanced mobility of the cervical spine, shoulders and respiration.

Point 2

Action: Pri-move applied to the brachial nerve plexus deep in the supraclavicular fossa. Action is bilateral (Fig. 6.19).

Resultant effect: Rapid reduction in tonus and relaxation of the general neck, shoulder and upper back musculature. Enhanced range of motion of the cervical spine generally. Enhanced respiration. Heart rate and blood pressure normalization.

Note: The phrenic nerves that innervate the diaphragm muscle originate largely from the cervical plexus but also receives some nerve supply from the brachial plexus.

In energetic terms, point 2 opens the frontal energy channel back to the diaphragm and sacrum.

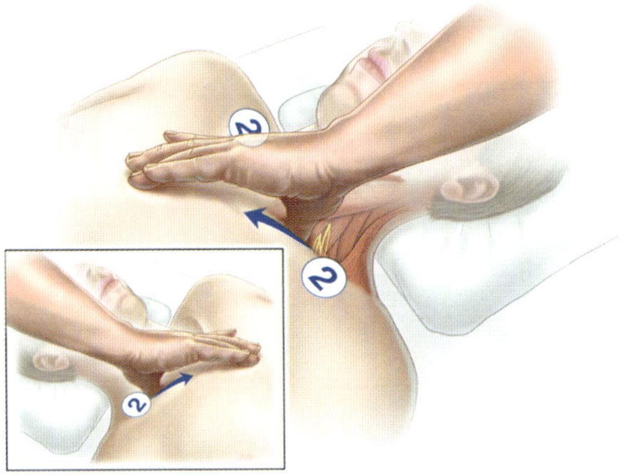

Figure 6.19 Pri-move applied to the brachial nerve plexus. Firstly left side and then right side. This powerful point typically achieves a rapid reduction in neck and shoulder muscle tension.

Relevant corollary point in TCM is the all-important Stomach 12 which in TCM is important for almost everything, as it has direct connections with most other meridians.

Point 3

Action: Oblique Pri-move is applied to the levator scapulae muscle adjacent to its insertion into the scapula and at the approximate level of spinal vertebra T2. Action is bilateral (Fig. 6.20).

Resultant effect: At this point of the DBB, this Pri-move is reinserted (previously inserted at point 4 in DBB2) to make sure that no twisting or torquing of the levator scapulae muscle has occurred, whilst the patient moved from a prone to supine position.

Note: In energetic terms, the reinsertion of the point at this juncture, is to ensure that the "gate" remains clear and open until final completion of the energy cycle is achieved with activation of point 4 from DBB3.

Relevant corollary points in TCM are bladder 11, governing vessel 14, small intestine 15 and 19.

Point 4

Action: Pri-move is applied to the origin of the upper trapezius muscle at the superior nuchal line of the cranium. Action is bilateral (Fig. 6.21).

Resultant effect: Often imperceptible in terms of noticing any direct muscle tonus reduction, but important mechanoreceptors are contained in the upper trapezius muscle's cranial tendon and activation of these points helps with cranial mobility, an important feature for the proper function of the Secondary Respiratory Mechanism - SRM. Patient may feel light-headed or dizzy.

It's also worthwhile considering the unbroken connection that the upper trapezius tendon shares with the nuchal ligament and the general cranial aponeurosis, in regard to neck and cranial conditions and SRM/SGS function.

Points 4 are also adjacent to the greater occipital nerve that penetrates the semispinalis capitis muscle on its way to the skin of the cranium that it innervates.

Although not directly traceable, it appears that activation of these points assists with gen-

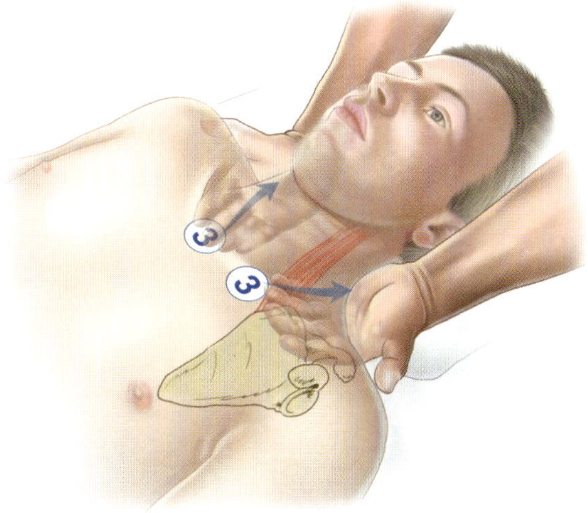

Figure 6.20 Pri-move applied to the insertion of the levator scapulae muscle into the scapula. Firstly left side and then right side. Ensures that levator scapulae muscle is fully released.

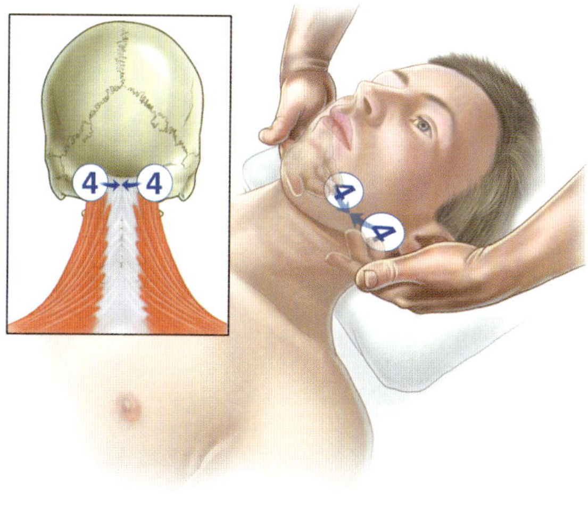

Figure 6.21 Medial bilateral Pri-move applied to upper trapezius muscle origin at the superior nuchal line of the cranium. Small but important points that assist with enhanced cranial mobility and the function of the SRM generally.

eral improvement of the range of motion of the neck, sinusitis, dizziness, visual disturbance and headaches.

Note: There is always a benefit in allowing the body to respond to the changes that follow activation of these four important points, as they can tend to be both of a cranial nature and whole body nature. After all this is the point where the sacrum and cranium finally meet. In short, there is a lot going on in terms of muscle, nerve and fascial releases, including intracranial releases.

In clinical practice, the practitioner gives a 1-2 minute pause after points 4, which can be achieved by working on the lower extremity if necessary.

In energetic terms, points 4 are the insertion points for Bowen's channel and are significant from a craniosacral energy flow perspective. Indeed, it is exactly at these points that the Primary Respiratory Mechanism – PRM is induced from (see Chapter 7, Cranial Procedure – 5 Steps).

Relevant corollary points in TCM are gallbladder 20, bladder 10, governing vessel 16 and 17.

Point 5

Note: Point 5 is simple an instruction for the practitioner to leave the head region allowing the patient to have a 1-2 minute pause and simply go to the knee on the left side ready to execute the next Pri-move (Fig. 6.22).

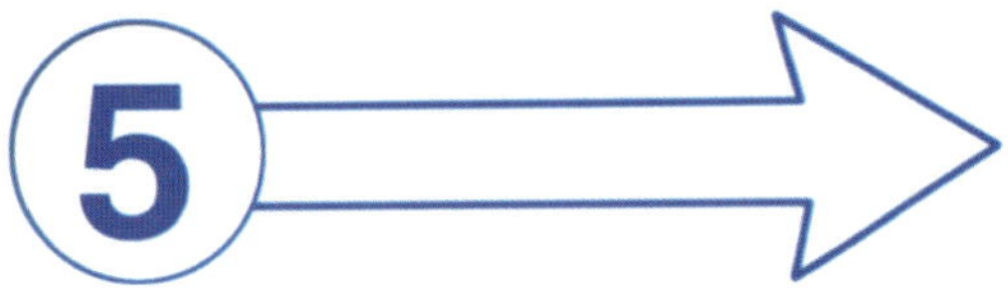

Figure 6.22 Arrow indicating that the practitioner now stops working at the cranium and moves to the left leg where either point 6 of DBB3 or the Knee procedure (see Chapter 7, Knee Procedure) should be performed.

Point 6

Action: Pri-move applied to the insertion of the vastus lateralis muscle at the superior lateral aspect of patella of the knee. Action is bilateral (Fig. 6.23).

Resultant effect: Rapidly improves articulation of the knee and reduces knee pain. Assists with pelvic, hip and sacral integration, and consequently has an overall positive effect on the integration and function of the SRM. Hamstring function also improves.

Note: This Pri-move must be performed very slowly to release effectively, and typically provides a strong "bump" as it releases.

There may be a noticeable difference in the volume of one vastus lateralis tendon to the other, and this is always regarded as being a good "reading point" for the general tensegrity of the lower extremity and also for the recent status of the pelvis.

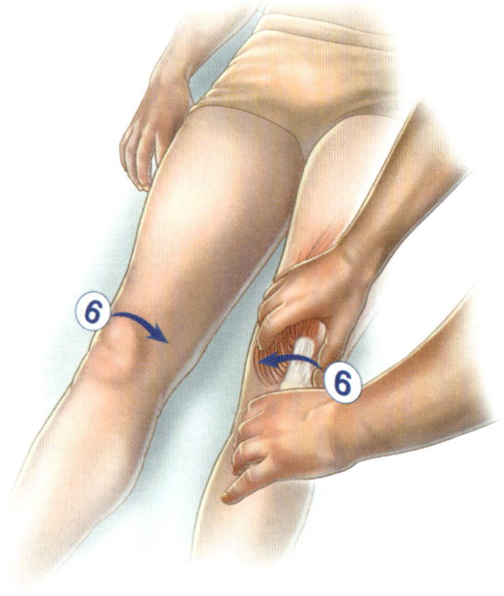

Figure 6.23 Medial Pri-move applied to the insertion of the vastus lateralis muscle at the superior lateral aspect of the patella. Firstly left side and then right side. Significantly improves knee articulation, pelvic girdle mobility and consequently function of the SRM.

Point 6 therefore is used at subsequent sessions to monitor patient progress, and is a reliable indicator for when the SRM generally is holding its integration or not.

While most points in the NST system are activated just once, or perhaps twice, points 6 may be activated several times as they function as dispersion points for the lower extremities and appear to further settle the SRM into rhythm.

To Bowen, this release was one of the most important points in his whole system of points. He claimed that it would release the pelvis, assist with shoulder release and restore the energy flows of the body's energy cycle. It must be remembered that Bowen had no knowledge of the SRM or PRM, yet his terminology frequently referred to their function both singularly and interactively.

Relevant corollary points in TCM are gallbladder 33 and stomach 34.

Point 7

Action: Pri-move applied to the origin of the upper trapezius muscle at the nuchal ligament at the level of spinal vertebrae C4-C5. Action is bilateral (Fig. 6.24).

Resultant effect: Relaxation of the upper trapezius muscle with possible enhanced range of movement in the cervical spine and shoulders. Respiration may also further improve.

Note: This Pri-move must be performed very slowly to release effectively, and typically provides a strong "deflection" when it releases.

There may be a noticeable difference in the volume of one upper trapezius point 7 to the other, and this is always regarded as being a good "reading point" for the general tensegrity of the neck musculature, and perhaps even the history of the patient's neck condition.

Point 7 therefore is used at subsequent sessions to monitor patient progress, for neck and shoulder conditions.

Whereas most points in the NST system are

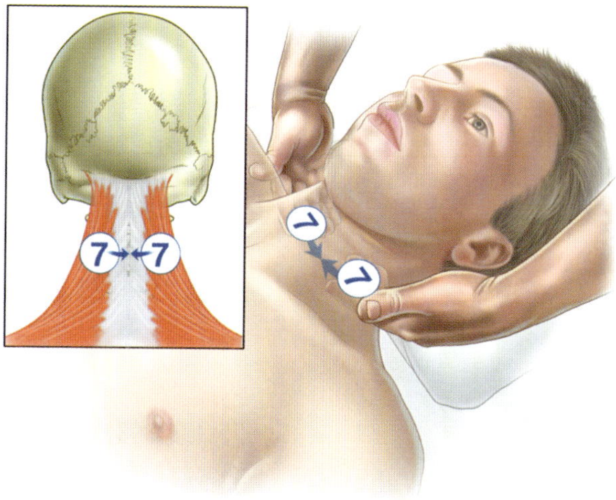

Figure 6.24 Medial bilateral Pri-move applied to upper trapezius muscle origin lateral to the nuchal ligament, at the level of cervical vertebrae C4-C5.

activated just once, or perhaps twice, points 7, like points 6, may be activated several times as they function as dispersion points for the cervical spine musculature and appear to help further settle the SRM into rhythm.

Relevant corollary points in TCM are gallbladder 14 and 15.

CONCLUSION

Dynamic Body Balance – Parts 1, 2, 3 – is the Essential Core of NST work, the "NST engine" if you will, and Dynamic Body Balance alone will move mountains therapeutically speaking, by bringing the components and the rhythm of the Secondary Respiratory Mechanism back into balance.

If the Dynamic Body Balance was the only structural and spinal intervention technique, that a practitioner had at his or her disposal to use, it would be a very effective correction strategy in and of itself.

To summarize things thus far and accustom ourselves to the flow of an NST session, here's how the Dynamic Body Balance would be performed.

PRONE SECTION

DBB1 ← *Pause for 5 minutes after point 5.*
DBB2
End of prone section ← *Pause for 2 minutes*

SUPINE SECTION

DBB3 → Points 1-4
5 → Go to the left knee
DBB3 → Point 6
DBB3 → Point 7
Optional - reinsert points 6 and 7
End of supine section ← *Pause for 2 minutes*

However, Dynamic Body Balance can also be added to with various specific procedures and protocols, to build a more detailed and tailored session for each patient, thereby creating deeper release of the spine and its structures, ultimately, leading to a more rapid and thorough elimination of symptoms and sustainability of corrections.

In reality, in modern day clinical practice, in dealing with the complex chronic structural and neuromuscular conditions that patients present with, tailoring a session with detail is the most desirable, efficient and effective way to proceed when applying NST.

Our next section, Chapter 7, will add further scope to building an integrated NST session, and will detail the specific procedures and protocols that may be added in the prone and supine positions, that will essentially add deeper unlocking to the core through the sacrum, diaphragm, pelvis, coccyx and TMJ. It will also introduce the procedures for symptoms contained in the extremities themselves.

Adding Depth and Specificity to the Session 7

INTRODUCTION

Adding depth and specificity to an NST session are done with two general objectives in mind. Firstly to enhance the level of musculoskeletal integration, and thereby bring the organism back to a point where it can hold the corrections.

Hence better integration leads to sustainability of corrections, and there is no better outcome for the patient than to know that they have been properly "reset", and barring accidents or sabotaging lifestyle practices, they will have every chance of holding their corrections!

Building a more tailored and integrated NST session is accomplished by adding further procedures and protocols that suit the patient's presenting condition, or that match soft tissue or structural indicators that the practitioner finds at the table throughout the session.

Tight ligaments, specific articulation restrictions, specific pain and range of motion conditions and leg length differences, are some of the most classical indicators that are evaluated when deciding on which other procedures or protocols to include in the session.

The second objective or reason to add further procedures would be for when a larger procedure, such as Coccyx, Pelvis or TMJ (all determined by assessment), requires that certain prerequisite procedures are performed firstly, such as sacrum for coccyx, knee for pelvis or shoulder for TMJ.

Adhering to recommended prerequisites in NST is what really creates the unlocking of deep and chronic compensations in the neuromuscular system, adding significantly therefore, to the sustainability of corrections achieved within the session.

As an NST session always commences in the prone position, all further potential procedures for the prone position are considered before any supine work is commenced. Once all prone work is completed, the patient moves into a supine position where additional procedures are considered. There is no "flip-flopping" the patient between prone and supine positions.

It's simply all of the prone work first, and then all of the supine work secondly.

And throughout this process certain procedures are woven into the fabric of the DBB, in a particular order that has proven over countless cases to be the most optimal.

Every NST session always commences (in the prone position) with DBB1 and DBB2, after which additional prone procedures may be included, such as:

- Sacrum procedure
- Iliolumbar ligament release
- Hip procedure
- Coccyx procedure
- Hamstring procedure

Once the patient moves into the supine position DBB3 is always added, then there are several more procedures that may also be added, and importantly, significant system procedures such as Lung, Pelvis and TMJ are always considered and/or tested for inclusion.

As with the NST prone position work, procedures in the supine position are done in a particular order as well, thus continuing the process of optimal musculoskeletal integration through the SRM and SGS.

Apart from DBB3, additional **supine** procedures that may be included are as follows:

- Lung procedure
- Knee procedure
- Hamstring procedure
- Ankle procedure
- Foot procedure
- Shoulder procedure
- Elbow and wrist procedure
- Hand procedure
- Pelvic procedure
- TMJ procedures
- Cranial procedure
- Final check cranium to body checks – sitting position

The above procedures and protocols are woven into the Dynamic Body Balance as required for each patient, to create what is essentially a very tailored and integrated osteospinal and osteopathic correction capable of being applied to any presenting symptom.

Whilst the above procedures represent the main body of structural NST work, there are still several more mini-protocols and specific points that can be added for more specialised indications.

These will no doubt become the subject of further publications on NST in the future.

Throughout the following pages all of the above procedures mentioned, will be detailed with basic indications, prerequisites, a short description of how each point is performed, and a specific image for that point.

PRONE POSITION PROCEDURES

Sacrum Procedure – 5 steps

Indications: Sacral pain, sacroiliac conditions, sciatica, sacral edema, back pain, pelvic conditions, knee conditions, occipital headaches, SRM and SGS integration.

Prerequisites: Dynamic Body Balance - Parts 1 and 2 must be completed.

Point 1

Action: Bilateral Pri-move applied to the lateral border of the iliocostalis lumborum muscle at the level of spinal vertebrae L3-L4 (Fig. 7.1).

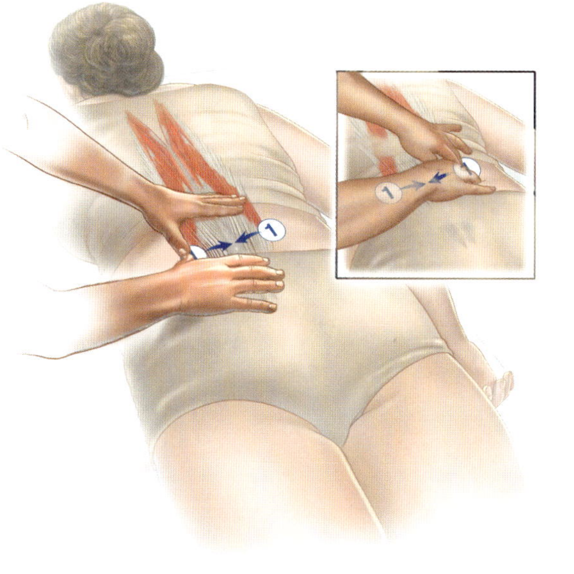

Figure 7.1 Medial bilateral Pri-move applied to L3-L4 level. Acts as a re-confirmation of point 1 in DBB1.

Points 2 and 2a

Action: Abrupt Pri-move applied directly over the Posterior Superior Iliac Spine (PSIS) on the left hand side followed by an abrupt Pri-move over the main angle of the sacral body (Fig. 7.2).

Note: Points 3 and 4 follow on directly after points 2 and 2a. All 4 points must be completed on the left side first.

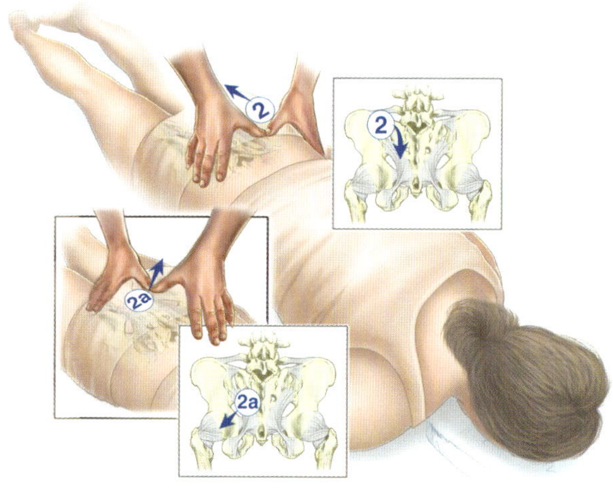

Figure 7.2 Abrupt Pri-move over the PSIS on the left and an abrupt Pri-move over main angle of the sacral body on the left. Assists in releasing the thoracolumbar aponeurosis around the sacrum.

Points 3 and 4

Action: Deep digital pressure is applied to the junction of the sacrotuberous and sacroiliac ligaments directly lateral to the main angle of the sacral body and maintained (Fig. 7.3).

Whilst "holding point" is maintained, a Pri-move is applied to the intersecting border of the gluteus maximus and gluteus medius muscles on a line consistent with the superior level of the gluteal crease.

Note: Repeat points 2, 2a, 3 and 4 on the right hand side.

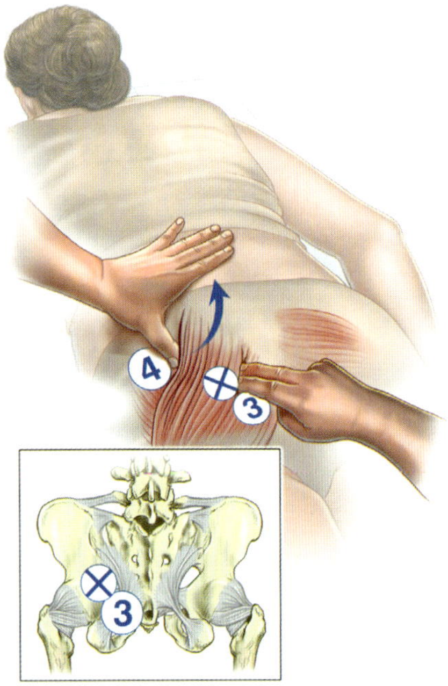

Figure 7.3 Point 3. Deep bi-digital pressure applied to the junction of the sacrotuberous and sacroiliac ligaments on the left and maintained until point 4 is completed. Point 4. Medial Pri-move applied to the intersection of gluteus maximus and gluteus medius muscles on the left. Note: Points 2, 2a, 3 and 4 are now performed on the right side. Assists in relaxing the deeper tissues of the sacrum and improves sacral mobility.

Point 5

Action: Deep lateral Pri-move applied to the common tendon of the iliotibialis (hamstring) muscle group immediately distal to the ischial tuberosity, followed by three posterior Pri-moves applied to the iliotibial tract in a distal to cranial direction. Action is bilateral (Fig. 7.4).

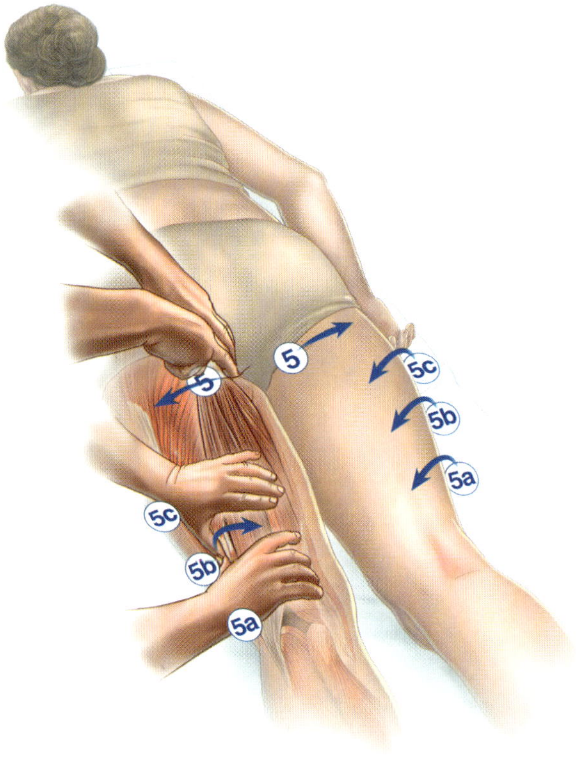

Figure 7.4 Lateral and medial Pri-moves applied to the common tendon of the hamstring muscles and the iliotibial band respectively. Firstly left leg and then right leg. Acts as a re-confirmation of point 5 in DBB1. Necessary at this point to ensure that sacral releases achieved with points 1 to 4 are maintained.

Iliolumbar ligament release – 1 step

Indications: When the ligament is still tight after the Sacrum procedure is completed as determined by palpation.

Improves sacral stability and integration, improves gait walking mechanism.

Prerequisites: Dynamic Body Balance - Parts 1, 2 and Sacrum procedure must be completed.

Point 1

Action: Deep slow Pri-move applied to the iliolumbar ligament in the space between the PSIS and transverse process of the 5th lumbar vertebra (Fig. 7.5).

Note: Typically one thumb is used on top of the other to exert the deeper pressure required to influence the ligament's mechanoreceptors. The iliolumbar ligament is deep, being covered by layers of skin, erector spinae muscle fibers and thoracolumbar fascia.

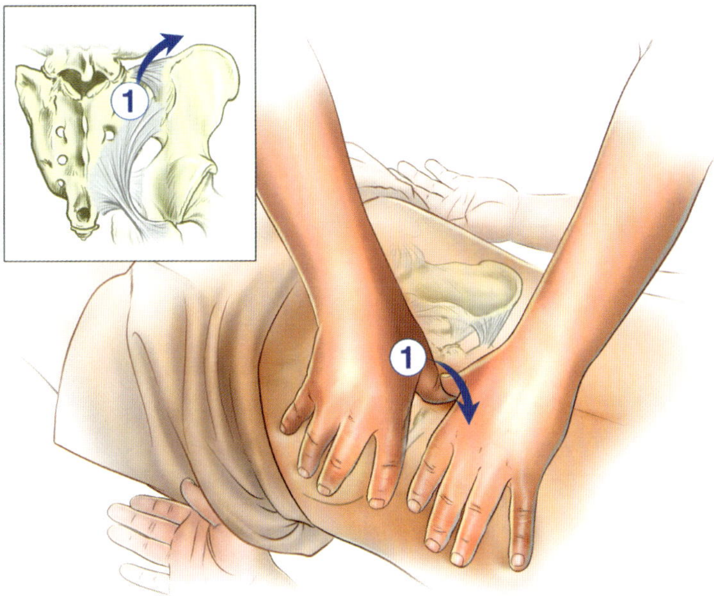

Figure 7.5 Deep slow Pri-move applied to the iliolumbar ligament in a lateral direction. Sufficient contact must be applied to release the iliolumbar ligament as it lies deep to the skin, erector spinae muscle fibers and the thoracolumbar fascia that overlay it. Applied to the tight side only. Assists with lumbosacral integration and improvement in the gait walking mechanism.

Indications: Sciatica, buttock pain, all sacral, pelvic and hip conditions, clicking hip, general leg conditions or for when a short leg persists prior to turning the patient into supine position.

Prerequisites: Dynamic Body Balance - Parts 1, 2 and Sacrum procedure must be completed.

Points 1 and 2

Action: With the hip externally rotated to relax the deep hip rotator muscles (1) a series of deep soft slow Pri-moves are applied to the insertion of the common tendon of the deep hip rotator muscles (2). Action is unilateral to the affected side (Fig. 7.6).

Note: The lower inset image shows that the insertion of the iliopsoas muscle may be crossed just superior to the lesser trochanter with a deep oblique Pri-move as the hip is held in an internally rotated position. Although optional, applying this additional Pri-move can have a very positive effect on restoring appropriate hip articulation and assisting to reduce deep hip pain.

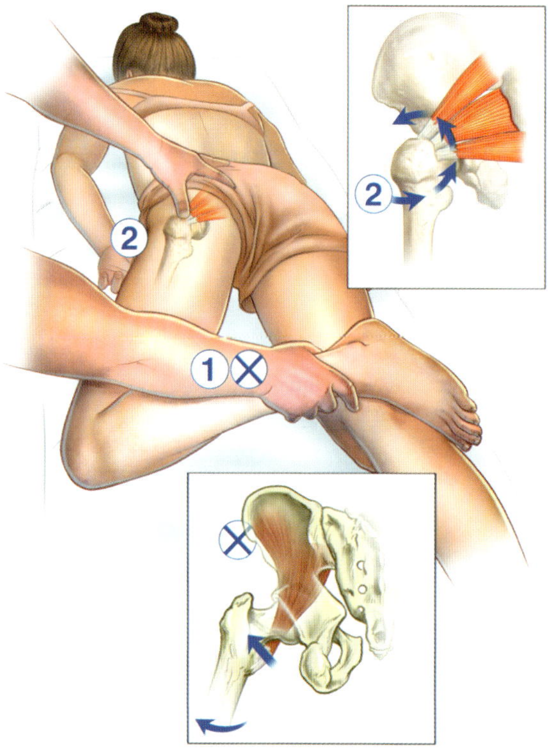

Figure 7.6 The leg is abducted and rotated posteriorly causing an external hip rotation. A series of deep short Pri-moves are applied around the circumference of the greater trochanter. Option: When hip articulation is compromised, the insertion of the psoas muscle may be released just superior to the lesser trochanter. Applied to the affected side only. Improves hip and sacral relationship and releases pressure on the sciatic nerve.

Points 3a and 3b

Action: The lower leg is now moved into a vertical position (3a) with deep thumb contact on the iliofemoral ligament. The leg is momentarily further elevated, then carried laterally and "dropped" as the iliofemoral ligament is crossed superiorly with a deep Pri-move. Action is unilateral (Fig. 7.7).

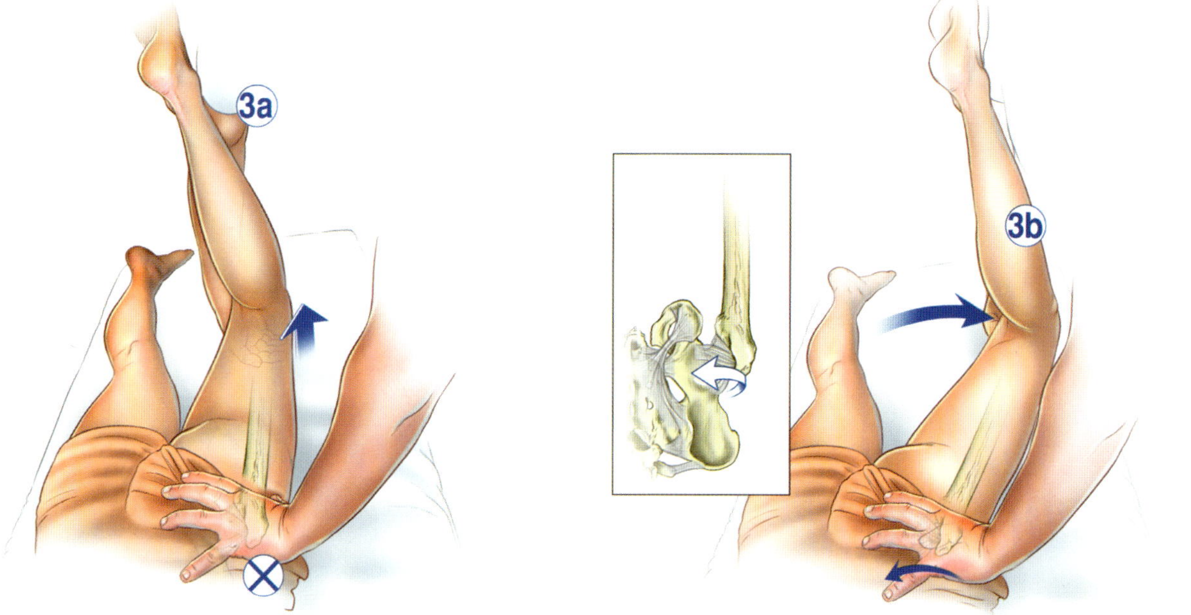

Figure 7.7 Deep slow Pri-move applied to the iliofemoral ligament immediately superior to the greater trochanter, simultaneously as the patient's leg is carried posterolaterally and returned to the table. Applied to the affected side only. This strategy can have a rapid re-setting effect on the hip capsule and consequently hip articulation generally.

Coccyx Procedure – 5 steps

Indications: Coccyx pain, menstrual disorders, male and female fertility conditions, menopausal and prostate conditions, digestive conditions, constipation, persistent headaches, migraine headaches, visual conditions, back problems that will not resolve, neck problems that will not resolve, groin problems that will not resolve, persistent hamstring and knee conditions.

Prerequisites: Dynamic Body Balance - Parts 1 and 2 and Sacrum Procedure must be completed before commencing Coccyx procedure.

Note: The coccyx, due to its location as the last vertebrae in the spinal system and its connection to the dural membrane system via the filum terminale, is regarded as significant part

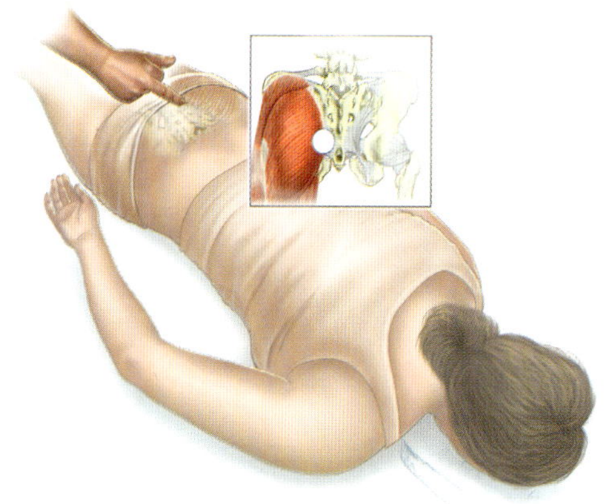

Figure 7.8 Digital pressure is applied lateral to the sacrococcygeal junction to determine if pain is evident on either side. The objective is to locate the painful or most painful side, which in turn determines the set-up for the leg positioning and correction.

of the NST system. Accordingly, it is assessed routinely at every session.

Further information on the coccyx can be found in Chapter 9 – System Procedures.

Assessment (Fig. 7.8): The coccyx is assessed by the practitioner by applying digital pressure into the connective tissue of the sacrococcygeal junction and muscle fibers of the gluteus maximus muscle adjacent to the angle of the coccyx body. This is typically a zone of inflammation normally associated with coccyx conditions.

The direction of pressure is lateral away from the coccyx itself. No pressure is applied to the coccyx bone per se.

If there is no pain on either side, the Coccyx procedure is not performed. When there is pain on one side or the other, the procedure is performed to the most painful side. If both sides are equally painful, the left side is nominated as the painful side.

Point 1

Action: Bilateral Pri-move applied to the lateral border of the iliocostalis lumborum muscle at the level of spinal vertebrae L3-L4 (Fig. 7.9).

Point 2

Action: The legs are crossed at the ankles importantly with the leg corresponding to the most painful side remaining on the table whilst it is crossed by the leg corresponding to the least painful side of the coccyx. The legs are flexed together and carried towards the buttocks (Fig. 7.10).

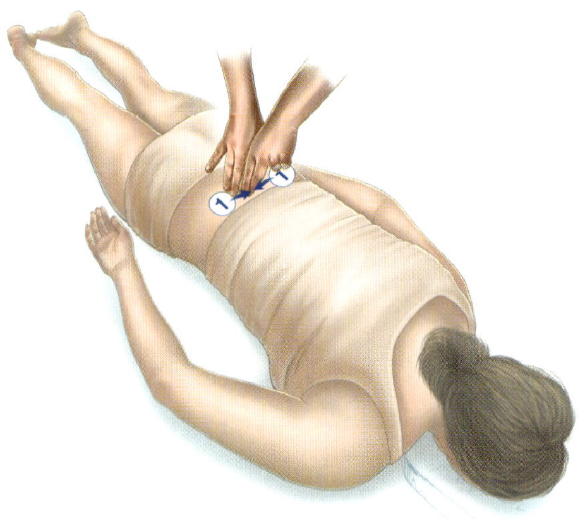

Figure 7.9 Medial bilateral Pri-move applied to L3-L4 level. Acts as a re-confirmation of point 1 in DBB1.

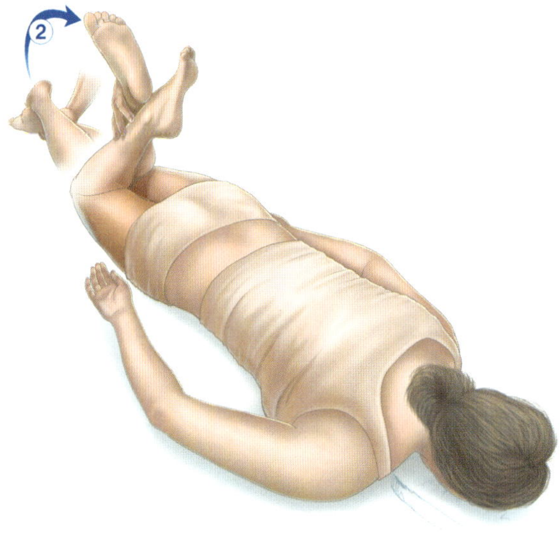

Figure 7.10 The leg corresponding to the painful coccyx side remains on the table. The other leg crosses the leg on the table at the level of the ankle. Both legs are carried toward the buttocks.

Points 3 and 4

Action: The practitioner's middle finger tip of the free hand makes contact with the patient's sacrococcygeal ligament and maintains contact as the patient's crossed legs are thrust in a cranial direction three successive times. Prior to each thrust, the patient is instructed to inhale and exhale. The patient's legs are then returned to the table and uncrossed (Fig. 7.11).

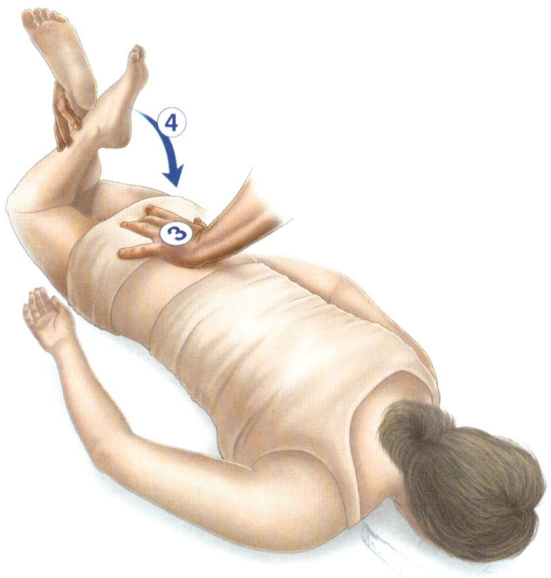

Figure 7.11 Practitioner's middle finger makes deep comfortable contact to the sacrococcygeal ligament, as the patient's crossed legs are slowly thrust towards buttocks three times, causing the finger to slide back and forth over the sacrococcygeal ligament. Assists in initiating the release of dural drag between the coccyx and the dura mater at S2 of the sacrum.

Point 5

Action: Deep lateral Pri-move applied to the common tendon of the hamstring muscles immediately distal to the ischial tuberosity, followed by three posterior Pri-moves applied to the iliotibial tract in a distal to cranial direction. Action is unilateral to the painful side leg only (Fig. 7.12).

Note: If the coccyx issue is ligament related the correction may be rapid. However, in all cases, the coccyx should be re-assessed at the following session, and if still painful, more advanced coccyx correction strategies should be considered, including the advanced Coccyx procedure and the coccyx lift technique, both detailed in other texts.

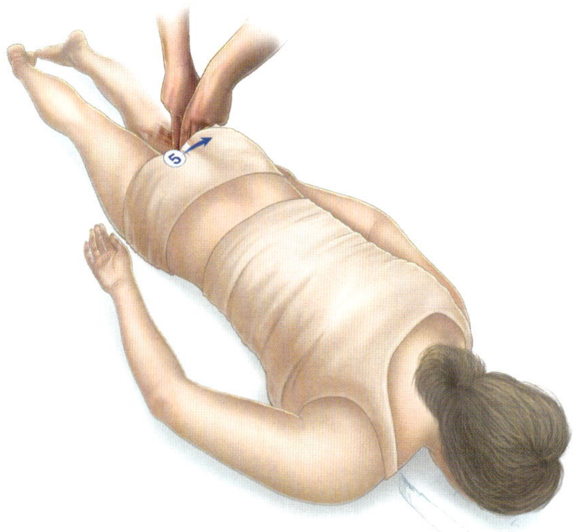

Figure 7.12 Lateral and medial Pri-moves applied to the common tendon of the hamstring muscles and the iliotibial band respectively. Applied to the leg that corresponds to the painful coccyx side only.

Hamstring Procedure – 6 steps

Indications: All hamstring muscle problems, back problems that will not resolve, knee problems that will not resolve, groin problems that will not resolve or hamstring muscles still tight after having completed all prone work.

Prerequisites: Dynamic Body Balance - Parts 1, 2 and Sacrum procedure must be completed.

Note: The Hamstring procedure is a two-part procedure with points 1-4 comprising the prone part and points 5-6 comprising the supine part. The supine part is completed after activation of point 7 from DBB3, or alternatively, the complete Knee procedure.

Point 1

Action: Bilateral Pri-move applied to the lateral border of the iliocostalis lumborum muscle at the level of spinal vertebrae L3-L4 (Fig. 7.13).

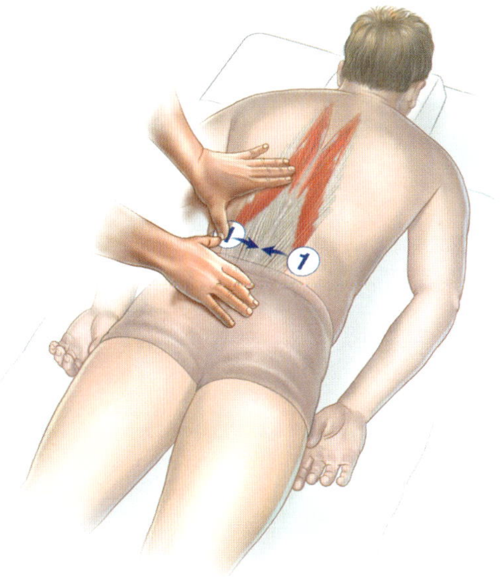

Figure 7.13 Medial bilateral Pri-move applied to L3-L4 level. Acts as a re-confirmation of point 1 in DBB1.

Point 2

Action: Leg is flexed into a right-angled position and the patient instructed to relax the hamstring muscle as much as possible. Action is unilateral to the affected side (Fig. 7.14).

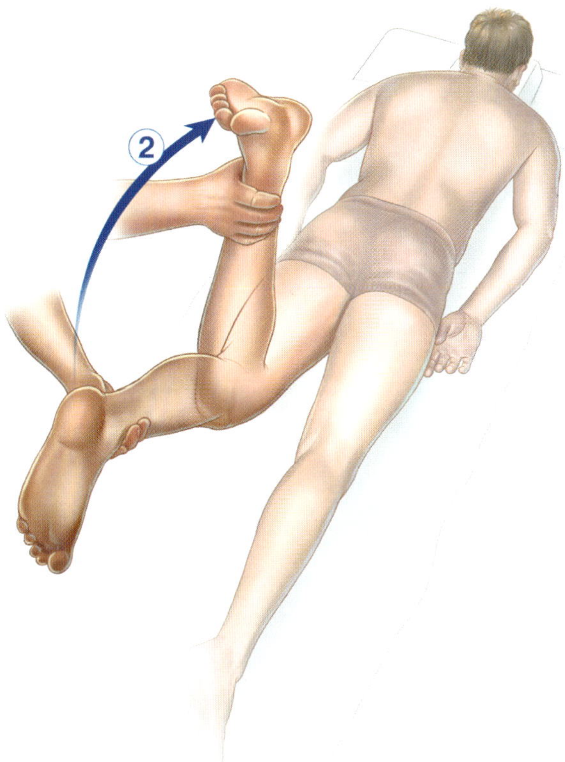

Figure 7.14 Practitioner flexes patient's leg into 90° position in preparation for point 3 release.

Points 3a and 3b

Action: Deep medial Pri-move applied to the common tendon of the hamstring muscles immediately distal to the ischial tuberosity (3a) directly followed by a deep soft and slow Pri-move crossing the median line of the popliteal fossa (3b). The intention is to cross the plantaris muscle and tibial nerve at the same time. Action is unilateral to the affected side (Fig. 7.15).

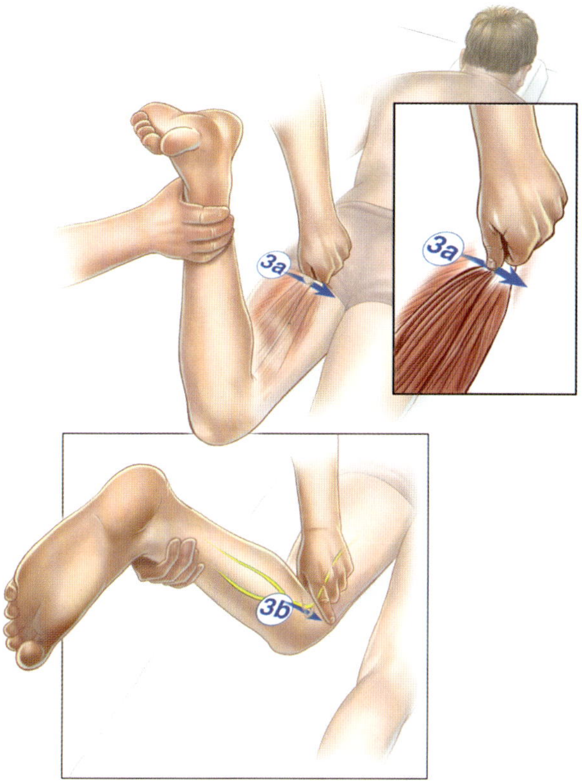

Figure 7.15 Deep medial Pri-move applied to the common tendon of the hamstring muscles followed by a soft-slow Pri-move deep in the popliteal fossa, crossing the plantaris muscle and tibial nerve simultaneously. Provides a rapid re-set of the hamstring muscles.

Point 4

Action: The patient's foot is now moved in a brisk "figure 8" fashion for 3 repetitions before being thrust abruptly towards the table (dorsiflexion) for 3 repetitions, thereby extending the Achilles tendon. Action is unilateral to the affected side (Fig. 7.16).

Note: In a tensegrity sense, the hamstring muscle represents one of the biggest "cables" acting on the skeleton, and its appropriate balance and integration cannot be underestimated, for the important role it plays in posture, locomotion and sacro-spino-cranial integration.

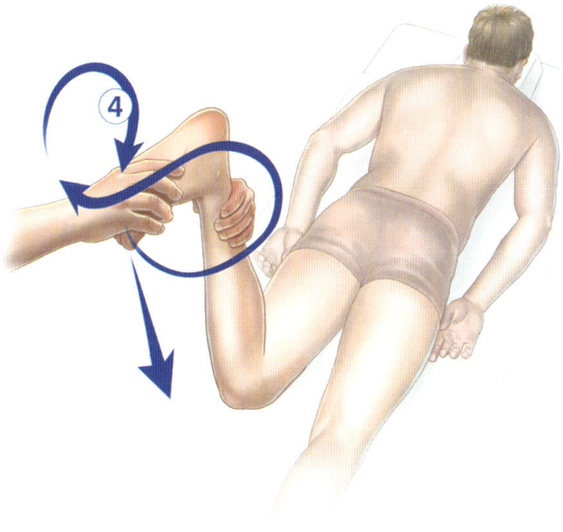

Figure 7.16 A brisk and thrusting release is applied to the foot and Achilles tendon. This action frequently improves foot articulation and assists the muscle train between the ischial tuberosity and calcaneus bone to re-establish appropriate tension.

Points 5 and 6

Action: With fingers positioned very deep between biceps femoris and semitendinosous muscles, bilateral Pri-moves are applied twice along the length of the muscles (5a and 5b), followed by an additional bilateral Pri-move deep in the popliteal fossa crossing the plantaris muscle and tibial nerve in opposite directions (5c).

Further deep slow bilateral Pri-moves are applied to the lateral and medial heads of the gastrocnemius muscle (6a) and its bellies (6b), followed by three medial Pri-moves to the Achilles tendon in a distal direction (6c, 6d, 6e) (Fig. 7.17).

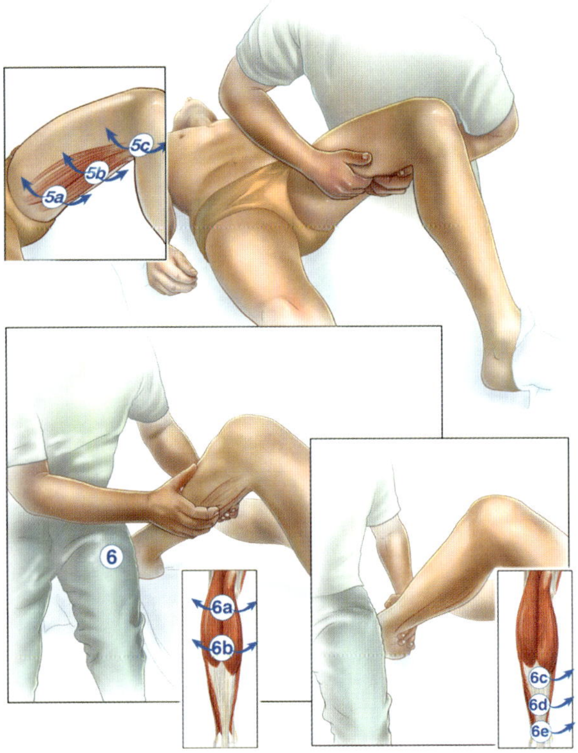

Figure 7.17 A series of Pri-moves are applied to the hamstring and gastrocnemius muscles respectively, and then onto the Achilles tendon. These addition points that are applied exclusively in the supine position, and typically after the release of the Knee procedure, will further enhance release of the hamstring muscles and general muscle train between the ischial tuberosity and calcaneus bone. Consequently collateral improvement can be observed in the function of the quadriceps, tibialis muscles and pelvic girdle generally. Further potential benefits for the spinal column, shoulder girdle and cranium must also be regarded as relevant considerations in an "integrated body" context.

SUPINE POSITION PROCEDURES – Lung and Lower Extremity

INTRODUCTION

The first of the supine procedures, prior to completing DBB3, is the Lung procedure, which is really just another name for the diaphragm release.

This is a strategic positioning of the diaphragm release prior to activating the first four points of DBB3, which all in one way or the other, positively affect respiration and hence the integration of the SRM.

Having completed the Lung procedure and points 1-4 of DBB3, the practitioner then moves to the leg on the left side and releases either point 6 from DBB3 or completes the full Knee procedure, which also contains point 6 - i.e., the release of the vastus lateralis tendon.

Once the practitioner is at the left leg, all

chosen procedures for the leg are completed. The minimum amount of work that can be performed is point 6 from DBB3. The other options are the Knee, Hamstring, Ankle and Foot procedures.

When the left leg is completed, the practitioner moves to the right leg and completes the chosen procedures for the right leg, which incidentally, do not have to match the procedures for the left leg.

Procedures for the lower extremity are chosen on the basis that they should correspond to the presenting symptom of the patient.

Further typical examples of how an NST session might be built appear at the end of this section.

Lung Procedure – 4 steps

Indications: Respiratory conditions, asthma, blood pressure, stomach and digestive problems, liver and gallbladder conditions, pancreas conditions, spleen conditions, ileocecal valve and valve of Houston conditions, hiatus hernia, distension, colic and projectile vomiting.

Prerequisites: Dynamic Body Balance - Parts 1 and 2 must be completed before commencing Lung procedure.

Point 1

Action: Deep soft digital pressure applied and maintained, at the insertion of the rectus abdominis muscle 2 cm below the xiphoid process. Pressure must be sufficient so that the patient experiences a mild shortening of the breath or the practitioner feels the aortic pulse, or both. The point should not cause pain (Fig. 7.18).

Note: The practitioner can also use the opportunity when working with the diaphragm, to discover whether or not there is any tension under the left or right costal margins. Tension or hardness in tissue under the left costal margin can often indicate a congested stomach or pancreas, whilst the same on the right side can indicate a congested liver or gallbladder. These important telltale signs might help explain why the patient has neck and shoulder pain, as all four organs share important neurovascular and neurolymphatic reflexive relationships with neck and shoulder muscles. Furthermore, and from a tensegrity perspective, if an organ is compromising a neck or shoulder muscle, then the spinal column will also be compromised, and it's not going too far to say that the whole "sacro-spino-cranial" system needs to adapt itself to this. Consequently, a discussion between practitioner and patient about the importance of diet, may be valid in such circumstances.

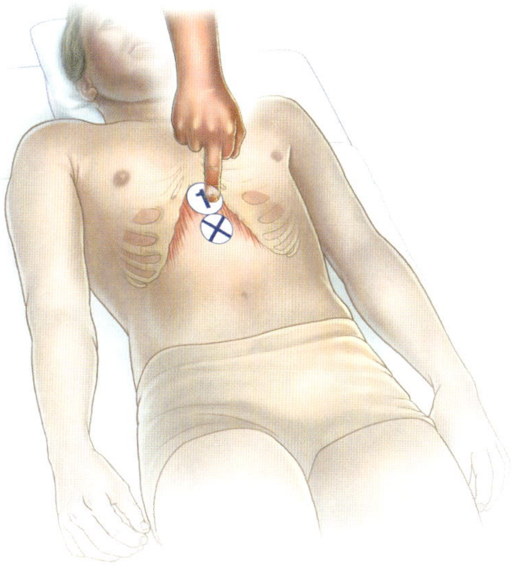

Figure 7.18 This important holding point 2 cm below the distal point of the xiphoid process, sets up the diaphragm for further release by temporarily impeding its natural rhythm. It's worth remembering that due to the attachments of the diaphragm onto the lumbar spine in particular, that much of the release of the diaphragm has already been achieved during the prone work throughout DBB1 and DBB2.

Point 2

Action: As point 1 is maintained, the patient is instructed to inhale and exhale, and whilst exhaled a series of short Pri-moves are applied along the left costal margin crossing the fibers of the external abdominal oblique, rectus abdominis, and onto the insertion of the diaphragm muscle under the costal margin, as much as is possible (Fig. 7.19).

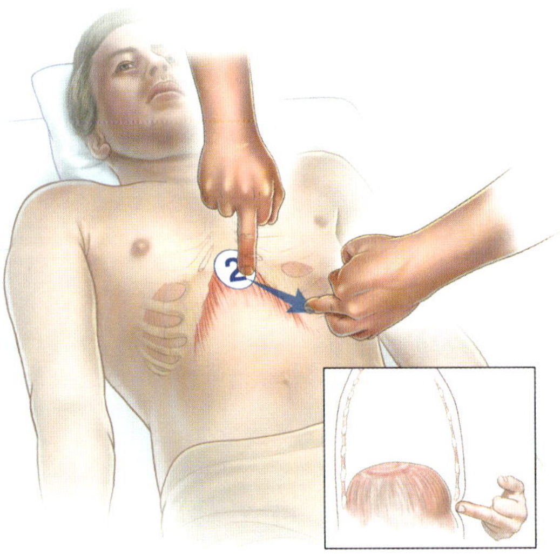

Figure 7.19 A series of lateral moving Pri-moves are applied deep under (access permitting) the left costal margin after the patient has fully exhaled. If the patient is too tight then "skin-deep" Pri-moves along the costal margin may be used.

Point 3

Action: As point 1 is maintained, the patient is instructed to inhale and exhale, and whilst exhaled a series of short Pri-moves are applied along the right costal margin crossing the fibers of the external abdominal oblique, rectus abdominis, and onto the insertion of the diaphragm muscle under the costal margin as much as is possible (Fig. 7.20).

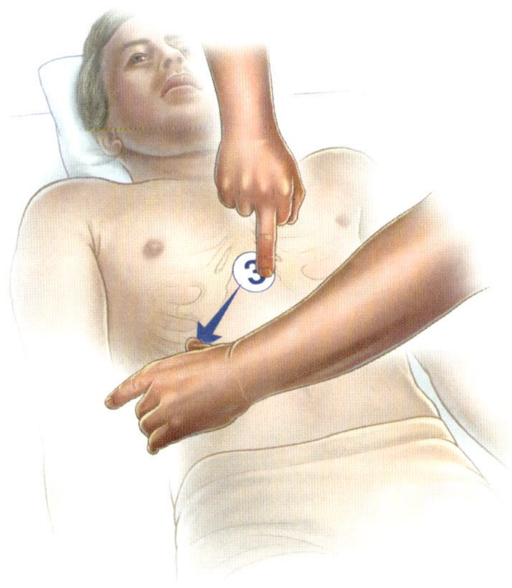

Figure 7.20 A series of lateral moving Pri-moves are applied deep under (access permitting) the right costal margin after the patient has fully exhaled. If the patient is too tight then "skin-deep" Pri-moves along the costal margin may be used.

Point 4

Action: The holding point is released and the patient instructed to once again inhale and exhale, and whilst exhaled a series of short Pri-moves are applied along the linea alba of the rectus abdominis muscle, from the xiphoid process to the umbilicus (Fig. 7.21).

Once complete, a continuous deep sliding release is applied three times, to the linea alba.

Covering the patient's abdomen with a soft towel throughout this final release will be more comfortable for them.

Note: Once point 4 is completed, the flow of the session continues with the release of DBB3 points 1-4 after which the practitioner moves to the left leg and activates either point 6 from DBB3 or the complete Knee procedure.

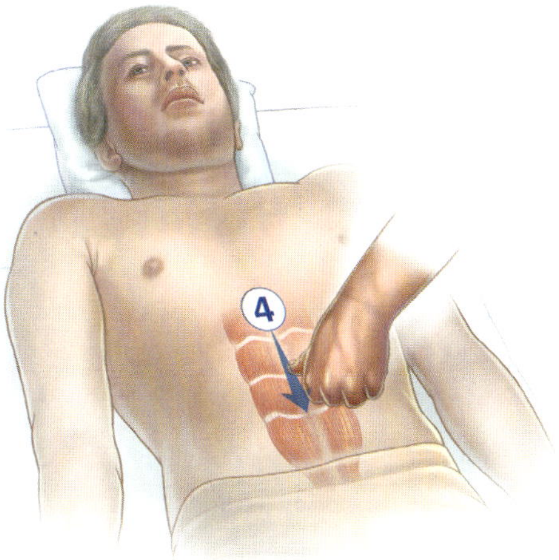

Figure 7.21 A series of Pri-moves along the linea alba of the rectus abdominis muscle are applied prior to applying a further deep sliding release, for three repetitions, along the linea alba. The deep sliding release can be done through light clothing or with the aid of a small amount of appropriate skin cream or oil.

Knee Procedure – 7 steps

Indications: Knee conditions, as an adjunct procedure to all lumbar, pelvic and hamstring conditions or if patella is still tight having completed point 6 from DBB3.

The Knee procedure is also a prerequisite for the Pelvic, Ankle and Foot procedures.

The Knee procedure is only applied to the painful knee or otherwise both knees when used as a prerequisite release for the pelvis.

Prerequisites: Dynamic Body Balance - Parts 1, 2 and points 1-4 from DBB3 must be completed before commencing Knee procedure.

Point 1

Action: Lateral Pri-move applied to common border of the sartorius and rectus femoris muscles at the approximate level of the pubic symphysis (Fig. 7.22).

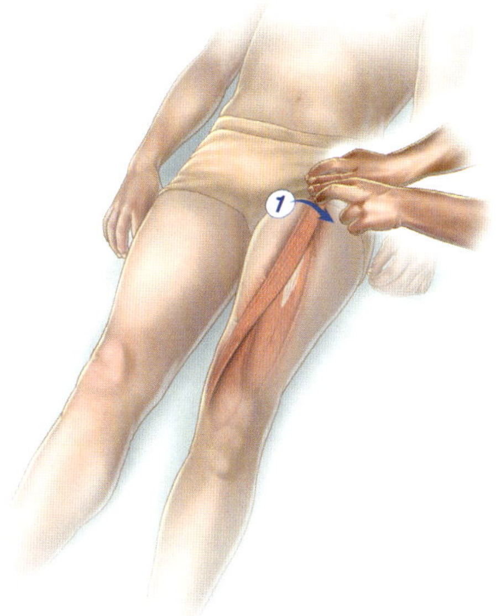

Figure 7.22 Applied to the common border of the sartorius and rectus femoris muscles, point 1 helps to sedate the sartorius muscle in preparation for knee release. In energetic terms, point 1 is an energy block for the knee.

Point 2

Action: Deep short Pri-move applied to posterior border of the iliotibial band where it crosses the vastus lateralis muscle approximately one hand width above the patella (Fig. 7.23).

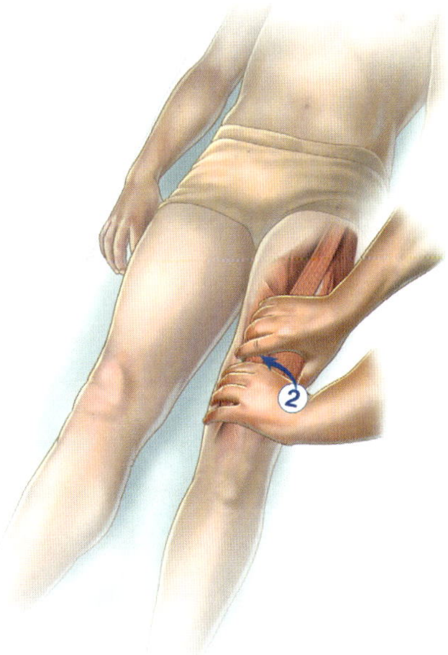

Figure 7.23 Applied to the iliotibial band approximately one hand-width above the patella. This Pri-move, like point 1, assists in the preparation of optimizing tensions around the knee, in preparation for the main knee release points – points 3 & 4 (see also point 6 in DBB3).

Point 3

Action: Pri-move applied to the insertion of the vastus lateralis muscle at the superior lateral aspect of patella of the knee (Fig. 7.24). The point is retained in its rotated position whilst points 4 and 5 are performed.

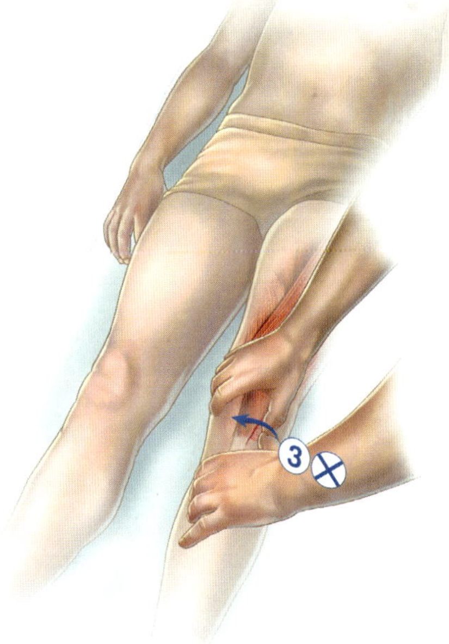

Figure 7.24 Applied to the insertion of the vastus lateralis muscle tendon and retained. Significantly improves knee articulation, pelvic girdle mobility and consequently function of the SRM. The retention assists points 5 to release more effectively.

Point 4

Action: Pri-move applied to the vastus medialis approximately 2 cm above the patella and in a lateral direction (Fig. 7.25). The point is retained in its rotated position with point 3 whilst points 5 are performed.

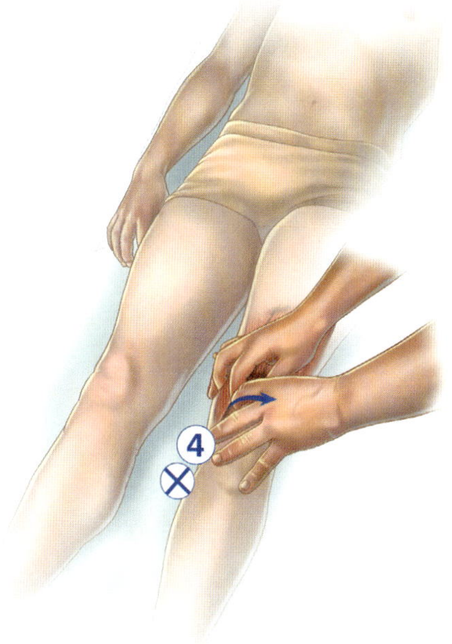

Figure 7.25 Pri-move applied to the vastus medius muscle and retained. The Pri-move further stabilizes the release achieved with point 3 and the retention assists points 5 to release more effectively as well.

Point 5

Action: Two short oblique Pri-moves applied to the patella retinacula, lateral then medial, directly distal to the patella.

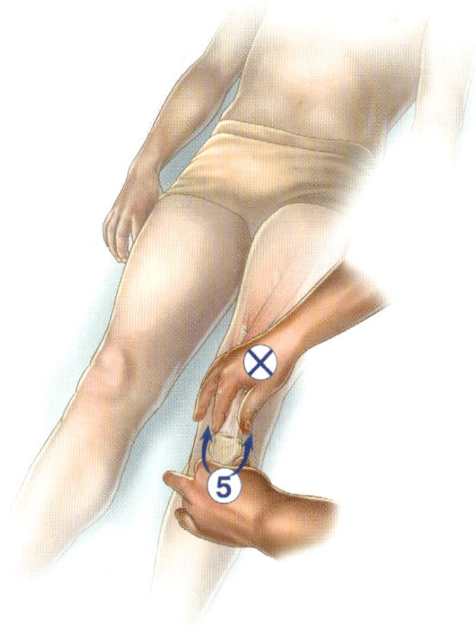

Figure 7.26 Two very small Pri-moves applied bilaterally to the patella retinacula that assist with general knee stability and mobility.

Point 6

Action: Deep bilateral Pri-move applied in the popliteal fossa crossing the plantaris muscle and tibial nerve in opposite directions (Fig. 7.27).

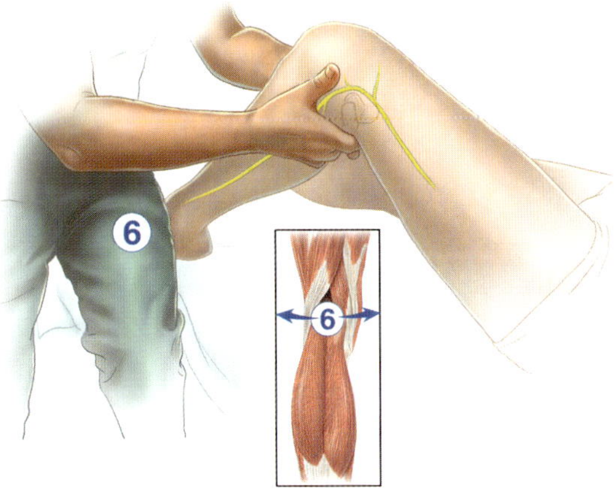

Figure 7.27 Deep bilateral Pri-moves applied to the plantaris muscle and tibial nerve deep in the popliteal fossa. Assist with knee articulation mobility and prepares gastrocnemius muscles for release.

Point 7

Action: Deep slow bilateral Pri-moves are applied to the lateral and medial heads of the gastrocnemius muscle (7a) and its bellies (7b), followed by three medial Pri-moves to the Achilles tendon in a distal direction (7c, 7d, 7e) (Fig. 7.28).

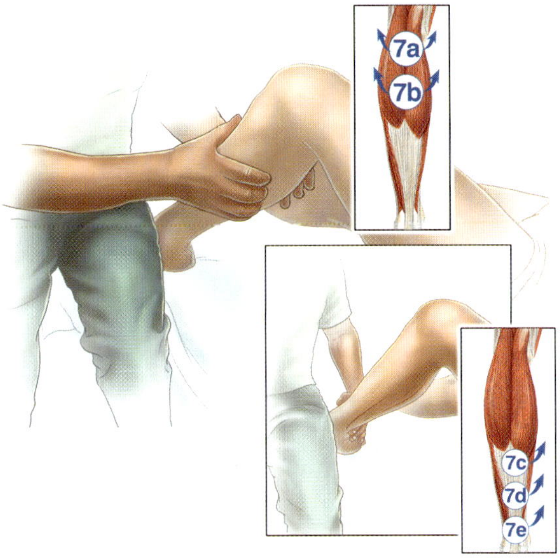

Figure 7.28 Series of Pri-moves applied to the gastrocnemius muscles and Achilles tendon respectively. Designed to release and integrate posterior musculature between the knee and the foot.

Ankle Procedure – 5 steps

Indications: All ankle conditions including lateral sprains, knee and groin conditions and combines well with Hamstring, Knee and Foot procedures, as a preventative or maintenance strategy for all athletes.

Prerequisites: Dynamic Body Balance - Parts 1, 2, 3 and Knee procedure must be completed before commencing Ankle procedure.

The Ankle procedure is also a prerequisite for the Foot procedure.

The Ankle procedure is only applied to the painful ankle.

Prerequisites: Dynamic Body Balance - Parts 1, 2 and points 1-4 from DBB3 and the Knee procedure must be completed before commencing Ankle procedure.

Point 1

Action: Series of deep short Pri-moves crossing the tibialis anterior, extensor digitorum longus and peroneus longus muscles on a line immediately distal to the head of the fibula (Fig. 7.29).

Crossing the lateral border of the peroneus longus will produce an abrupt "bump".

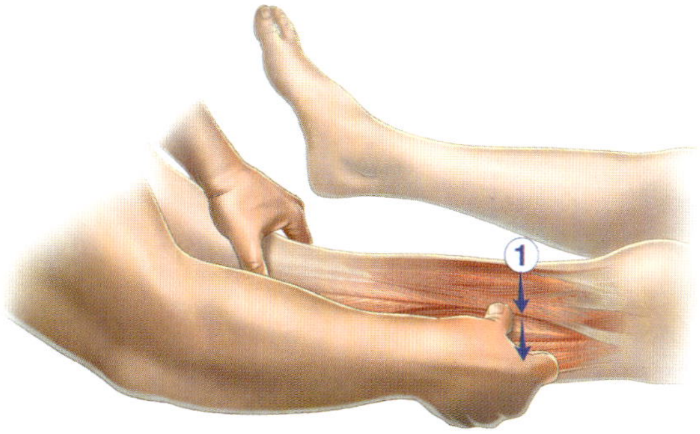

Figure 7.29 Three sequential Pri-moves applied to the tibialis anterior, extensor digitorum longus and peroneus longus muscles, that act as both a sedation and release of those muscles. Designed to release in integrate anterior musculature between the knee, ankle and foot.

Point 2

Action: Series of short deep Pri-moves around the distal aspect of the lateral malleolus crossing the anterior talofibular and calcaneofibular ligaments (Fig. 7.30).

Once Pri-moves are complete, reapply one more time.

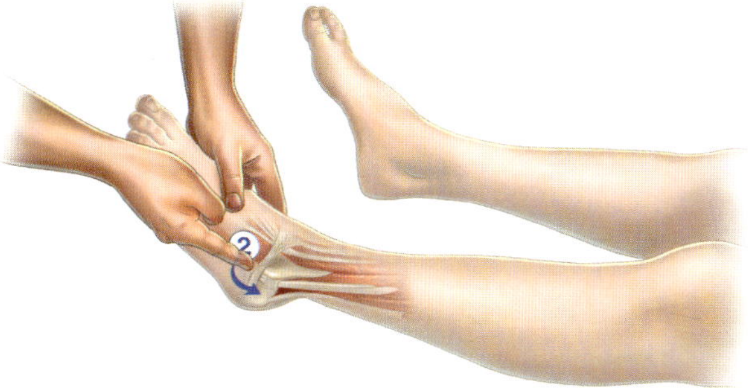

Figure 7.30 A series of deep short Pri-moves applied to the lateral ligaments of the ankle. Improves articulation of the talocrural and talocalcaneal joints.

Point 3

Action: Series of short deep Pri-moves around the distal aspect of the medial malleolus crossing the deltoid ligament (Fig. 7.31).

Once Pri-moves are complete, reapply one more time.

Note: Figure 7.31 shows the right foot for ease of viewing but Pri-moves are to the left side.

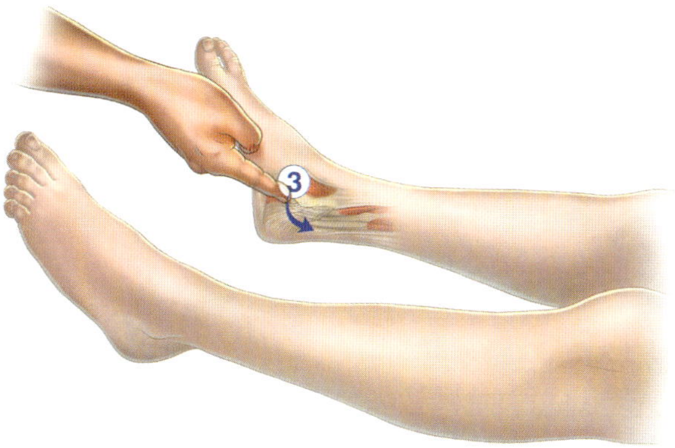

Figure 7.31 A series of deep short Pri-moves applied to the medial ligaments of the ankle. Improves articulation of the talocrural and talocalcaneal joints.

Points 4

Action: Invert patient's foot and stretch skin over the extensor retinaculum in preparation for Pri-move application (4a) (Fig. 7.32 a).

Evert patient's foot and, simultaneously, apply Pri-move crossing both the extensor retinaculum and the tendon of the extensor digitorum longus muscle and rolling onto the medial margin of the tibialis anterior muscle's tendon. Firmly clamp the tibialis anterior muscle's tendon and retain (4b) (Fig. 7.32 b).

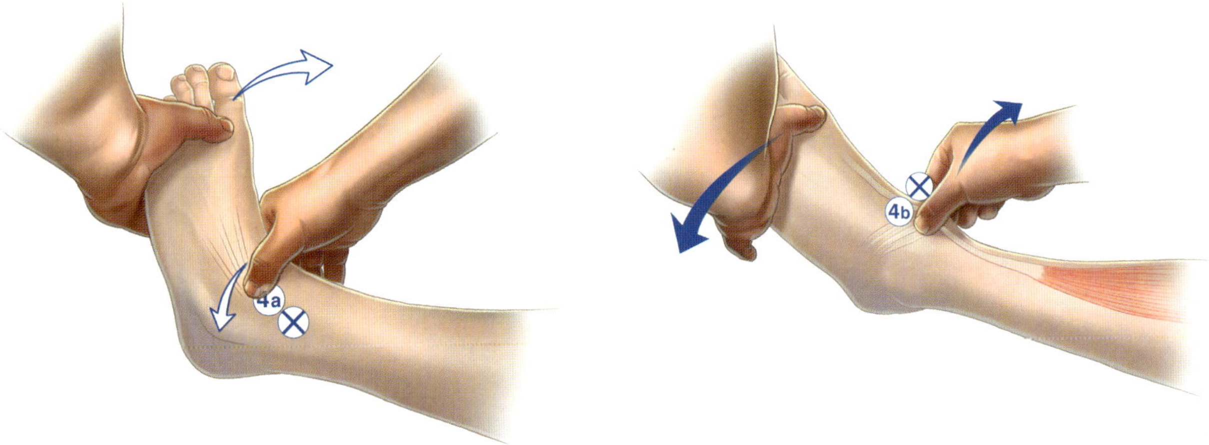

a b

Figure 7.32 This combination release has two parts. (**a**) A release crossing the extensor tendons of the foot at the extensor retinaculum. (**b**) Firm digital contact applied to the talocrural fossa simultaneously with a retention "clamp" of the tibialis anterior muscle's tendon. Although a release of the dorsal foot musculature in itself, this move also prepares the foot for a final thrusting release in point 5 following.

Point 5

Action: Whilst firmly clamping the tendon of the tibialis anterior muscle, rotate the patient's foot bilaterally 2-3 times and then dorsiflex the foot 2-3 times, ensuring that the holding thumb thrusts onto the extensor retinaculum.

The shallow talocrural fossa should be perceptible throughout the thrusting action (Fig. 7.33).

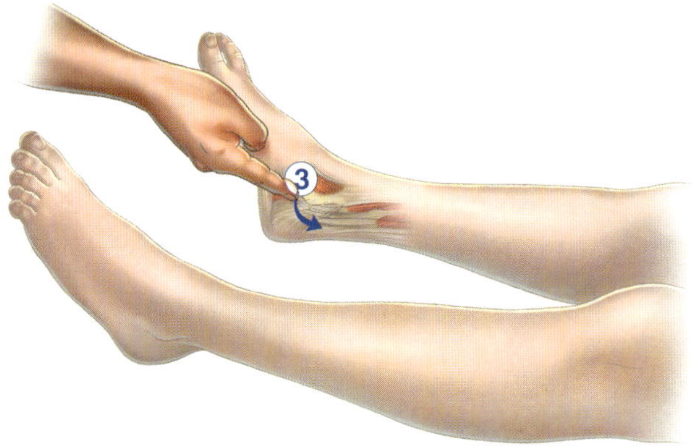

Figure 7.33 With the tibialis anterior muscle's tendon firmly clamped, the foot is vigorously rotated in both directions 2-3 times prior to being thrust into dorsiflexion 2-3 times. The final point in the Ankle procedure takes advantage of the releases achieved in the preceding four points, and typically achieves a remarkable liberation of the general talocrural joint and foot musculature. Benefits for the whole body in terms of enhancement in postural stability must be considered a realistic derivative of the Ankle procedure, and the Foot procedure that follows.

Indications: Pain, lack of mobility or stiffness in the feet or toes. Especially useful for sports people who frequently use their feet (runners, tennis players, footballers, hockey players, etc.). Excellent for supporting pelvic, SRM and SGS corrections.

Prerequisites: Dynamic Body Balance - Parts 1, 2 and points 1-4 of Part 3, Knee Procedure and Ankle Procedure.

Pre-check (Fig. 7.34): Prior to applying the Foot procedure, the tissue around the head of the fibula is palpated for pain.

If pain to palpation is evident, a series of short deep Pri-moves are applied around the circumference of the fibula head crossing the insertion of the biceps femoris on its superior aspect and common ligament of the peroneus longus and extensor digitorum longus muscles at its inferior aspect. This series of Pri-moves should be performed twice.

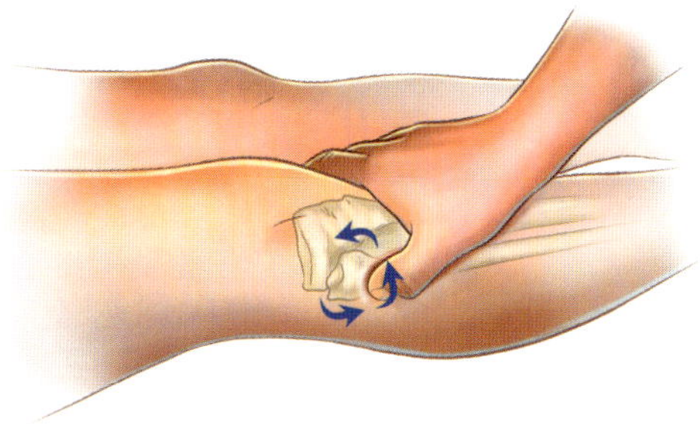

Figure 7.34 The pre-check for the Foot procedure is performed to ascertain if there is any sensitivity in the tissues surrounding the proximal tibiofibular joint. Sensitivity in the tissues generally indicates that the head of the fibula may be slightly displaced. If positive, a series of Pri-moves are performed around the head of the fibula to help improve its articulation and assist its partner, the distal tibiofibular joint, in their common job of load-bearing. Assists foot articulation.

Point 1

Action: Short Deep "finger-tip" Pri-move applied to the tibial nerve and the flexor digitorum longus tendon simultaneously, immediately posterior and slightly distal to the medial malleolus (Fig. 7.35).

The patient should feel an electric discharge into the foot.

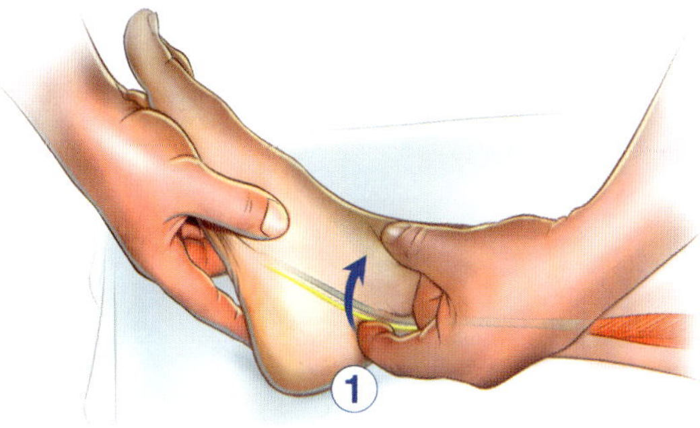

Figure 7.35 A short "finger-tip" Pri-move to the tibial nerve helps prepare the muscles of the foot for release by creating a temporary sedation of the nerve itself.

Point 2

Action: Deep digital pressure applied to the extensor retinaculum and underlying extensor tendons and the Achilles tendon at the same time and retained (Fig. 7.36).

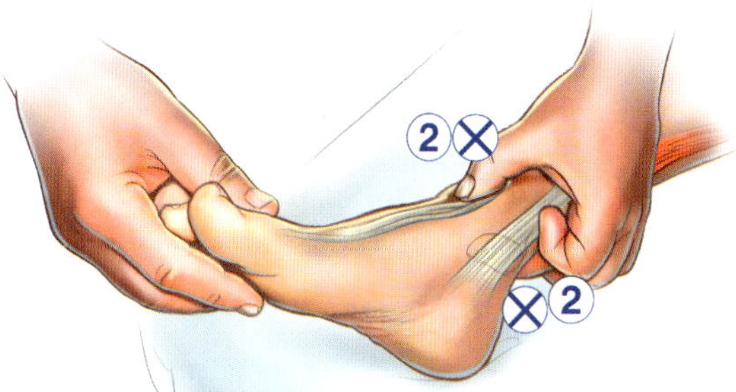

Figure 7.36 Using deep digital contact to retain the extensor and Achilles tendons of the foot, creates an altered tensional context, for the optimal release of the extensor tendons in point 3.

Point 3

Action: Whilst points 2 are retained, a series of bilateral Pri-moves are applied to the common extensor tendons of the foot until the surface tension in the skin, of the foot softens (Fig. 7.37).

The Pri-moves should produce "micro bumps" as the tendons are crossed.

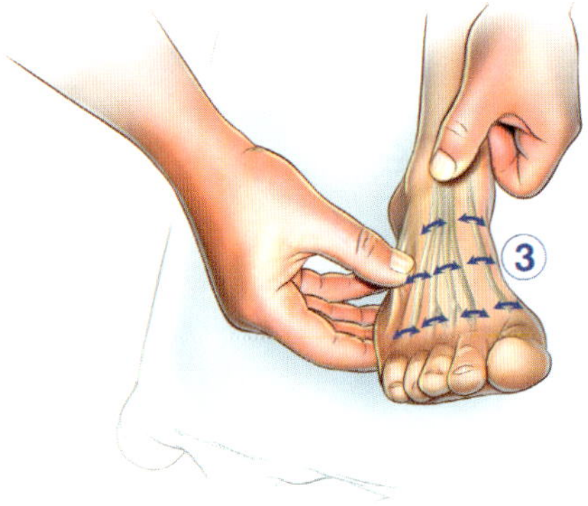

Figure 7.37 Applying a series of random Pri-moves to the extensor tendons of the foot until they soften ensures better access and release to the structures on the plantar surface of the foot, to be attended to in points 4, 5 and 6.

Point 4

Action: Series of deep short Pri-moves applied to the deep plantar ligaments of the foot (Fig. 7.38).

The series of Pri-moves should be performed twice.

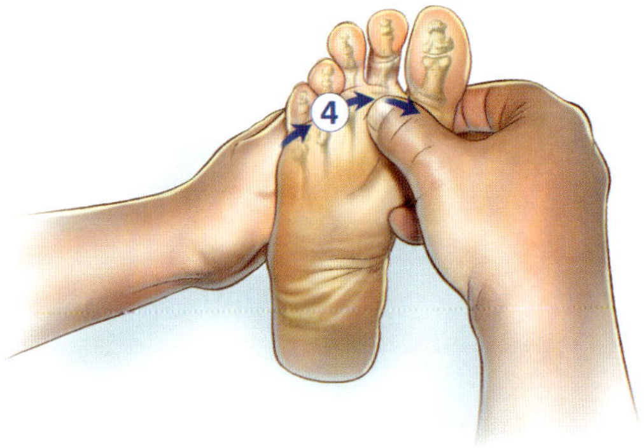

Figure 7.38 Pri-moves applied to the deep plantar transverse metatarsal ligament quickly improve metatarsophalangeal joint capsule articulation.

Point 5

Action: Series of deep short "finger-tip" Pri-moves applied to the abductor hallucis and abductor digiti minimi muscles (Fig. 7.39).

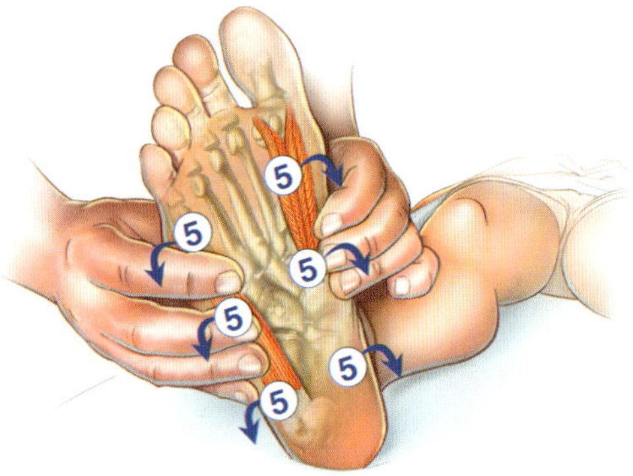

Figure 7.39 Pri-moves applied to the abductor hallicus and abductor digiti minimi muscles generally, facilitate a deep relaxation of the plantar surface of the foot and improvement of the medial arch.

Point 6

Action: Series of Pri-moves applied to the adductor hallucis transverse muscle in the direction of the heel (Fig. 7.40). This series of Pri-moves should be performed twice.

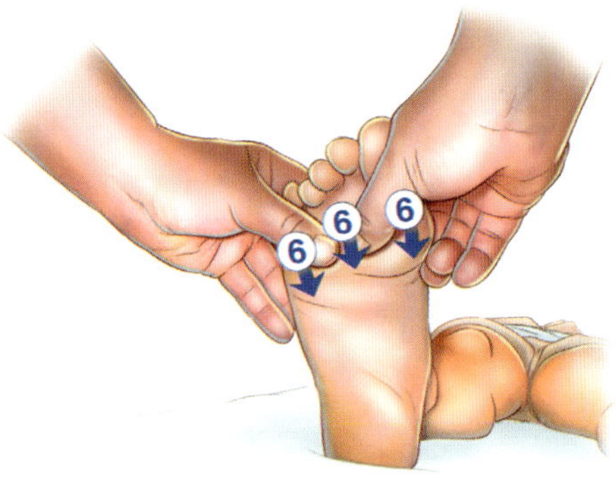

Figure 7.40 Pri-moves applied to the adductor hallucis transverse muscle trigger enhanced integration between the metatarsals, phalanges and general plantar area of the foot.

Point 7

Action: Medial and lateral ligaments are firmly clamped, immediately distal to both the medial and lateral malleolus, as the foot is "thrust" abruptly into dorsiflexion three times (Fig. 7.41).

Lower Extremity - Summary

Once all procedures have been completed for the left leg, the right leg is addressed. Procedures for the right leg do not have to mimic those utilized on the left leg but should reflect symptoms within the right leg.

After procedures for both legs have been completed, the practitioner moves back to the upper body and inserts point 7 from DBB3 before adding procedures for the upper extremities.

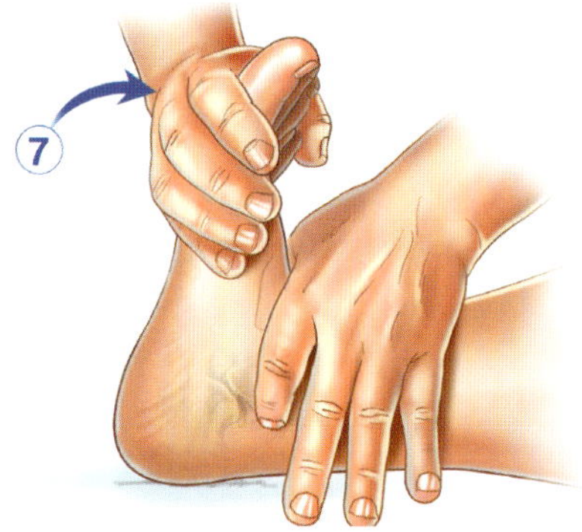

Figure 7.41 With medial and lateral ligaments of the foot firmly clamped, a final repetitive thrusting of the foot into dorsiflexion, takes advantage of points 1-6 in delivering an enhanced articulation of the foot generally, and a reduction in pain symptoms.

This illustrates the typical "flow" of an NST session in the supine position that not only optimizes spinal unlocking and integration, but indeed SRM integration.

SUPINE POSITION PROCEDURES – Upper Extremity

INTRODUCTION

Having completed point 7 from DBB3, the upper extremities may now be approached. Following this rule provides for optimal results in releasing conditions of the shoulders, elbows, wrists and hands as they are significantly influenced by the status of the cervical spine.

To summarize, once the patient turns into a supine position, the steps for the "flow" of the session are as follows:

1. Lung procedure
2. Points 1-4 of DBB3
3. Lower extremity procedures
4. Point 7 of DBB3
5. Upper extremity procedures

Shoulder Procedure – 3 steps

Indications: Shoulder injury, tight, stiff or frozen shoulders, neck problems that will not resolve, TMJ problems that will not resolve, elbow problems that will not resolve, thoracic back problems that will not resolve.

Prerequisites: Dynamic Body Balance - Parts 1, 2 and 3 must be completed before commencing Shoulder Procedure.

Always release both shoulders starting with the least affected shoulder, as the source of shoulder pain may be originating from the least affected side. Shoulder conditions may also be generated via faults in the "gait" walking mechanism and/or pelvic girdle.

Point 1

Action: With patient's hand resting on the abdomen to relax deltoid muscles, a deep and slightly quick Pri-move is applied the posterior margin of the posterior deltoid muscle, in an anterior direction (1a) (Fig. 7.42).

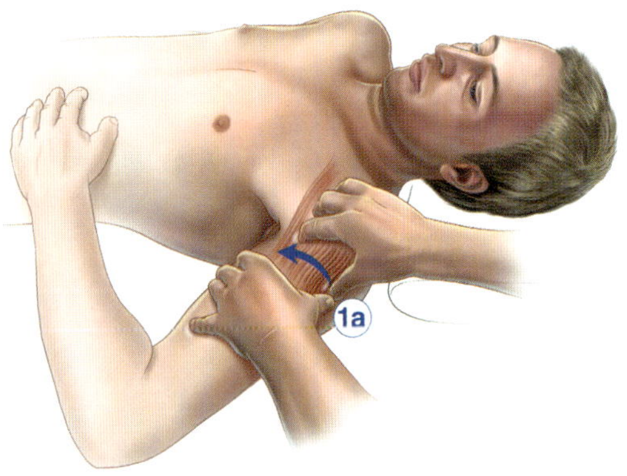

Figure 7.42 This deep quick Pri-move, applied to the proximal posterior border of the posterior deltoid muscle, is designed to commence the process of release for the general shoulder articulation. The Pri-move creates a temporary sedation of the shoulder capsule assisting in pain relief as well.

Note: If this Pri-move is performed too slowly, the posterior border of the posterior deltoid will not be released effectively.

Once point 1a is completed, the patient's arm is carried across the chest where firm pressure is applied to the distal aspect of the humerus, resulting in a mild traction being applied to the deltoid muscles, and the axillary nerve plexus being compressed at the same time.

The patient's arm is retained in this position, whilst the practitioner, using the soft heel of their free hand, applies 2-3 mild "bumps" to the patient's shoulder capsule, indicated by the large blue arrow (the bumps are designed to excite the firing activity of the axillary nerve plexus) (Fig. 7.43).

Once the bumps have been completed, the patient's arm is carried back to an open position and a deep, soft and slow Pri-move is applied to the anterior border of the anterior deltoid muscle at its proximal aspect (1b) (Fig. 7.44).

Note: Points 1a > "Bumps" > 1b are designed to be performed as a slow sequential release.

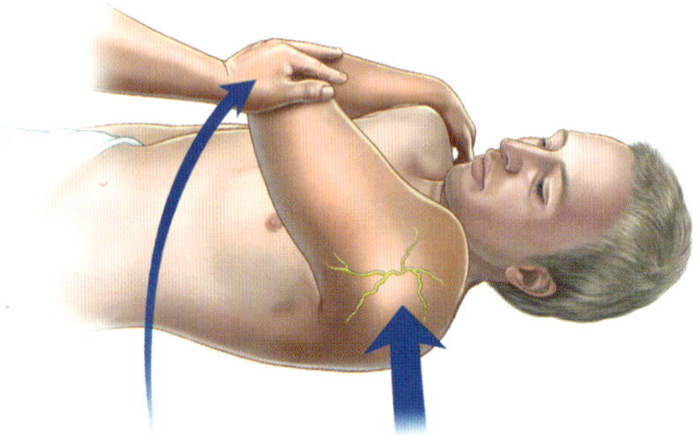

Figure 7.43 After 1a is completed, the arm is carried across the patient's chest and compressed whilst 2-3 mild impact "bumps" are applied to jolt the shoulder capsule with the intention of stimulating the axillary nerve plexus into normal functional status.

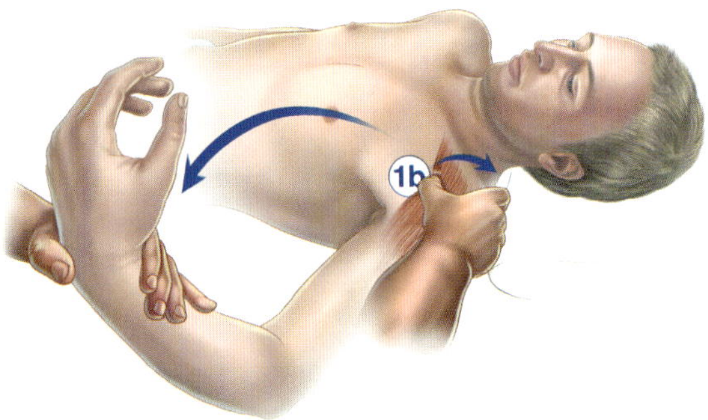

Figure 7.44 Completing the capsular release, the arm is opened and a Pri-move applied to the proximal anterior border of the anterior deltoid muscle, adding further release to the shoulder articulation.

Point 2

Action: Deep slow lateral Pri-move applied to the distal aspect of the common triceps muscle tendon (Fig. 7.45).

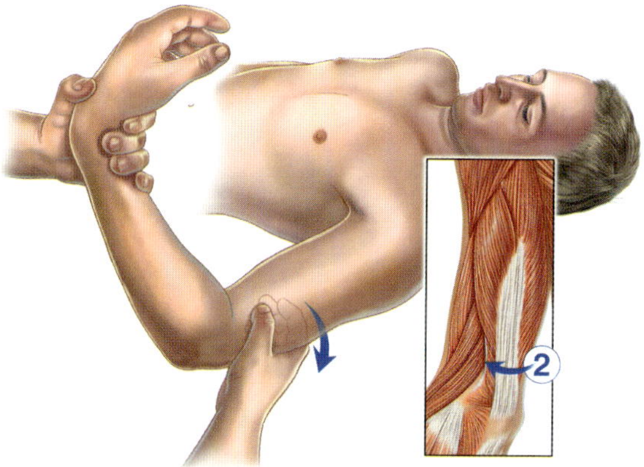

Figure 7.45 This deep slow Pri-move across the triceps muscle tendon is designed to reset the length of the triceps muscle, improving articulation of the shoulder and elbow articulations.

Point 3

Action: Three slow deep lateral Pri-moves applied to the intermuscular space of the biceps brachii muscle. Direction is from proximal to distal (3a, 3b, 3c) (Fig. 7.46).

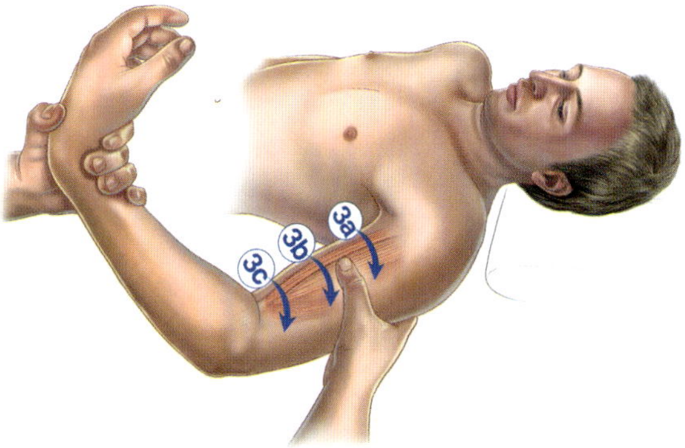

Figure 7.46 A series of Pri-moves between the biceps brachii muscle bellies, designed to reset the length of the biceps brachii muscle, improving articulation of the shoulder and elbow articulations.

Elbow and Wrist Procedure – 7 steps

Indications: Elbow and wrist pain, tennis elbow, repetitive strain injury, tingling sensations in elbow, wrist or fingers.

Prerequisites: Dynamic Body Balance - Parts 1, 2 and 3 and Shoulder procedure, must be completed before commencing Elbow and Wrist procedure.

It is only necessary to do the Elbow and Wrist procedure on the affected side.

Point 1

Action: Deep slow lateral Pri-move applied to the distal aspect of the common triceps muscle tendon (Fig. 7.47). The point is retained for approximately 1 minute in combination with point 2 that follows.

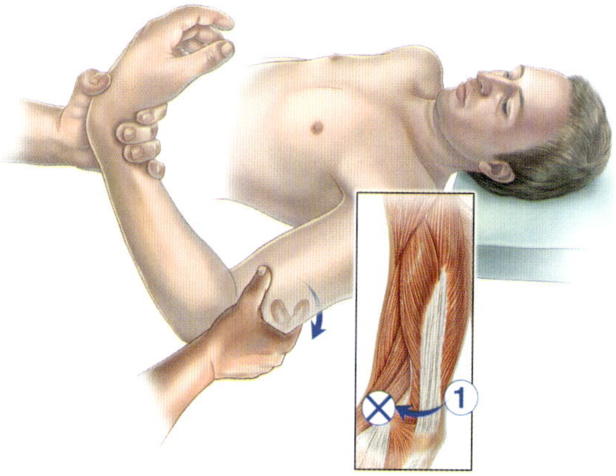

Figure 7.47 This "retained" Pri-move across the triceps muscle tendon is combined with point 2 to sedate and relieve pain in and around the elbow articulation.

Point 2

Action: Pri-move applied to the soft head of the brachioradialis muscle (Fig. 7.48). The point is retained for approximately 1 minute in combination with point 1.

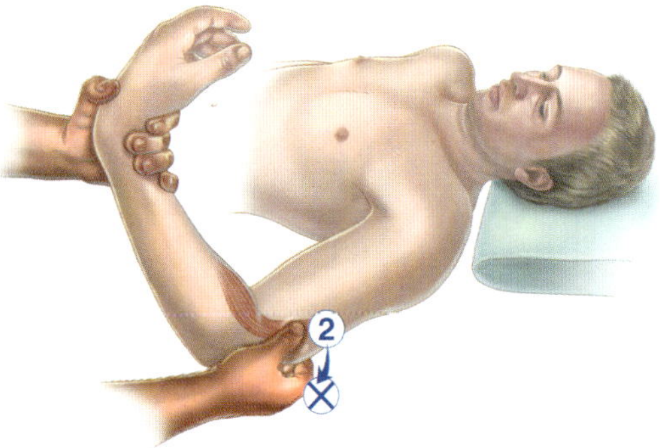

Figure 7.48 This "retained" Pri-move across the brachioradialis muscle is combined with point 1 to sedate and relieve pain in and around the elbow articulation.

Point 3

Action: Points 1 and 2 are now released, and the patient's arm is rotated with a circular and lateral movement for 3 rotations, and then fully extended into a straight position. The elbow articulation may be gently extended at the same time (Fig. 7.49).

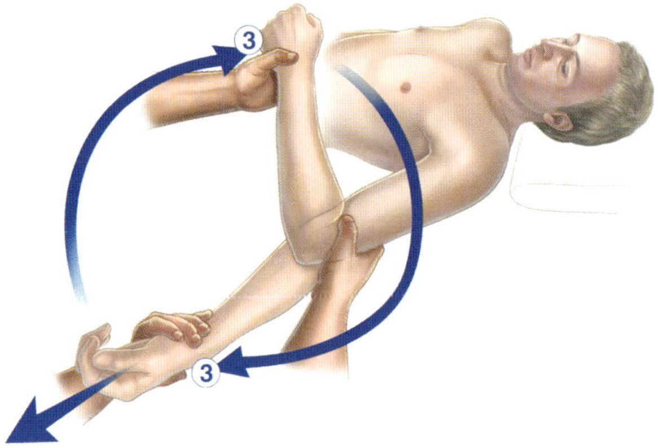

Figure 7.49 This combination release of lower arm rotation and full arm extension is designed to naturally re-establish appropriate articulation of the elbow articulation prior to releasing the wrist articulation.

Point 4

Action: Pri-move applied to the extensor digitorum muscle in a lateral direction. The middle finger should noticeably extend in response to this Pri-move (Fig. 7.50).

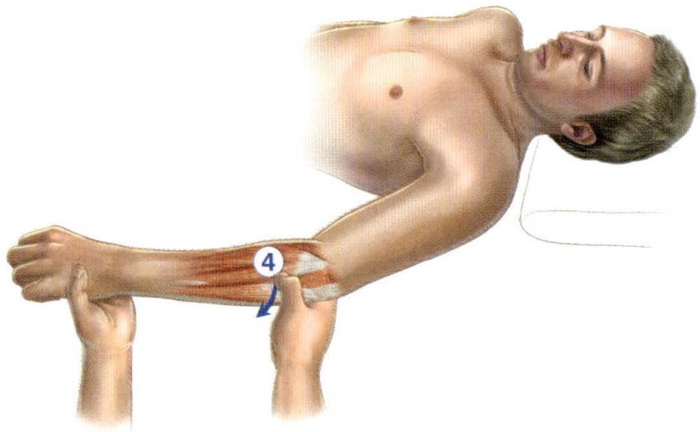

Figure 7.50 Pri-move applied to the extensor digitorum muscle is designed to reset its length, thereby improving both elbow and wrist articulation, and any pain symptoms in either articulation.

Point 5

Action: Pri-moves applied to the flexor car pi radialis and flexor carpi ulnaris muscles in a lateral direction. The palmaris longus muscle may consequently be crossed at the same time (Fig. 7.51).

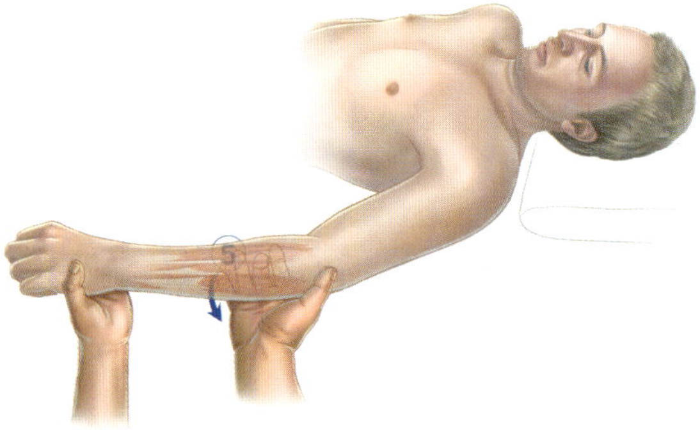

Figure 7.51 This Pri-move crossing both the flexor carpi radialis and flexor carpi ulnaris muscles is designed to reset their respective length, thereby improving both elbow and wrist articulation, and any pain symptoms in either articulation.

Point 6

Action: Deep slow Pri-move crossing the extensor retinaculum and extensor tendons of the metacarpals from lateral to medial direction (Fig. 7.52).

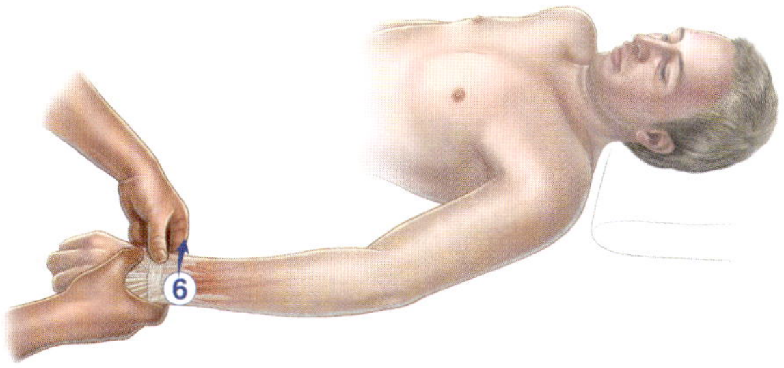

Figure 7.52 Applied simultaneously to the extensor retinaculum of the wrist and the collective extensor tendons, this broad Pri-move is designed to gently reposition the extensor tendons and also to relieve any tension in the extensor retinaculum itself, and consequently the palmar carpal ligament, which it is continuous with.

Point 7

Action: Using thumbs and fingers, the practitioner applies traction and a squeezing hold to the wrist articulation. The patient's fingers should abduct in response (Fig. 7.53).

The traction and squeezing hold are maintained as a slow "figure 8" movement of the wrist articulation is applied, followed by a slow flexion of the wrist articulation.

The "figure 8" movement and flexion of the wrist articulation may be repeated a second time.

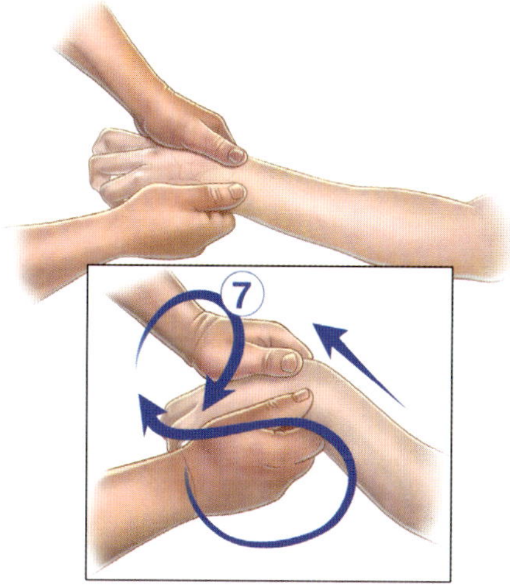

Figure 7.53 With the collective benefits that the preceding six points have contributed to the release of the wrist articulation, now established, this final combination release for the wrist is designed to simply gently and naturally assist with the repositioning of the bones of the wrist, thereby further optimizing its articulation.

Indications: Hand pain conditions, lack of mobility or stiffness in the hand, fingers or thumb. Especially useful for piano players, tennis players, keyboard operators or any activity that requires extensive usage of the hands, involving either gross or fine motor control.

Application of the Hand procedure also induces calmness and relaxation and may therefore be used as a stress defusion strategy.

It is only necessary to treat the affected hand.

Prerequisites: Dynamic Body Balance - Parts 1, 2 and 3, Shoulder Procedure and Elbow & Wrist Procedure, should be completed prior to commencing the Hand procedure.

Point 1

Action: Deep pressure applied to the abductor pollicis longus and extensor pollicis brevis tendons, immediately distal to the styloid process of the radius and retained whilst points 2 are performed (Fig. 7.54).

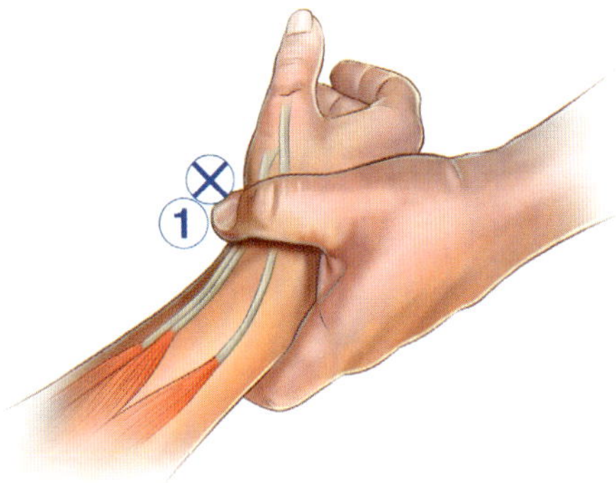

Figure 7.54 The static block applied here is simply designed to increase tension in the general extensor and abductor tendons of the thumb in preparation for their release with point 2.

Point 2

Action: Random series of bilateral "micro" Pri-moves applied to the abductor pollicis longus and extensor pollicis brevis tendons along their length, causing "micro bumps" as they are crossed (Fig. 7.55).

Similarly "micro" Pri-moves may be applied to the articular capsule at the distal end of the metacarpal.

Note: The number of Pri-moves and the order in which they are performed is not set; however, the outcome should be that the skin along the dorsal aspect of the thumb should noticeably soften when completed.

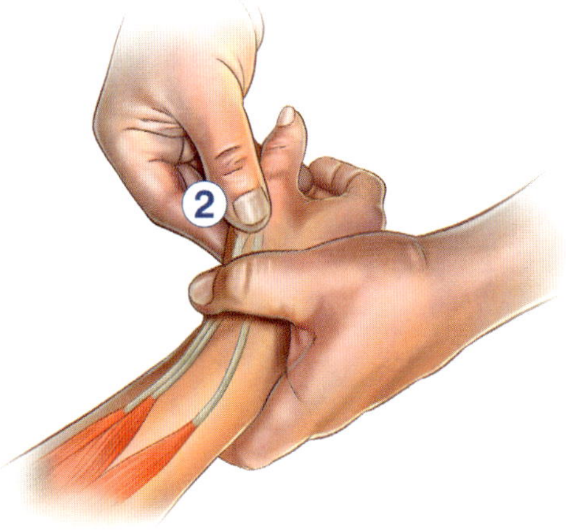

Figure 7.55 A series of "micro" Pri-moves is applied to the abductor pollicis longus, extensor pollicis brevis and longus muscle tendons, causing them to "bump" as they are crossed. The response of the tendons is to soften and therefore lengthen very slightly. The effect is sufficient to release micro tension in the tendons, and consequently improve articulation of the collective articulations of the thumb.

Point 3

Action: Sufficient digital pressure is applied to the dorsal aspect of the wrist to compress the fibers of the extensor retinaculum and extensor digitorum tendon onto the capitate bone (Fig. 7.56). The point is retained whilst points 4 are completed.

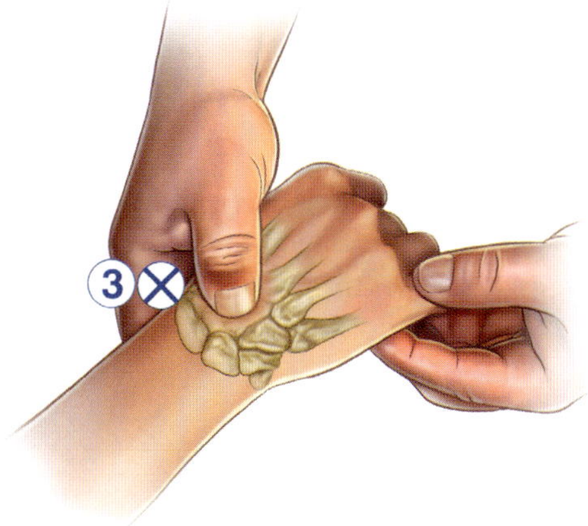

Figure 7.56 The static block applied here is simply designed to increase tension in the general extensor tendons of the hand in preparation for their release with point 4. It may also facilitate general pain relief of the hand.

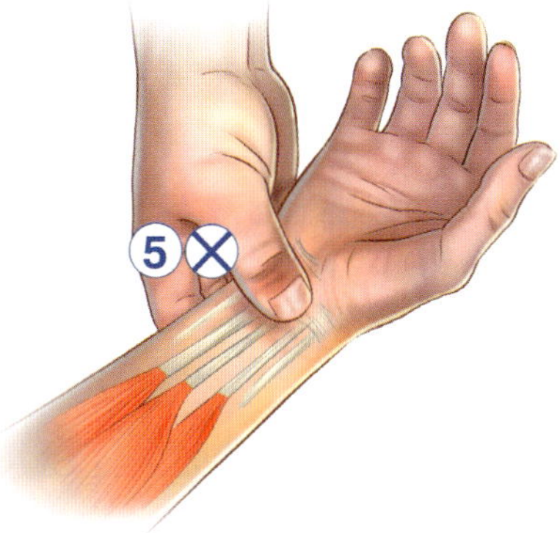

Figure 7.58 The combined static block applied here, and its subsequent sedation of the median nerve, is designed to increase tension in the general flexor tendons of the hand, and also to relax the palmar aponeurosis in preparation for deeper release with point 6.

Point 4

Action: Whilst point 3 is retained, a random series of bilateral "micro" Pri-moves applied to the extensor tendons of all fingers and to their articular capsules at the heads of their respective metacarpals (Fig. 7.57).

Note: The number of Pri-moves and the order in which they are performed is not set; however, the outcome should be that the skin covering the dorsal aspect of the hand should noticeably soften when completed.

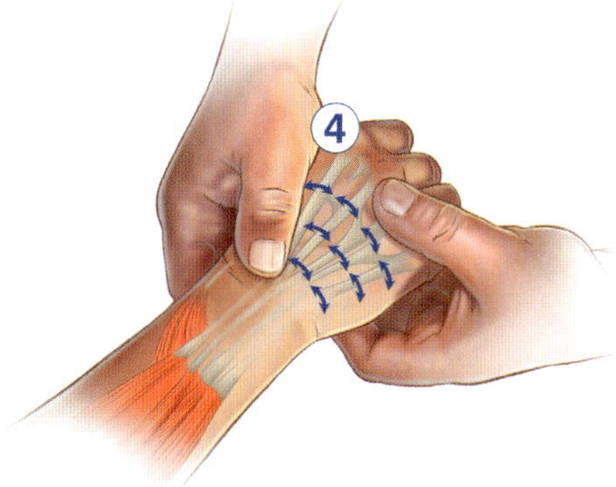

Figure 7.57 A series of "micro" Pri-moves is applied to the collective extensor tendons of the hand, causing them to "bump" as they are crossed. The response of the tendons is to soften and therefore lengthen very slightly. The effect is sufficient to release micro tension in the tendons, and consequently improve articulation of the collective articulations of the hand.

Point 5

Action: Sufficient digital pressure is applied to the palmar aspect of the wrist to compress the fibers of the flexor retinaculum, palmaris longus tendon, flexor tendons and median nerve, so that the patient experiences a temporary mild numbness in the hand (Fig. 7.58).

Point 6

Action: Whilst point 5 is retained a firm bidigital clamp is applied to the adductor pollicis muscle and held for approximately 15 seconds and then released. A second firm bidigital clamp is applied to the palmar fascia and held for a further 15 seconds (Fig. 7.59).

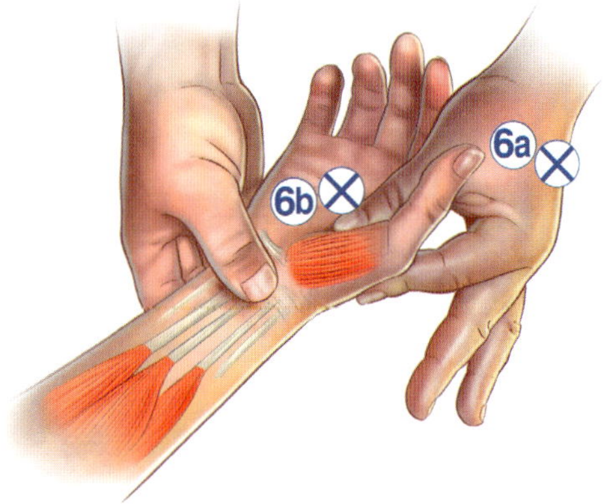

Figure 7.59 The effect from point 5 with additional contact to the adductor pollicis muscle 6a, releases tension between the muscle's three origins on the capitate bone, third and second metatarsals respectively, and the proximal phalanx of the thumb to which it inserts. This is yet another valuable release and strategic step in preparing the palmar aponeurosis of the hand for final release, which is achieved by applying deep bidigital pressure with point 6b.

Point 7

Action: Series of short deep Pri-moves applied to palmar aspects of all articular capsules (Fig. 7.60). Action may be repeated until the skin covering the palmar aspect of the hand becomes noticeably softer when completed.

Option: Using the thumbs, the practitioner deeply slides through palmar surface of patient's hand, and in a continuous motion, crosses the palmar base and then along the sides of the hand. Repeat 2-3 times.

Note: Additional optional detailing work using micro Pri-moves around the circumferences of all finger articulations may be added to further improve flexion and extension and reduce pain when necessary.

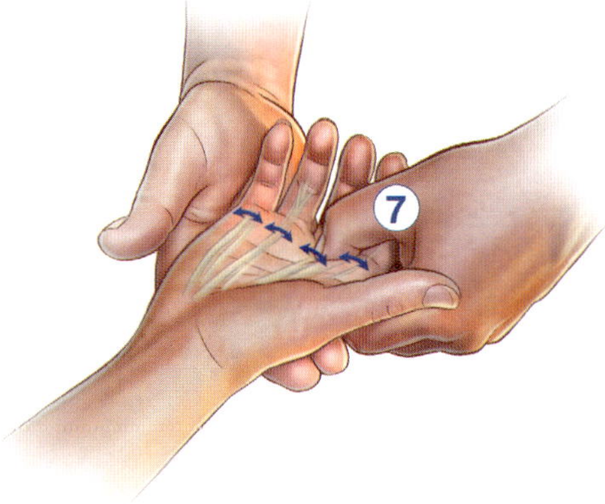

Figure 7.60 The series of Pri-moves to the palmar aspects of the articular capsules extends the release from the palmar aponeurosis into the digits thereby completing the hand release.

CONCLUSION

Once the upper extremities work is completed, the patient is generally given a 1-2 minute pause so that changes can be assimilated. This pause is recommended but not mandatory.

After the pause and with the body now largely in a state of vastly improved "tensegrity", the timing is ideal for returning to the "Core" to check whether or not the Pelvic or TMJ procedures need to be performed.

Along with the Coccyx both of these important procedures relate intimately to the Stomatognathic System and its function, and both are frequently indicated in over 50% of clinical cases.

The other possibility is to add the "cranial integration release" at the end of all supine body work to better induce the Primary Respiratory Mechanism.

Furthermore, when the patient comes into a sitting position prior to leaving the treatment table, and becoming load-bearing through the sacroiliac joints, further opportunity exists to perform some final releases for the neck and therefore the body's "Micro to Macro system" relationship.

All of these final procedures, along with the coccyx, can be considered as part of adjusting the Super Core in NST terminology. The Base Core having been dealt with, by way of corrections achieved utilizing the Dynamic Body Balance, Sacrum and Lung (diaphragm).

However, before we move into our final Super Core adjustments, let's summarize the work thus far, by looking at an integrated session that includes DBB1, 2, 3, the Sacrum, Lung and some of the extremities work.

The session below is just an example of typical NST flow, and which procedures come first, and where to give the pauses. Note: the prerequisites provide the keys to determining the steps.

PRONE SECTION

DBB1 ← *Pause for 5 minutes after point 5*
DBB2
Sacrum + iliolumbar ligament release
Hamstring procedure – prone part
End of prone procedures ← *Pause for 2 minutes*

SUPINE SECTION

Lung procedure
DBB3 → Points 1-4
Knee procedure
Hamstring procedure – supine part
DBB3 → Point 7
Shoulder procedure
End of supine procedures ← *Pause for 2 minutes*

The above "hypothetical example" obviously does not contain all of the procedures covered up to this point with the hips and coccyx omitted in the prone position and the ankles, feet, elbow & wrists and hands omitted in the supine position.

Naturally, we could have included some or all of those procedures had the patient presented with symptoms that warranted their inclusion. And their actual positioning in the above example would be determined by the prerequisites given for every procedure.

However, for the purpose of this "hypothetical example" we are simply imagining that this integrated session fitted our imaginary patient's symptom pattern as presented.

Importantly, the example shows the order and flow of things according to how an integrated NST session is built. Once our final section containing the Pelvic, TMJ, Cranial and sitting position work is completed, a further more integrated session will be provided.

SUPINE POSITION PROCEDURES – Super Core

INTRODUCTION

In Chapter 3, NST Operating Systems, we covered the topic of the Stomatognathic system detailing how its components sit predominantly at either end of the vertebral spinal column, in the cranium and pelvic girdle respectively.

This final section of procedures often referred to as NST's Super core work, will detail procedures for the pelvis, TMJ and cranium. It is important to keep in mind that the coccyx, already covered earlier in the prone procedures section, also belongs to the Super core. It's just that it's timing for inclusion always comes in the prone position, directly after the Sacrum procedure has been completed.

In this final section, the procedures below will be covered, followed by a typical example of how to include them with the Dynamic Body Balance along with some of the other procedures already covered thus far as well.

- Pelvic procedure
- TMJ procedure
- Cranial procedure
- Final cranium to body checks – sitting position

Pelvic procedure – 4 steps

Indications: Pelvic back conditions, hip problems, groin problems, adductor muscle pain, leg pain and edema, shin pain, menstrual disorders, male and female fertility problems, back problems that will not resolve, knee problems that will not resolve, ankle problems that will not resolve, pain under ball of foot, neck problems that will not resolve, jaw problems that will not resolve, headaches that will not resolve, and lymphatic drainage problems.

Prerequisites: Dynamic Body Balance - Parts 1, 2, 3, Sacrum and Knee procedures must be completed before commencing Pelvic procedure.

Test: Such is the importance of the pelvic girdle's integration to the whole body, that the patient is tested at every session to determine if the Pelvic procedure is required or not.

The typical test employed is the FABER test referring to Flexion – Abduction – External – Rotation of each leg to determine if any groin, sacrum, hip, knee or back pain result as a consequence of doing the test (Fig. 7.61).

If there are any of the above results on either leg, the patient is said to be "positive" and the Pelvic procedure should be performed.

Due to "gait" walking mechanism involvement in pelvic function, both sides of the pelvis are always treated, and always starting with the least affected side. This rule is also applied to the Shoulder procedure for the same reason.

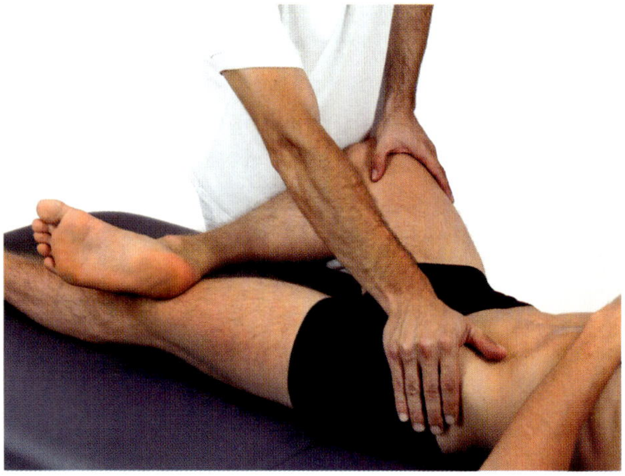

Figure 7.61 The FABER test is a test for the pelvic girdle. FABER is an acronym for Flexion – Abduction – External – Rotation and describes how the test is performed. Each leg is checked to determine if any groin, sacrum, hip, knee or back pain result as a consequence of doing the test. The patient determines which side is the more painful or restricted. And the Pelvic procedure commences on the least affected side. If both sides are equally affected the Pelvic procedure is started on the left side. If neither side is painful or restricted the Pelvic procedure is deemed unnecessary.

Point 1

Action: Practitioner's fingers are positioned deep under the common border of the gracilis and adductor longus muscles directly inferior to the pubic symphsis (Fig. 7.62).

The patient is instructed to inhale and exhale three times prior to a deep slow Pri-move being applied. Action may be repeated a second time without respiration.

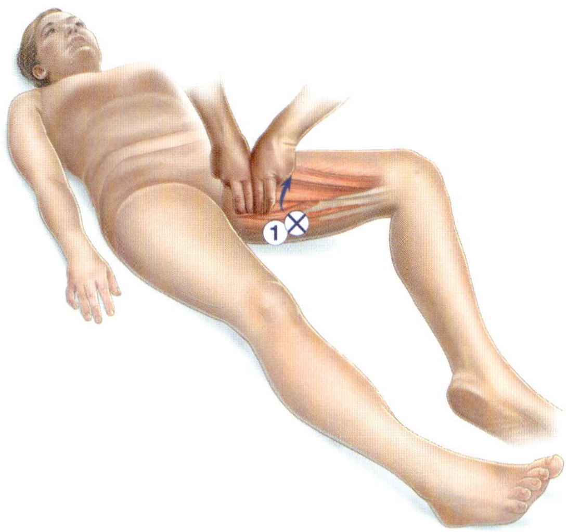

Figure 7.62 As with the Hamstring procedure, the Pelvic procedure contains some big "cables" that can also influence the pelvic girdle and therefore the "sacro-spino-cranial" system as a whole. Point 1 targets the gracilis and adductor longus muscles to assist in restoring proper tensegrity between the tibia, femur and pubic bone of the pelvic girdle. The three successive rounds of respiration prior to executing this important Pri-move, help to induce some pelvic flare designed to facilitate the release and deeper integration.

Point 2

Action: The patient is instructed to inhale and exhale once before a Pri-move applied to the head of the sartorious muscle directly inferior to the anterior superior iliac spine (ASIS).

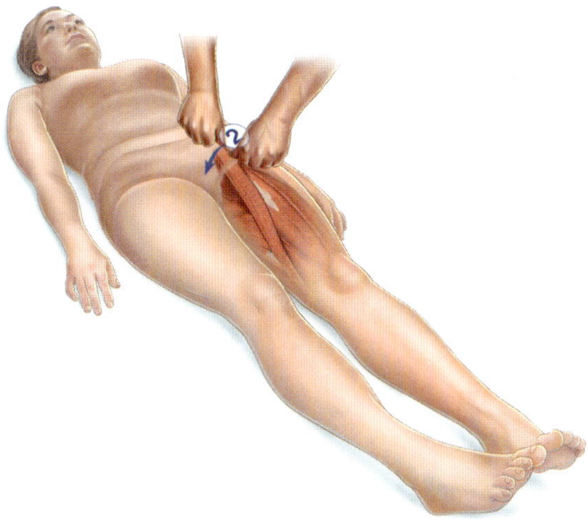

Figure 7.63 The release of the sartorious muscle directly after the gracilis-adductor release in point 1 ensures further improvement in the tensegrity of yet another big cable that shares its insertion with the gracilis and semitendinosous muscles. The conjoined tendons of three muscles (often referred to as the "goose foot" or pes anserinus) insert onto the anteromedial surface of the proximal extremity of the tibia. Given the three muscles cross the knee joint, it should come as no surprise that knee conditions often improve with pelvic release and vice-versa. In NST the Knee procedure is stipulated as a prerequisite procedure for the Pelvic procedure.

Point 3

Action: Practitioner's index and middle fingers are abducted and carefully moved around the patient's inguinal ligament approximately in the middle of the ligament.

The patient's leg is flexed towards the contralateral shoulder and retained in this position (Fig. 7.64).

The patient is instructed to inhale and exhale once before a Pri-move is applied successively to the inguinal ligament 2-3 times.

The patient's leg is extended and returned to the treatment table.

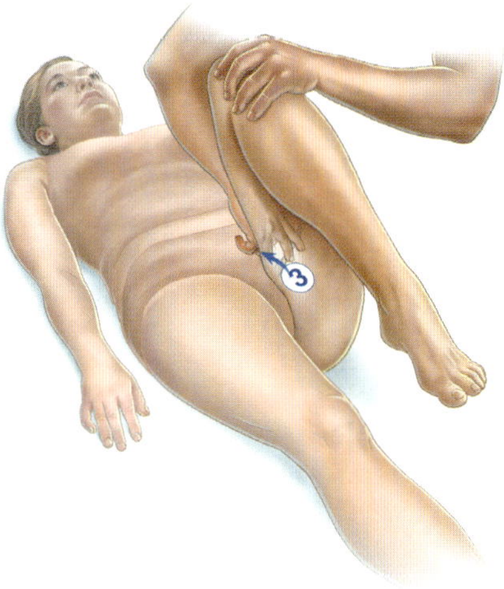

Figure 7.64 This Pri-move, performed directly on the inguinal ligament, is designed to free any contact between the inguinal ligament and the psoas major muscle that passes directly under it. Also intended to release any contact to the psoas minor muscle if it exists (psoas minor is absent in around 50% of people) and the iliac fascia. In particular the psoas major muscle may be pushing anteriorly onto the inguinal making it feel tight and in some cases painful. Point 3 helps prepare the way for point 4 which is applied directly to the iliacus muscle.

Point 4

Action: Patient's leg is fully abducted, as the practitioner positions thumb directly medial to the ASIS, and deep through the external oblique muscle inferior fibers and its aponeurosis, onto the iliacus muscle. Pressure is now applied towards the ASIS (Fig. 7.65).

The patient is instructed to inhale and exhale once, as the practitioner commences to adduct the patients leg. Approximately midway through adduction, a deep Pri-move is applied to the iliacus muscle in a superolateral direction.

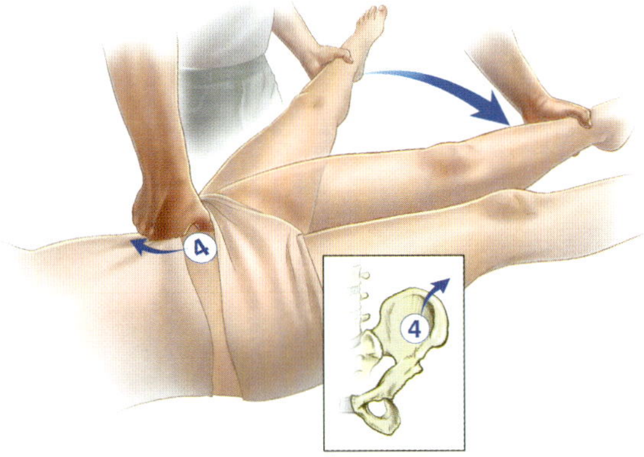

Figure 7.65 This dynamic release involves fully abducting the patient's leg and then adducting it as the iliacus muscle is stimulated with a superolateral Pri-move, directly medial and deep to the ASIS. The release literally helps complete muscular integration from below the knee to the lumbar spine, where all structures involved are considered in a tensegrity sense. It's worth remembering that the psoas muscle in particular is positively affected by the work done in DBB1, as are the nerve supplies to both the psoas major and iliacus muscles that originate from L1-L3 and L2-L4 respectively. In other words, DBB1 has already prepared the pelvic girdle for release and integration, and the addition of the Pelvic procedure completes this. Note: Once the four pelvic points have been completed on the least affected side, they are immediately released on the affected side.

Indications: Painful or clicking jaw, orofacial pain, facial pain, tinnitis, ear conditions, eye conditions, headaches, migraine headaches, neck pain, shoulder pain, pins and needles in the fingers, throat problems, thyroid problems, lower and mid back pain, menstrual disorders, chronic fatigue, immune regulation, adrenal conditions, autoimmune conditions, emotional depression, sinusitis, influenza, travel sickness, balance conditions, glandular fever, lymphatic drainage conditions, learning conditions, any problem that will not resolve using other procedures.

Prerequisites: Dynamic Body Balance - Parts 1, 2, 3, Sacrum and Shoulder procedures must be completed before commencing TMJ procedure.

Note: In Chapter 3 (NST Operating systems, Stomatognathic System – SGS), we learned that the SGS indeed exerts a hierarchical structural influence over the Secondary Respiratory Mechanism (SRM) and therefore the whole body.

Importantly, the TMJ (Fig. 7.66) were identified as being one of the integral components of the SGS Micro system, and it's worth reflecting on the significance of this every time we work with the TMJ, as their balance can literally be the difference between creating short-term, unstable corrections or long-term very sustainable corrections for our patients.

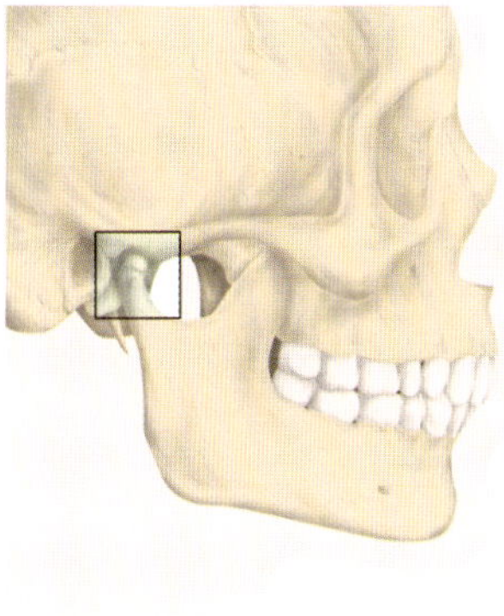

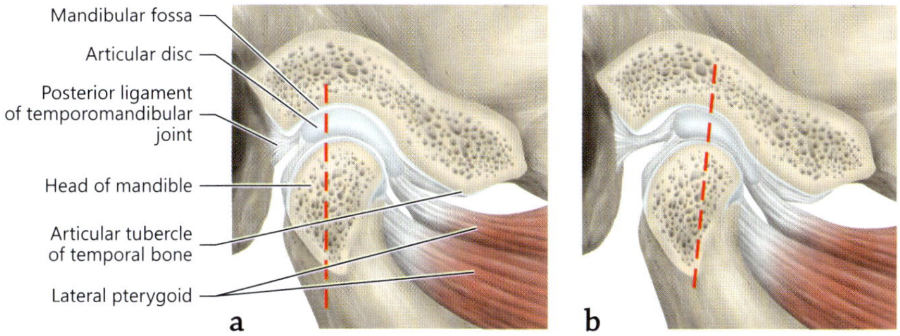

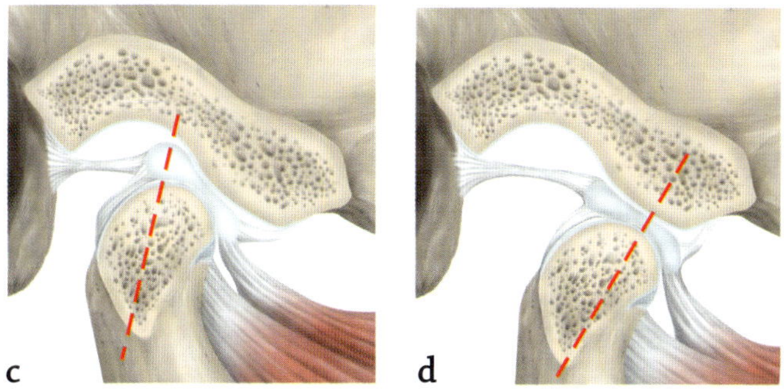

Figure 7.66 Temporomandibular joint (TMJ) highlighting four different positions of the mandibular head axis: (**a**) with mandible raised prior to opening – vertical – swallowing position, (**b**) initial stage of opening – rotation – lips together, (**c**) approximately half open – rotation & slight translation – speech and eating position, (**d**) fully open – full translation & depression – cheering and yelling position. Apart from the bony structures of the mandibular condyle and temporal fossa, the TMJ consists of a mobile soft tissue capsular joint that contains an intracapsular meniscus, that sits between an upper and lower synovial cavity complete with synovium. There is also a rich blood supply servicing the posterior portion of the meniscus rendering it capable of regeneration. The lateral pterygoid muscle is attached to the anterior portion of the capsule, and is responsible for ensuring that the capsule and its meniscus remain cushioned between the bony surfaces throughout slight opening (rotation) or fully opening (translation and depression) and the reverse when closing. As the mouth closes the responsibility for maintaining the appropriate position of the meniscus, largely falls to the elastic retracting ligament that is firmly attached to the posterior aspect of the TMJ capsule. In other words, throughout closing the lateral pterygoid muscle is inhibited, and the natural elasticity of the retracting ligament performs the task of ensuring the appropriate position of the meniscus.

In addition to the information provided on the SGS in Chapter 3 (NST Operating Systems), in Chapter 9 (System Procedures), we will consider further important practical information on the TMJ and their effects, and considering the information in both these sections will go a long way to developing a deeper working relationship with the TMJ.

For now we are going to look at how to assess the TMJ for imbalance, and how to correct them and finally how to stabilize them if necessary by the usage of simple intraoral appliances that every practitioner working with the TMJ, structure and the spine should be familiar with.

Throughout a thirty year period treating tens of thousands of individuals with structural and spinal conditions, using various treatment strategies, I was fortunately taught long ago, that the TMJ and the SGS system to which they belong, need to be dealt with correctly and specifically in order to achieve the best results.

Maintaining "attention to detail" and "thoroughness" are therefore the working mantras that should accompany every good effort in dealing with the TMJ.

In NST, the fundamental treatment plan consists of three important steps, and is applied to every patient at every session, as determined by each patient's presenting symptoms and indications, ultimately ensuring that no patient "slips through the net"!

The three important steps are as follows:

- Assessment
- Correction
- Stabilization

ASSESSMENT

Proper and thorough assessment needs to be carried out to determine whether or not the patient indeed has a TMJ imbalance or not, and each and every patient receives the three quick tests at every session. Collectively the tests will take no more than 1-2 minutes to perform.

Logically and practically, the tests are carried out from gross to fine, or the most obvious potential indication to the next most obvious indication to the least most obvious.

If the patient is positive to any of the tests, they will need to receive the 13 step TMJ correction detailed below.

If they are not positive to any of the tests, TMJ correction is not warranted and not applied.

Test 1 – Articulation

The most obvious indication of a TMJ condition is a clicking or clunking TMJ, which indicates displacement and/or degeneration of the intracapsular disc, of one or both of the TMJ.

The TMJ have three modes of movement: from Rotation > Translation > Depression and back.

As we speak, the head of the mandible simple rotates around its axis and remains within the confines of the perimeter of the temporal fossa. When we open our mouth to shout or place food in the oral cavity, the head of the mandible literally leaves the temporal fossa and moves forward and also downwards (translation > depression) at the same time. Closing simply is a reverse of this situation back into rotation.

A normal occurrence is for the practitioner to feel a "smooth gliding bump" (mandibular condyle) as the patient opens and closes the mouth. What is abnormal, is when instead of the "smooth gliding bump" the TMJ clicks, cracks, pops or grinds its way through opening and closing the mouth.

Instructions: The practitioner places conjoined middle and index fingers directly over the TMJ, the position for which is directly anterior to the tragus of the ear (Fig. 7.67).

The patient is instructed to swallow and then open the mouth as wide as they can and close.

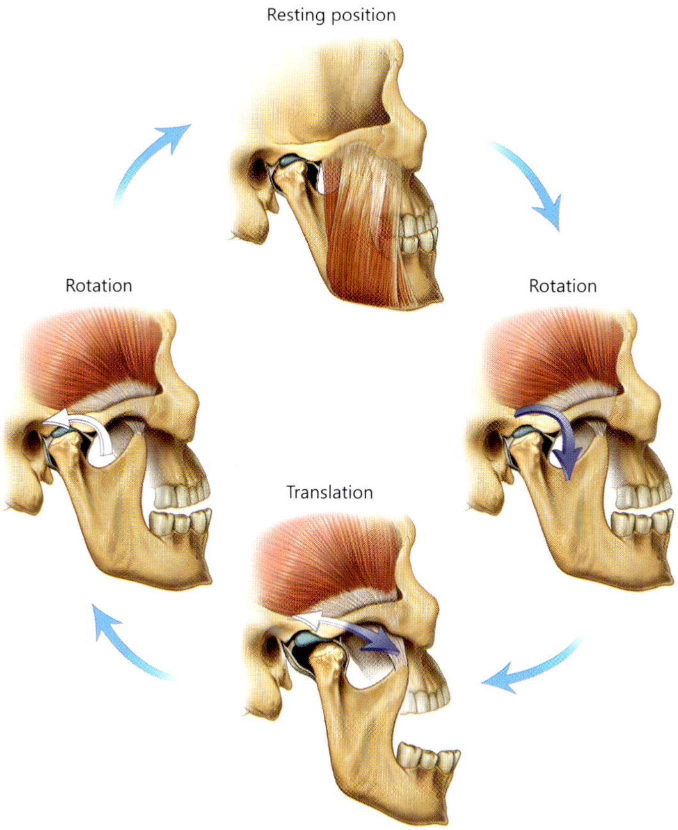

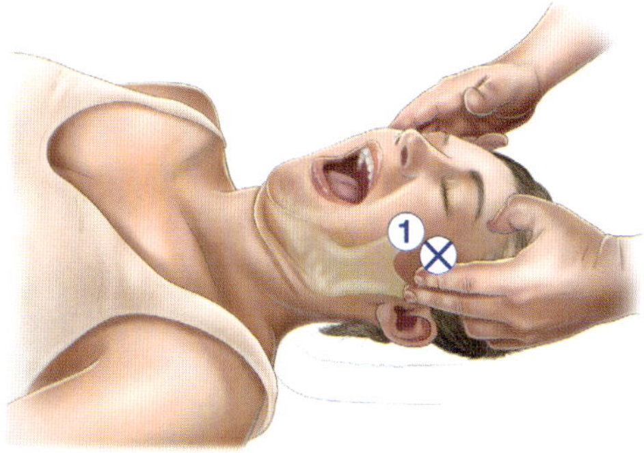

Figure 7.67 The image on the left shows the different positions of the mandibular head when the mouth is slightly opened (rotation) and fully opened (translation/depression). The practitioner needs to distinguish between the smooth bumps that the condylar heads of the mandible provide, as they transition between rotation and translation, and the otherwise dysfunctional signs that a TMJ in need of assistance can give. In assessing the TMJ for dysfunction, the practitioner is firstly looking for the most obvious indications, when the patient opens their mouth fully. Clicking, clunking and popping sounds, deviation of the mandible, a limited opening are all common indicators. The practitioner may also feel the joint is "gritty" almost as if there were coarse sand in it. A limited opening is yet another indication and of course pain and discomfort should always be regarded as obvious signs, indicating that attention is required. If the patient has any of the indications above, the TMJ procedure should be carried out. The image on the right shows the position that the practitioner's fingers need to be in for assessment, with two fingers placed directly anterior to the tragus of the ear, at the junction of the movable and immovable parts of the joint. The patient's mouth must be fully opened, as a partial opening will not reveal the full range of potential TMJ issues.

Outcome: If there is any clicking, cracking, popping or grinding felt by the practitioner the test is deemed positive. Furthermore, if there is any deviation of the mandible through opening and closing, this is also a positive indication. And if there is a noticeable restriction in the amount of opening that the patient enjoys, this is also a positive indication; the patient should be able to place index, middle and ring fingers stacked together between the top and bottom teeth, to determine full and appropriate opening. Average opening for adults should be 45-60 mm.

If the patient is positive to any of these tests, further testing is not necessary and the patient now receives the 13 step TMJ correction detailed below.

If the patient was negative to all tests above, the assessment procedure is nevertheless continued, as there could still be a TMJ condition in the making. And this is determined by palpating certain muscles and zones that are typically sensitive when a TMJ condition is "brewing" or indeed already established.

Test 2 – Tissue

Instructions: The practitioner now slowly and deeply palpates four specific areas for tissue inflammation or discomfort (Fig. 7.68). The outcome is determined solely by the patient.

The areas are: i) directly over the masseter muscles and around the TMJ themselves, ii) along the length of the sternocleidomastoid muscles, iii) directly behind the posterior border of the mandible, iv) over the temporalis muscles. First check one side, then the other.

Outcome: If the patient experiences any pain, discomfort or difference in sensation between one side and the other, the test is deemed positive.

If the patient is positive to any of these tests,

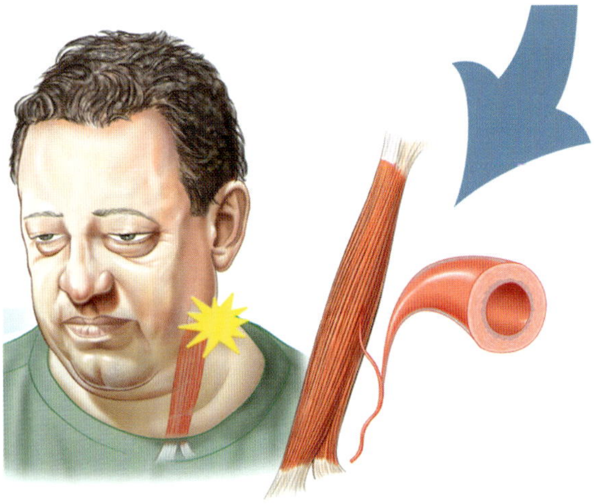

Figure 7.68 If the first test is negative, the practitioner proceeds to the second test of palpation of typical zones where inflammation may be occurring. The inflammatory phase of dysfunction precedes the first phase, and indicates that a TMJ condition is brewing. The zones for palpation are the masseter muscles and TMJ itself, strernocleidomastoid muscles and area directly behind the posterior border of the mandible and the temporalis muscles. If any of these zones are sensitive to deep slow palpation the patient is deemed positive and the TMJ procedure should be carried out.

further testing is not necessary and the patient now receives the 13 step TMJ correction detailed below.

If the patient was negative to all palpation tests above, the assessment procedure is nevertheless continued, as there could still be a TMJ condition in the making, at its very earliest beginnings, as indicated by "tensegrity" imbalances at the level of the SGS Micro system musculature.

Test 3 – Muscle

The final test is performed with the aid of an Applied Kinesiology test, preferably using the psoas muscle as an indicator muscle, as the psoas has a strong affinity with, and is therefore sensitive to, imbalances in the sacrum and pelvic girdle (Fig. 7.69).

Both the sacrum and pelvic girdle can be quickly disturbed by irregular dural torsions, initiated via the dura mater's attachments at the upper cervical vertebrae, and the second sacral segment of the sacrum, respectively.

The dura mater is a 95% non-elastic tough tissue that really acts as a direct link between cranium, cervical spine and sacrum. Nor should we overlook the additional connectivity and influence that longitudinal spinal ligaments can impose on this relationship.

However, the fundamental principle to keep in mind here is, that we are testing a closed system that is not load-bearing. In other words, the patient is in a supine position and the sacroiliac joint are unloaded. This simply provides for a bit more ease and clarity within the test.

It's also important to keep in mind the Macro-Micro system relationships of the SGS at this point, as indeed what we are testing is this relationship.

Specifically, the collective Micro system muscles consist of the muscles of mastication, the tongue, swallowing muscles, hyoid muscles, facial muscles, eye muscles and cranial muscles.

In simple terms, if the SGS is balanced the collective "tensegrity" of the Micro system musculature should be balanced against the collective "tensegrity" of the general musculature of the head on the neck.

If there are any imbalances in this relationship, resultant irregular tensional forces will act on the short suboccipital muscles at the base of the cranium, including the rectus capitis posterior major and minor, and the obliquus capitis superior and inferior, all on the posterior aspect of the cervical spine (occipital base, C1-C2). The capitis longus muscles on the anterior aspect of the cervical spine (C3-C6 and basilar part of occipital bone) will also be affected.

It is these short muscles that connect the upper cervical vertebrae to the cranium, and since the dura mater is firmly connected to the internal circumferences of the 2nd and 3rd cervical vertebrae, and the anterior portion of the second sacral segment of the sacrum, this distortion of the upper cervical vertebrae quickly transfers into distortions or "drag" in the dura mater, ultimately resulting in faults at the sacrum and within the SGS and SRM generally (Fig. 7.70).

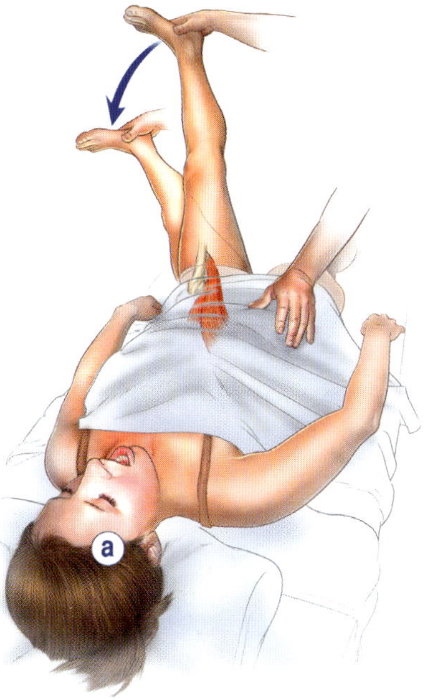

Figure 7.69 If the first and second tests are negative a third test using the psoas muscle is utilized. The image shows the patient opening the mouth as the practitioner tests if the psoas muscle can hold. If the psoas muscle is unable to hold strong on both sides the test is deemed positive and the TMJ procedure should be carried out. Instructions on how to perform the psoas muscle test are provided in the text in this section.

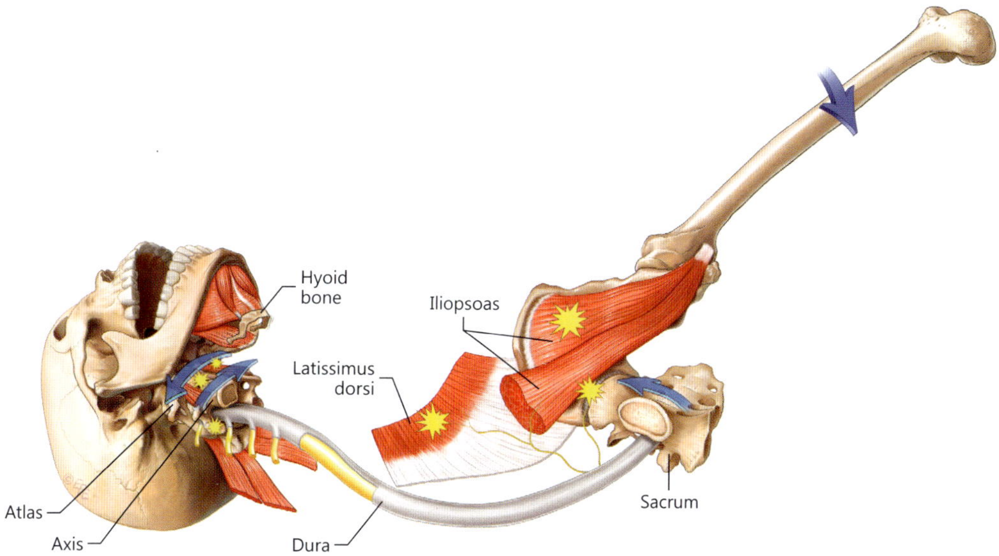

Figure 7.70 The image illustrates the mechanism that underlies the "mouth open psoas muscle test". When the mouth is open, any irregular tensions in the "Micro" system of neck and cranial muscles will be reflected in a tensegrity sense, into the short suboccipital muscles at the base of the cranium. Here they distort the upper cervical vertebrae to which the dura mater is firmly attached, and in doing so quickly disturb the status if the sacrum, via dural drag. As the patient is supine, in a non-load-bearing state, there are predictable muscle responses in the hamstring, psoas, quadratus lumborum, latissimus dorsi and erector spinae muscles. Further faults may also appear in the SGS and SRM. More specific information regarding the mechanism of the test is provided throughout the text of this section.

When this happens, there are predictable postural muscular imbalances in the hamstring, psoas, quadratus lumborum, latissimus dorsi and erector spinae muscles.

Realistically any of these muscles could be used as our indicator muscle, but the psoas muscle test will be described, as it is typically clearly "off" or "on" in response to this test and arguably easier to test as well.

Instructions: To test the psoas muscle, the patient is laying supine with feet together, and relaxed. The practitioner raises the patient's relaxed leg approximately 35-45 degrees off the table, then moves it about 20 degrees lateral to the midline. The patient's foot is then everted. The practitioner stabilizes the pelvis to the contralateral side at the ASIS (see Fig. 7.69).

The psoas muscle is now ready to be tested.

The practitioner asks the patient to open their mouth wide and push their leg vertically upwards. The practitioner applies an opposing vertically downward testing pressure and asks the patient to hold.

If the patient is unable to hold the leg up against the practitioner's testing pressure, this indicates a fault within the "tensegrity" of the patient's Micro system musculature, and the TMJ correction is equally as warranted, as it was with the preceding two tests when positive.

Conversely, a crisp clear response to the command "push vertically upwards" or "hold" is deemed as negative.

Importantly, the same psoas test also needs to be performed on the other leg as well, and a negative response is when both legs hold strong.

Note 1: It is important to keep in mind that the test itself is a test of the psoas muscles ability to lock to an opposing force. In other words, it is a test of the muscle's neurological integrity.

The test is not intended to be a test of physical strength, as the practitioner has a massive mechanical advantage in the leverage of the leg length over the patient's much shorter psoas muscle.

Note 2: If the patient is unable to use the psoas muscle because of a lumbar spine lesion, then the latissimus dorsi muscle is a reliable alternative. The latissimus dorsi is tested by having the patient maintain a straight arm and internally rotating the arm so that the back of the patient's hand is against the side of the leg. The patient is instructed to open their mouth, hold the arm firmly against the leg as the practitioner applies a mild pull in the direction of abduction.

If the patient is able to hold the arm firmly against the body, the test is negative. If the patient is unable to hold the arm strong against the body, the test is positive. As with the psoas, the latissimus dorsi test is bilateral.

CORRECTION

Point 1

Action: The practitioner contacts TMJ bilaterally and the patient swallows and opens and closes their mouth (Fig. 7.71). **Note**: This is designed to provide sensory input to the somatosensory cortex.

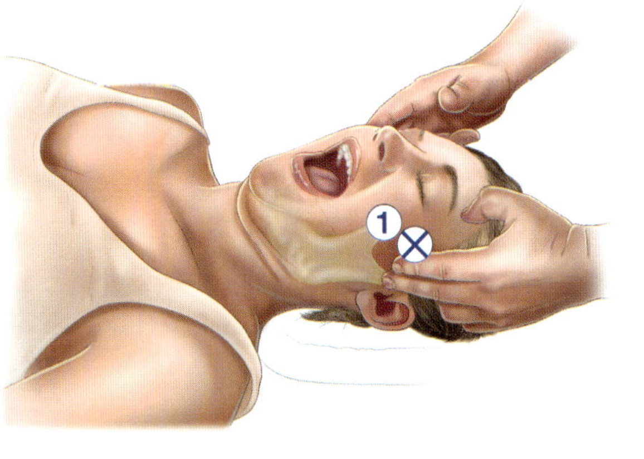

Figure 7.71 Image showing the practitioner contacting both TMJ, immediately anterior to the tragus of the ear, as the patient has a fully opened mouth, preceded by a single swallow. The combination of swallowing, opening and closing the mouth, and the practitioner's digital contact to the receptor-rich TMJ, in a "bio-computer" context, ensures a "burst" of sensory information is transmitted to the somatosensory cortex, alerting the brain to further impending releases in the SGS Micro system.

Point 2

Action: Oblique Pri-move is applied to the levator scapulae muscle adjacent to its insertion into the scapula and at the approximate level of spinal vertebra T2. Action is bilateral (Fig. 7.72).

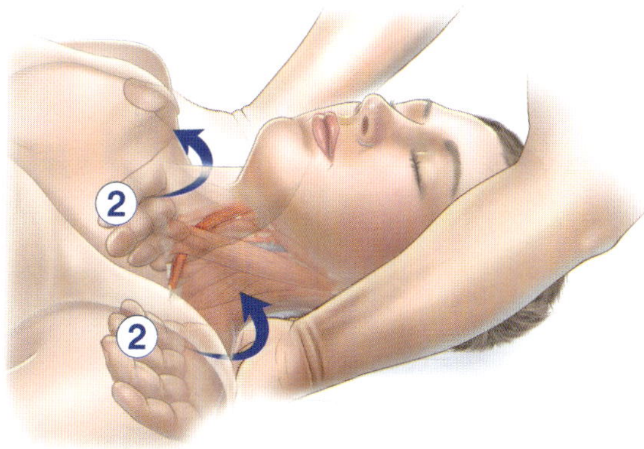

Figure 7.72 Pri-moves applied to the insertions of the levator scapulae muscles – left then right, ensure that there is no tension from these muscles acting on the cervical vertebrae.

Point 3

Action: Pri-move applied to the sternocleidomastoid muscle at its lateral clavicular aspect in a medial direction crossing both the clavicular and sternal heads. Action is bilateral (Fig. 7.73).

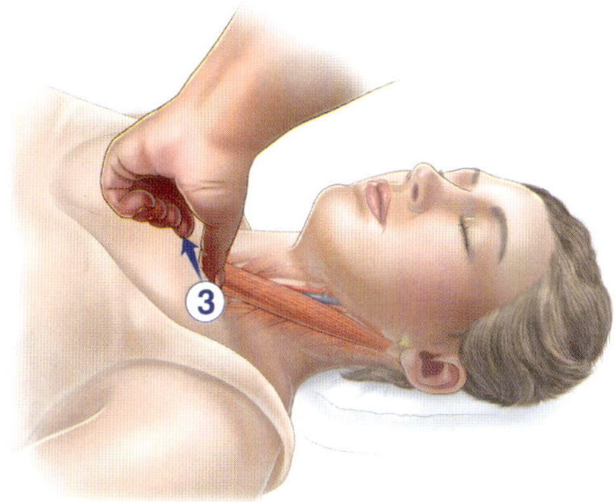

Figure 7.73 Pri-moves applied to the clavicular and sternal heads of the sternocleidomastoid muscles – left then right, eases torsion at the sternoclavicular joints and prepares the sternocleidomastoid muscles for deeper release in point 4.

Point 4

Action: Approximately four Pri-moves applied to the sternocleidomastoid muscle (SCM) from distal to cranial and finishing directly on the insertion of the SCM at the mastoid process. Action is bilateral (Fig. 7.74).

Note: There are important structures directly under and around the sternocleidomastoid muscles, which may positively affect a range of physiological activities after the muscles are released. The structures are a neurovascular bundle containing the common carotoid artery, the internal jugular vein, the vagus nerve and the ansa cervicalis of the cervical plexus.

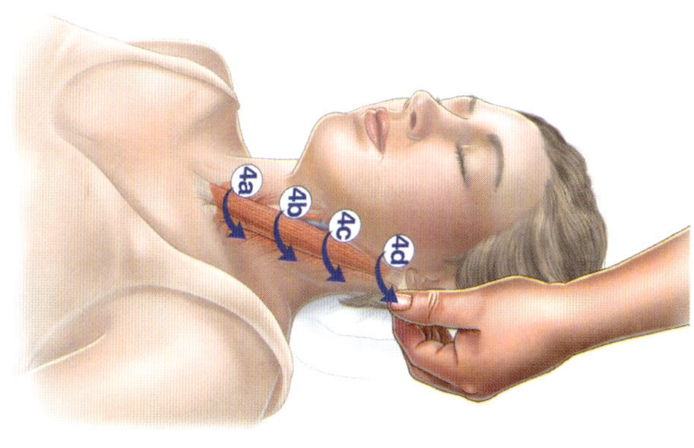

Figure 7.74 Series of Pri-moves applied to the sternocleidomastoid muscles – left then right, ensure that there is no tension from these important muscular cables acting on the mastoid processes, temporal bones or occipital bones. The Pri-moves also coincide with, and may influence, important trigger points along the muscles.

Point 5

Action: Practitioner softly contacts the hyoid bone and briskly moves it from side to side for 5 repetitions (Fig. 7.75). **Note**: This is designed to provide sensory input to the somatosensory cortex.

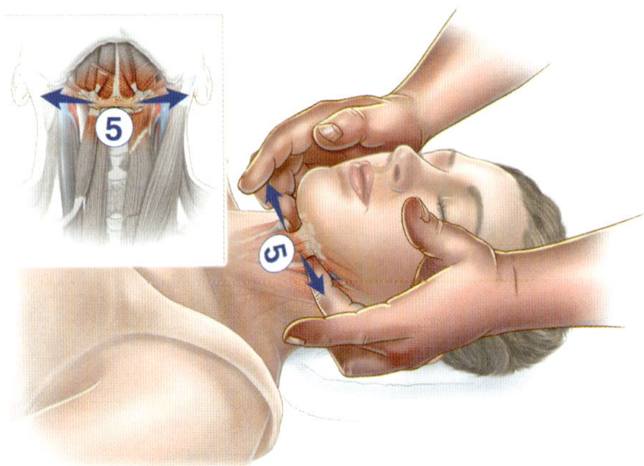

Figure 7.75 Practitioner locates the hyoid bone and applies contact to the lateral aspects of its greater horns. The bone is moved briskly from side to side about five times, providing micro stimulation to the many infra and supra hyoid muscles attached to its surfaces. **Note**: The hyoid muscles contain a high percentage of sensory nerve fibers that provide instant input to the somatosensory cortex when stretched. The hyoid bone and muscles may also be considered as somewhat of a gyroscope in the context of locomotion, providing the brain with reliable sensory input about posture, generated by the contralateral swing of the arms and shoulder girdle, during activation of the gait walking mechanism. Yet again, in this context, we see the relationship between Micro and Macro systems at play.

Point 6

Action: Pri-moves applied to the lateral aspect of the thyroid cartilage of the larynx crossing the omohyoid, sternohyoid and thyrohyoid muscles on the surface of the thyroid cartilage (Fig. 7.76).

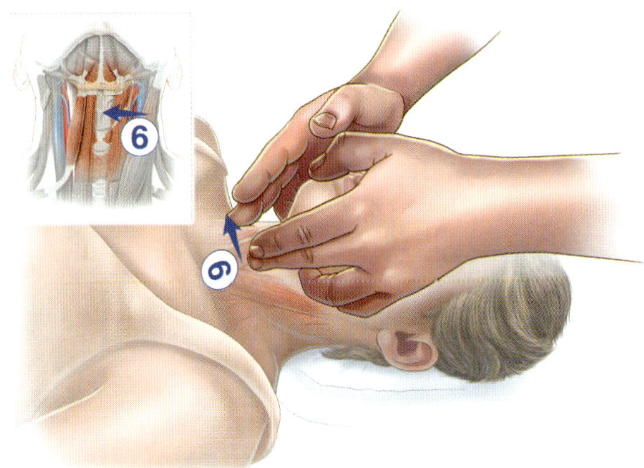

Figure 7.76 Mini Pri-moves applied to the omohyoid, sternohyoid and thyrohyoid muscles on the surface of the thyroid cartilage, ensure that tensions in the infrahyoid muscles are released.

Point 7

Action: Series of short Pri-moves crossing the mylohyoid muscle from the posterior border of the mandible to the mental protuberance crossing the origin of the anterior belly of the digastric muscle (Fig. 7.77).

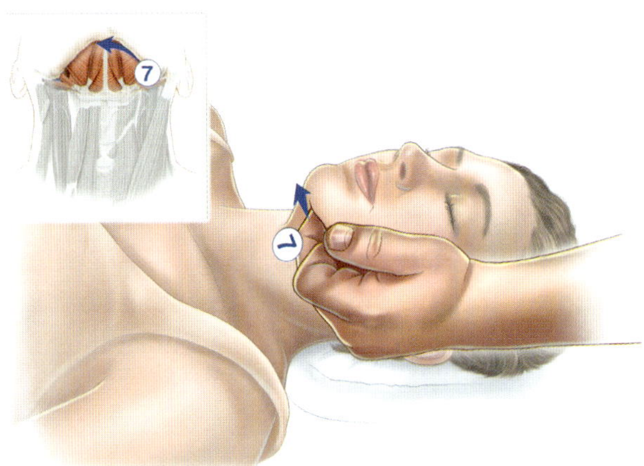

Figure 7.77 Mini Pri-moves applied to the mylohyoid and anterior digastric muscles ensure that tensions in the suprahyoid muscles are released.

Point 8

Action: The practitioner contacts TMJ bilaterally and the patient swallows and opens and closes mouth (Fig. 7.78). **Note**: This is designed to provide sensory input to the somatosensory cortex.

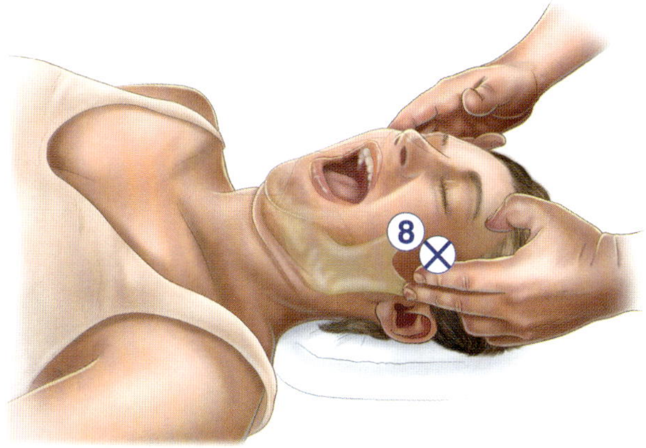

Figure 7.78 As with point 1, the combination of swallowing, opening and closing the mouth, and the practitioner's digital contact to the receptor-rich TMJ, in a "bio-computer" context, ensures a "burst" of sensory information is transmitted to the somatosensory cortex, alerting the brain to further impending releases in the SGS Micro system.

Point 9

Action: Patient is instructed to place their index finger between the teeth and bite gently. It is important that the patient keeps the finger in the mouth until the complete TMJ procedure is completed (Fig. 7.79). **Note**: This may induce swallowing which is part of the correction.

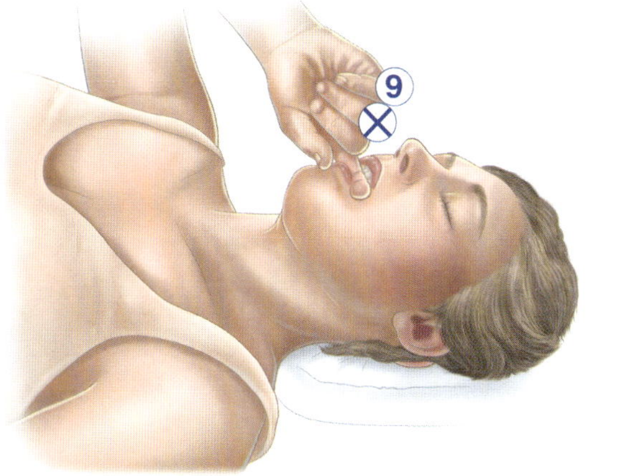

Figure 7.79 The patient is instructed to place a finger between their teeth to create an altered biomechanical relationship between the mandible – TMJ, and the posterior digastric, masseter and temporalis muscles, which will ensure their more immediate release, when carried out in points 11, 12 and 13.

Point 10

Action: Universal Pri-move applied to the TMJ by moving anterior to posterior and cranial to caudal. Action is bilateral (Fig. 7.80).

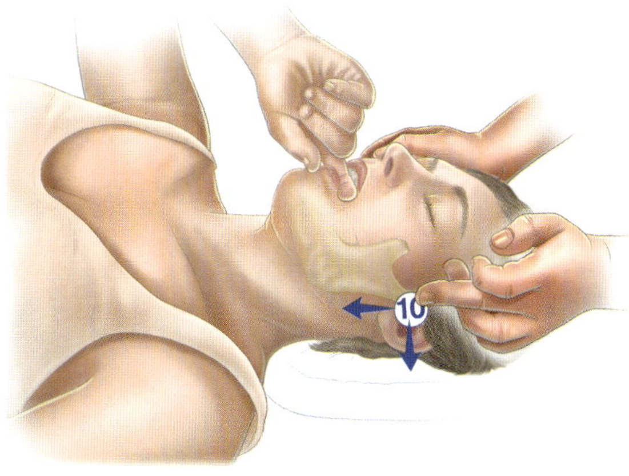

Figure 7.80 The universal Pri-move applied directly to the TMJ capsules is designed to stimulate the high density of mechanoreceptors that lay at the periphery of the joint but also within the joint meniscus. The afferent discharging that occurs when these mechanoreceptors are stimulated alerts the central nervous system of impending injury, which under normal circumstances would be averted through muscular reflex mechanisms. The effect in terms of this procedure however, is to use the reflex to create a relaxation of the surrounding muscles.

Point 11

Action: Series of delicate Pri-moves applied to the deep tissue at the posterior portion of the mandible crossing the posterior digastric muscle belly. Action is bilateral (Fig. 7.81).

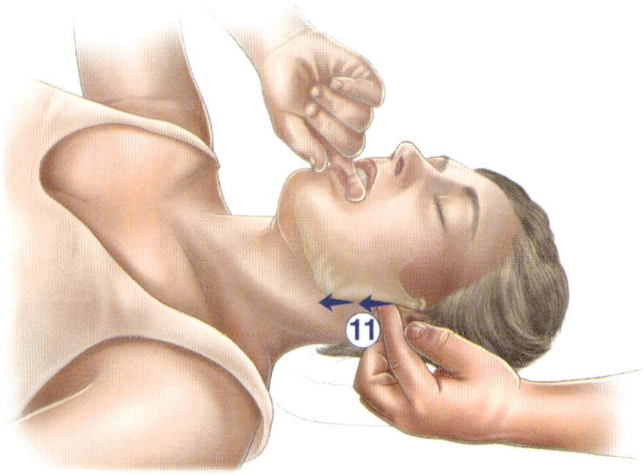

Figure 7.81 Pri-moves applied to the posterior digastric muscle belly, designed to relax and reset the muscle's length.

Point 12

Action: Pri-move applied to the anterior border of the masseter muscle rolling into the shallow fossa in its belly where digital pressure is applied for 5 seconds. Action is bilateral (Fig. 7.82).

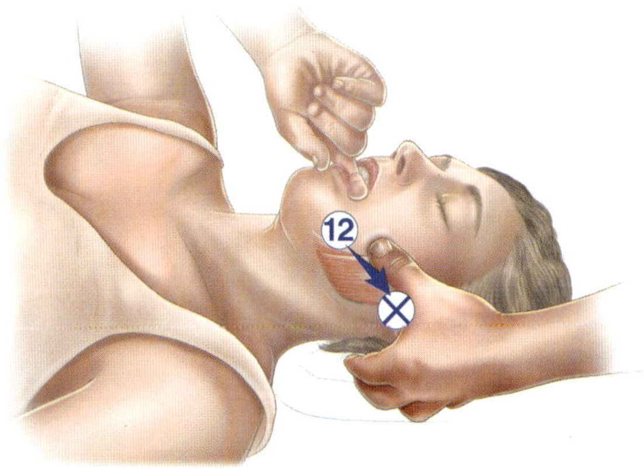

Figure 7.82 Pri-move applied to the masseter muscle belly, designed to relax and reset the muscle's length. The brief holding point utilized after the Pri-move, takes advantage of the fact that the jaw is open, which creates a slight indentation at the posterior border of the masseter muscle. Pressure applied to the indentation is designed to release the reflex point, that in turn has a direct influence on the masseter and pterygoid muscles, and therefore the TMJ.

Point 13

Action: Series of Pri-moves applied to the temporalis muscle from anterior to posterior, ultimately crossing its posterior border under the pinna of the ear (Fig. 7.83).

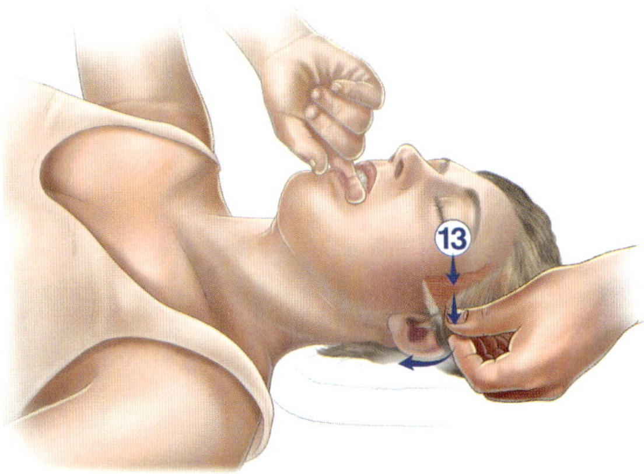

Figure 7.83 Pri-move crossing the fibers of the temporalis muscle and its belly, designed to relax and reset the muscle's length.

The TMJ procedure will very effectively reset the vast majority of TMJ and their Micro system support structures, within the two or three minutes it takes to perform the procedure, and of course, providing that the prerequisites (DBB1, 2, 3, Sacrum and Shoulder) have been attended to beforehand.

However, just as there are varying degrees of TMJ imbalance, from muscular imbalance to degeneration of the capsule, disc and articulating surfaces of the bones, there are varying degrees of balance achieved.

Indeed, while a patient is lying supine on the treatment table, having just had their body's "tensegrity" corrected to a large extent; structurally speaking we can assume that they will be well aligned.

But as soon as the patient stands up and becomes load-bearing again, thereby reinstating postural tone, the true outcome of how and where their "tensegrity" will "settle" will soon become apparent. And it may take some few days before the full extent of the body's capacity to hold its corrections or otherwise is fully known.

Add to this, the fact that the patient is very shortly going to go back to chewing, biting and swallowing again, and thereby exert forces back on the muscles, nerves, teeth and TMJ again, and if there is any "resident" weak link in the body's Micro system it will be found out sooner rather than later, leading to an incremental return to imbalance as each day passes.

What is guaranteed is that when a patient has degeneration or chronic inflammation within the body's system of articulations, and particularly the TMJ, the capacity of the body to hold its corrections is noticeably diminished, unless we take action by using "stabilization" strategies.

The rule that governs the body's Micro system general operation, and its capacity to stay balanced, therefore, is simply that its capacity to function and stay balanced is directly proportional to the integrity of its weakest link or part.

Just the same as the strength of any chain is determined by its weakest link!

And a clicking, cracking or popping TMJ is going to be an unwelcome impediment to the process of a full return to balance, and indeed a state where the body can hold its corrections achieved on the table; unless we do something about it.

As practitioners, it's useful to keep in mind that the body's tendency towards integration is far stronger than its tendency towards disintegration, so there's no doubt that we are working with a powerful force for the good!

But the body is designed to manage disintegration as well, and a truer picture of the facts regarding the human organism generally, is that it is constantly integrating and disintegrating in response to so many of life's abundant stressors.

In simple terms, what we know is that long periods of integration equate to feeling pain free, vital and healthy. Conversely, long periods of disintegration equate to pain, low energy becoming unhealthy.

Obviously, our goal is to maximize "post-session" integration and sustainability of corrections as much as we can, and attending to the final and tremendously important aspect of our TMJ treatment plan will give the patient every chance to do this, when and if applicable.

STABILIZATION

Stabilization refers specifically to stabilizing the TMJ after an NST session has been performed, if in fact there is a need to do so.

And the need to attend to stabilization is fully evident and confirmed when a patient has one or two clicking, cracking or popping TMJ or if the psoas or latissimus dorsi muscle test applied in assessment, still tests weak after the TMJ procedure has been completed.

These are our two simple NST rules for determining which patients will need stabilization and which patients will not.

And if you use these two simple rules judiciously, you will quickly be able to identify who is a candidate for stabilization and who is not.

As a guide, and from a personal statistical point of view, in my own patient observations both in Australia and around the world, I discover that regardless of the presenting condition be it back, neck, shoulder, knee pain to headaches, to menstrual disorders, digestive disorders, to respiratory conditions, chronic fatigue, etc., about 80% of individuals present with a TMJ dysfunction at one level or the other, from mild muscular to degenerative osteoarthritis.

Women outnumber men patients by approximately 2:1 and in younger patients, generally, there is a prevalence of more muscular and disc displacement type of TMJ issues whereas the older the patient, the more the prevalence of the more degenerative osteoarthritis types.

Of that 80% of patients who have a TMJ dysfunction over all age groups and sexes, about 45% will require stabilization.

In simple mathematical terms, 80 patients in every 100 will present with some sort of TMJ dysfunction. And 45% of these 80 patients (36 patients) will require stabilization to hold their corrections long term. The others (44 patients) will not require stabilization.

So what is stabilization?

In simple terms, stabilization of the TMJ refers to the usage of intraoral appliances such as an NST MOJO to stabilize and support the TMJ so that they can repair themselves (Fig. 7.84). And the fact that the TMJ can repair themselves is one of nature's and the body's small miracles.

Briefly, the TMJ capsule, disc and articulating surfaces consist of a highly specialized form of fibrocartilage that is capable of rapid regeneration under the right conditions.

The intracapsular disc itself possesses a very high percentage of collagen, not only giving it great rigidity, but also the capacity for rapid regeneration.

Inside the TMJ capsule there is the disc as noted, and above and below the disc there are synovial cavities containing synovial fluid, that brings nutrition to the disc and capsule itself.

Much of the disc depends on the synovial fluid containing valuable micronutrients and regenerating mesenchymal stem cells in which it is bathed, for nourishment and ongoing repair. However, the retro portion of the disc has its own rich vascular supply and nerve innervation.

In fact, it is highly likely it is this nerve innervation that ironically causes the local pain in the TMJ, when the disc has slipped anteriorly and the retro portion is being compressed inappropriately.

The disc itself is curved concavely on its underside, to sit on top of the curve of the condyle of the mandible while its upper surface is curved convexly, to suit the temporal fossa that it must articulate with (Fig. 7.85).

Both ends of the disc are thicker but more cushioned than its central "intermediate" portion that is thinner, but made of tougher fibrocartilage, and consequently capable of withstanding greater direct compressive forces.

The anterior portion of the disc is woven into the capsule and lateral pterygoid muscle's superior head, that pulls it forward and downwards through the phases of rotation, translation and

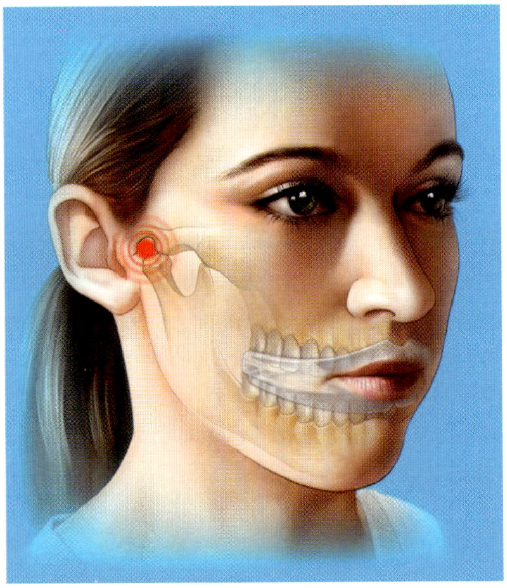

Figure 7.84 Image showing an intraoral TMJ appliance in position. This particular appliance is an NST MOJO appliance. MOJO is an acronym for "mandibular – orbicularis – joint – optimizer" and it is designed to rapidly repair the TMJ and retrain associated musculature.

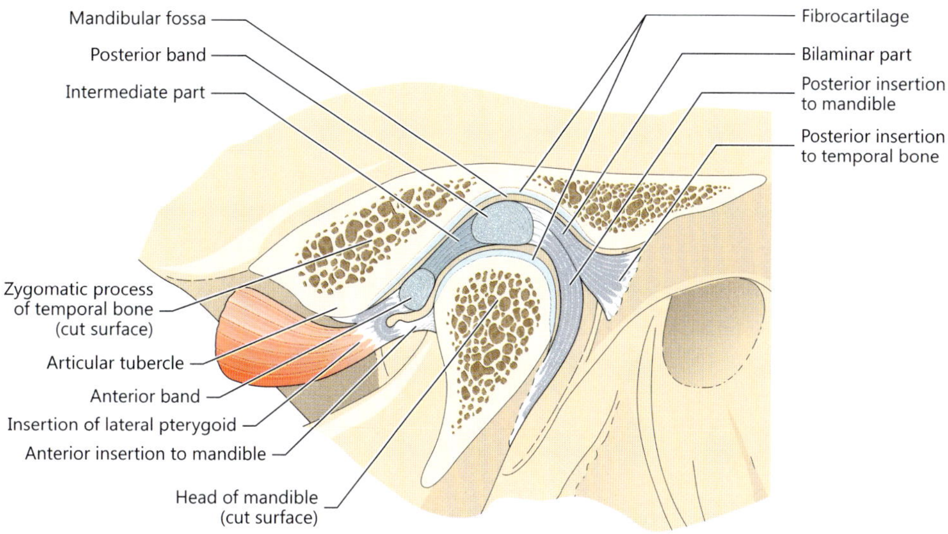

Figure 7.85 Image showing a cross-section of a TMJ highlighting several aspects of the joint.

depression of the mandible. The posterior portion of the disc is woven into the capsule and a fibroelastic ligament, that acts as a counter strain device, effectively pulling the disc and capsule back into position when the mandible is closing.

In considering the general strategy of using stabilization by employing intraoral appliances, we firstly need to make one small additional step in our understanding, and ask how does disc displacement and then degeneration occur?

The simple answer is, that when an individual clenches or grinds the teeth over many months or years, during sleep and/or throughout the day, the muscles of mastication loose their calibration or "tensegrity".

The consequences are firstly misplaced disc and sore muscles, but later this situation turns into degeneration or osteoarthritis, as the condylar heads of the mandible repeatedly apply pressure to the disc with every chew, bite swallow, clench and grind.

A popular theory as to why some individuals clench and grind their teeth (particularly during sleep) while others don't, is simply that clenching and grinding are activities that the body uses to rid itself of built up stresses that it has not been able to resolve at a conscious level (Fig. 7.86).

In other words, clenching and grinding can be seen as a survival mechanism of sorts, but like many survival mechanisms that are overused, the costs become prohibitive.

The further additional complication with grinding the teeth is simply that, the occlusal surface of the teeth may to greater or lesser

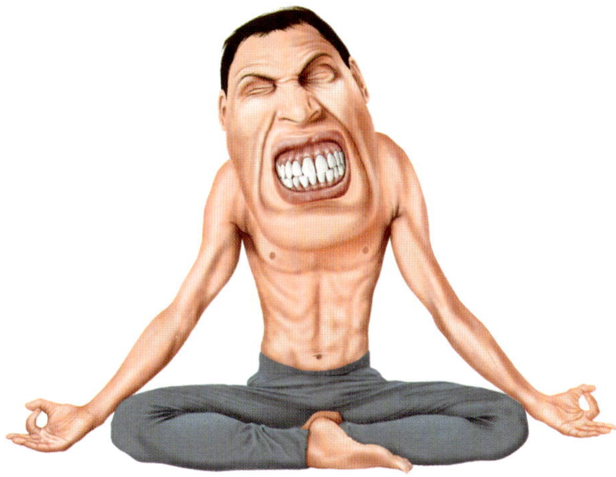

Figure 7.86 This cartoon image emphasizes how tricky it can be to stay balanced in the modern world. One of the reasons, behind why some individuals clench and grind their teeth, can be simply explained in terms of the individual using it as a survival mechanism to relieve unwanted accumulated stress at a conscious and subconscious level. Over time, clenching and grinding wreak havoc on the TMJ.

extent become worn, leading to cross bite and overbite situations, and an imprecise and unreliable foundation therefore, against which swallowing chewing and biting muscular functions must be performed.

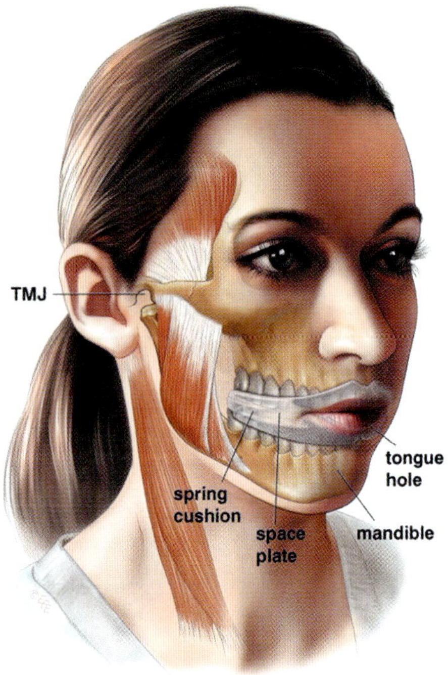

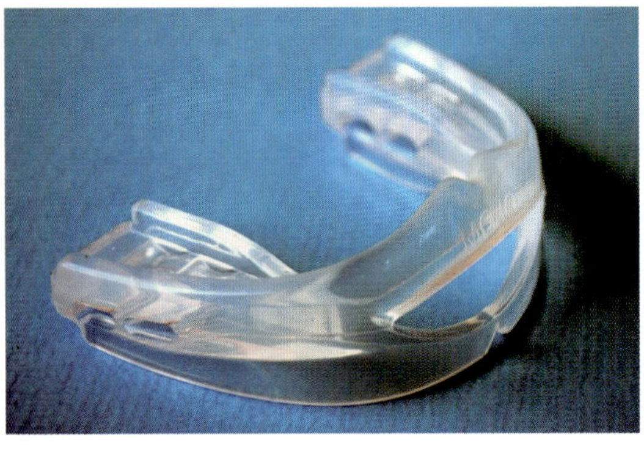

Figure 7.87 Image showing the MOJO in more detail with its tongue hole, space plate and spring cushion. The tongue hole and spring cushion, have been designed to be used as part of some optional but highly recommended accelerator exercises, described in detail on every MOJO brochure. Notice that there is no frontal channel for the teeth to grip onto, a feature that essentially obliges the orbicularis oris muscle to perform the task of holding the MOJO in place, thereby strengthening its closing power and improving the function of other facial and cranial muscles.

This simply leads to further miscalibration of the Micro system musculature, compounded by a position of the mandibular heads that are now constantly pressing on the capsule and disc.

When patients present as described above, the practitioner simply must accept and anticipate, that a highly probable predisposition to slipping back into this faulty position is going to occur, once the patient leaves the clinic, even though the corrections achieved at the table have been very positive.

About the MOJO Appliance and how it works

Firstly the name MOJO is an acronym for Mandibular Orbicularis Joint Optimizer and summarizes to some extent what the appliance is designed to do and how (Fig. 7.87).

- Mandibular is obviously in reference to the mandible.
- Orbicularis is in reference to the orbicularis oris muscle (lips) that really must work to keep the appliance in place.

  This is a unique feature of the MOJO that other TMJ appliances do not have, and provides a huge neuromuscluar advantage, in that it strengthens the orbicularis oris muscle, which in turn has a very direct and positive impact on many of the other facial muscles, including the buccinators whose fibers it blends with. In turn, this helps "set the tone" for proper tongue and swallowing muscle activities, that are so vital to the proper integrity of the SGS Micro system's musculature.

  Significantly, the buccinator muscle originates from the alveolar process of the maxilla, mandible, and pterygomandibular raphe and inserts at the corners of the mouth where it decussates with the fibers of the orbicularis oris muscle. The buccinator-pterygoid link is yet another important facet of the retraining capacity the MOJO affords.

  Strengthening the orbicularis oris muscle appears to have a very positive effect on facial nerve and cranial nerve function generally, which may have more to do with the muscles intimate relationship with the somatosensory and motor cortices.

As a collateral benefit, regular usage of the MOJO and its prescribed exercises will also noticeably improve facial muscle tone and facial appearance.

- Joint refers to the TMJ itself.
- Optimizer because the TMJ function are optimised through tissue repair of the TMJ, a reduction in local symptoms (TMJ pain) and also global symptoms (back pain).

Once the MOJO is in the oral cavity and the patient's lips are closed, three important changes take place, namely:

1. The TMJ are decompressed.
2. The mandible is repositioned forwards.
3. Facial and neck muscles relax.

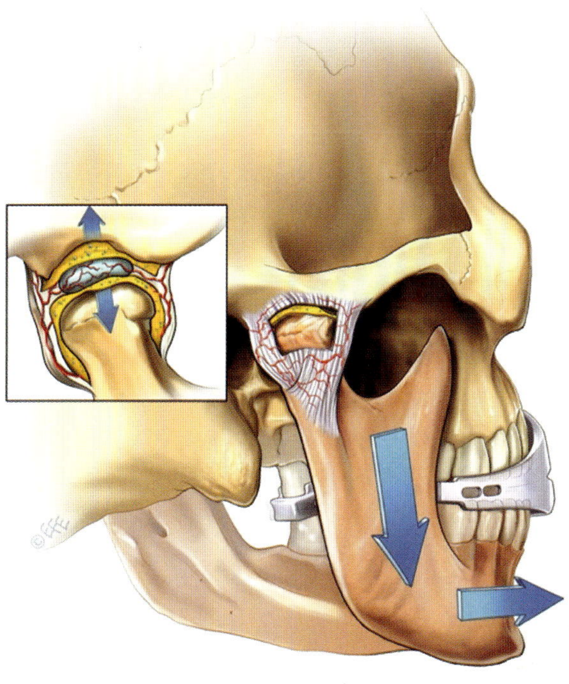

Figure 7.88 The MOJO achieves decompression of the TMJ and repositioning of the mandible into a forward position, and both actions are intended to take pressure off the TMJ and to create space in and around them. When pressure is taken off the TMJ and its intracapsular meniscus, the blood supply servicing the meniscus along with synovium are able to facilitate tissue repair and regrowth.

Benefits of TMJ stabilization

Taking pressure off the TMJ and intracapsular disc by "decompression and repositioning" of the mandible, provides for enhanced blood flow to the disc, better nerve innervation, an opportunity for inflammation of tissue in and around the TMJ to reduce, and muscles to reset (Fig. 7.88).

Importantly, the cranial nerves that sit directly posterior to the TMJ, namely the hypoglossal, glossopharyngeal, accessory, facial, trigeminal and vagus are able to function with greater ease due to the reduced pressure and inflammation on them, and this perhaps accounts for one of the most significant benefits of all in using an intraoral appliance.

Autonomic Nervous System (ANS) function noticeably improves delivering a myriad of positive physiological benefits.

The tendency for the short muscles at the base of the cranium (rectus capitis posterior major, obliquus capitis and capitis longus muscles) to interfere with the upper cervical vertebrae is also eliminated or reduced, leading to better integration of the SGS and SRM generally, and therefore sustainability of corrections.

In addition, the MOJO Appliance provides protection of tooth enamel and a reduction in the tendency to clench and grind.

Other benefits that may be expected as a result of using a MOJO Appliance

Every individual's TMJ dysfunction is in someway unique, and there is no hard and fast rule about how or when to use a MOJO, however, going slowly at the outset has proven to be a great bonus in clients maintaining ongoing usage.

The general recommendation that I give all of my patients is to start with 5-10 minutes of usage, and if this feels confortable repeat as often as feels comfortable throughout the first few days.

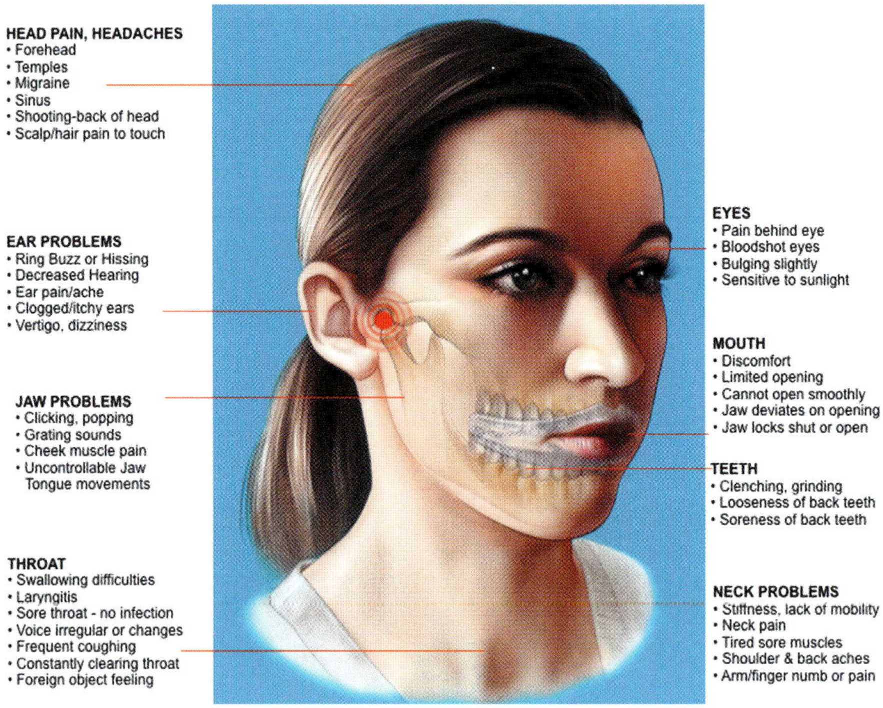

Figure 7.89 The benefits of using a MOJO are not just confined to the TMJ and associated musculature. The chart indicates many symptoms and conditions that may benefit from using a MOJO.

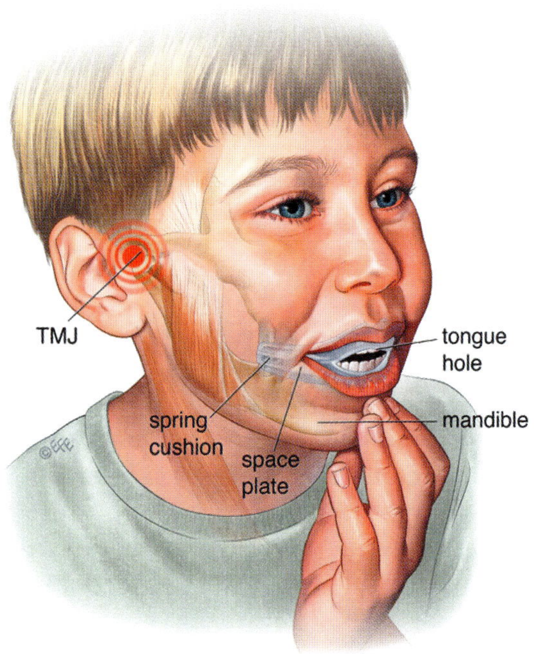

Figure 7.90 Image showing a children's MOJO in position and its various parts. The children's MOJO is identical to the adult MOJO but smaller in size to suit the oral cavities of children aged between 6-12 years.

It is quite normal for the MOJO appliance to feel bulky in the mouth to begin with; however, this soon subsides with ongoing usage.

Using the appliance at night is an added bonus but not essential. MOJO is an ideal strategy to employ when driving long distances, as it keeps neck and back muscles more relaxed and enhances alertness. For this reason alone many truck and taxi drivers use a MOJO.

Office workers may also benefit when working long hours at a computer, as neck and shoulder discomfort is vastly reduced as well.

As a general rule, if total daily usage equates to about one to two hours or even more, this is ideal and positive results will be noticed very soon (Fig. 7.89).

The time period that a patient should maintain is directly dependent on the state of their TMJ condition, and typically, the more chronic and degenerative, the longer the overall usage period. However, a month of regular daily usage for a less severe condition will produce very pleasing results, whereas several months, even

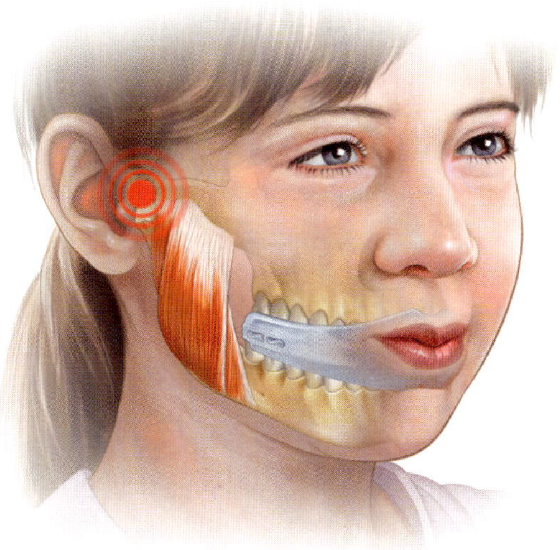

Figure 7.91 Image showing a child with MOJO in place and lips closed.

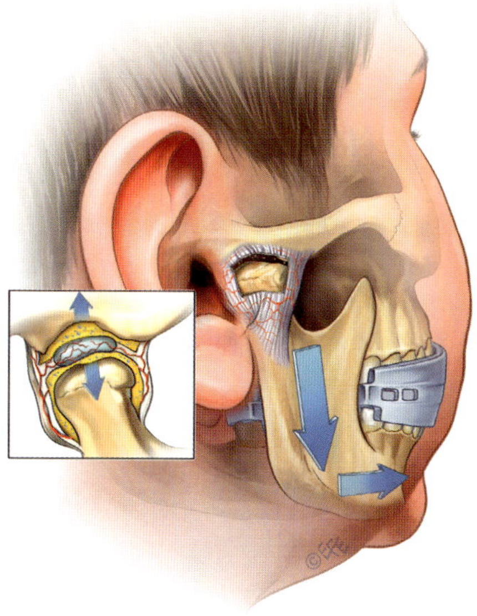

Figure 7.92 Image showing decompression and repositioning of the TMJ with a MOJO being used by a child.

up to 12 months, would be a typical usage period for a more chronic case.

The definitive point for stopping usage is simply when all symptoms have abated.

Of course, having maintenance NST sessions in conjunction with MOJO usage, is even more desirable and will continue to accelerate results even further. Maintenance NST sessions are typically given on a monthly basis, once all major symptoms (apart from the TMJ dysfunction) have settled.

MOJO's are made for both adults and children and sizes vary accordingly (Figs. 7.90-7.92). Children's appliance is used from 6-12 years of age, after which adult size is typically used. MOJO's are made according to a universal size design and generally adapt to all oral cavity sizes without fuss.

Indications: Used as an optional finishing strategy in any NST session, to integrate the Primary Respiratory Mechanism (PRM) with all other corrections attained in the SRM or SGS, respectively. May also be utilized as a stress defusion strategy for patients who are in a state of distress.

Prerequisites: When all other NST prone and supine sequences have been completed.

Note 1: Please refer to the section Primary Respiratory Mechanism discussed in Chapter 3.

Note 2: This technique has been adapted from DeJarnette's Cranial Respiratory Impulse Technique used for the same purpose. Although Bowen had no such direct technique for inducing the cranial and body rhythms, he claimed that his body work alone would "bring the cycle of the body" back into balance.

Although terminologies vary, the fundamental principle is that this craniosacral or sacro-occipital flows are being induced.

Pre-check: Using bidigital contact (conjoined index and middle fingers), the practitioner palpates the bilateral cranial origins of the upper trapezius muscles, immediately inferior to the superior nuchal line of the cranium, and makes a comparative assessment regarding their volume.

If one upper trapezius origin has more "volume" than the other, the volume needs to be equalized prior to starting the cranial correction.

On the side that has more volume, the practitioner applies firm bidigital traction and retains this position. While maintaining traction to this point, the patient is instructed to inhale and exhale slowly for three repetitions.

The practitioner now re-assesses both upper trapezius origins for volume, which should be the same. If a volume differential is still perceptible, the equalization correction is performed for a second time.

Step 1

Action: With patient's cranium "cupped" in practitioner's hands, using bidigital contact (as in pre-check), practitioner contacts both upper trapezius muscle origins and simple holds for 30 seconds with gentle pressure (Fig. 7.93).

Note: A vascular pulse of 60-70 beats per minute may be discernable and may vary in speed and intensity at each point. Some practitioners feel it and others not. Regardless the technique works in any case.

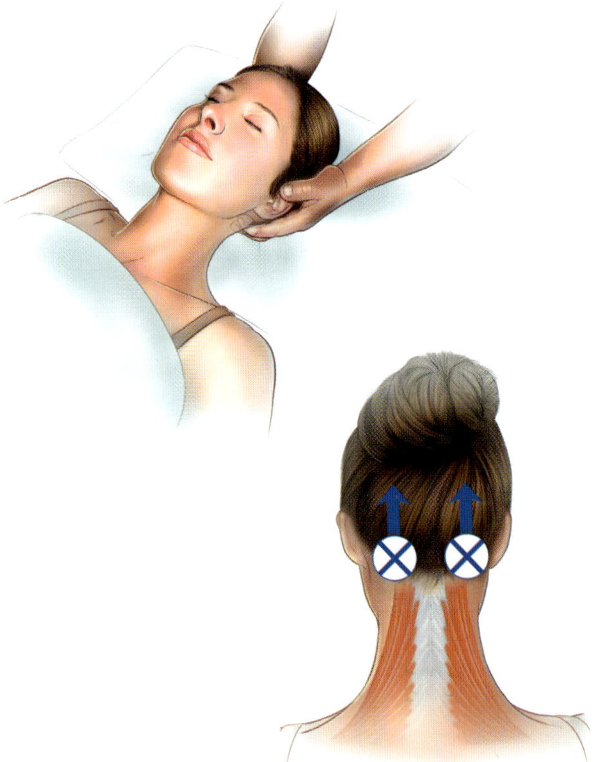

Figure 7.93 The top image shows the position that the practitioner's hands need to be in, while the botton image shows a clearer view of the actual points (upper trapezius muscle origins) that are contacted by the fingers. The points are immediately inferior to the superior nuchal line of the cranium. The arrows indicate the direction of gentle traction that the practitioner makes during contact.

Step 2

Action: Practitioner now releases contact for 5 seconds and waits (Fig. 7.94).

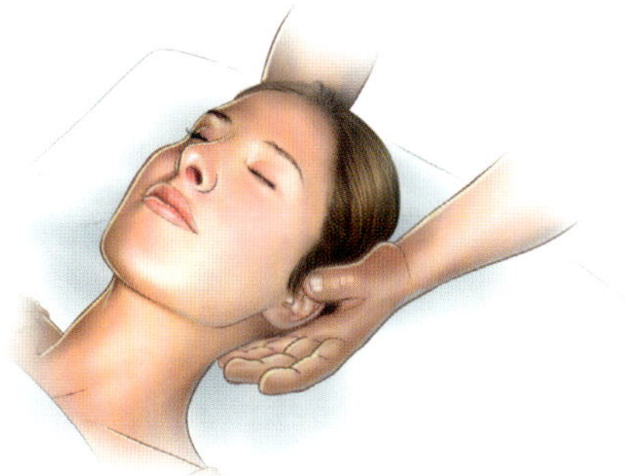

Figure 7.94 The image shows that although the practitioner's hands are in place, digital contact to the upper trapezius muscle origins has been released.

Step 3

Action: Practitioner now recontacts the upper trapezius points and this time holds for just 10-15 seconds (Fig. 7.95).

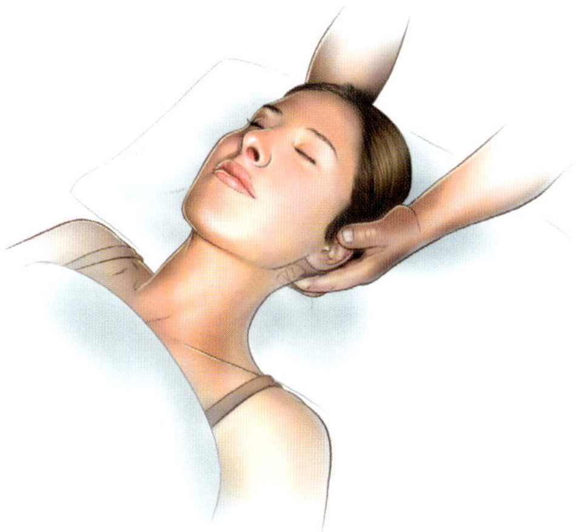

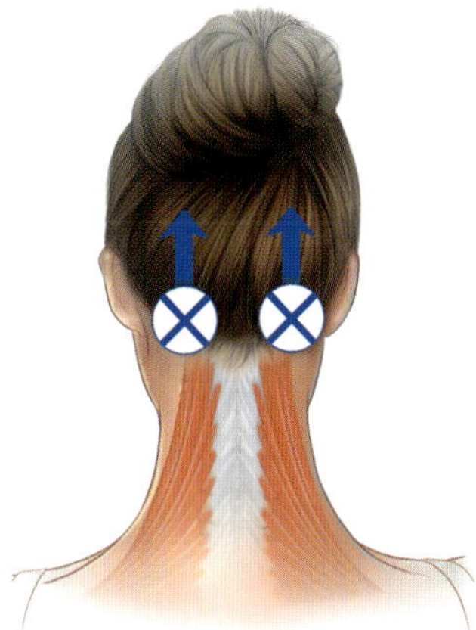

Figure 7.95 The image on the left shows the upper trapezius muscle origins being contacted once again by the practitioner's fingers. The image on the right shows a clearer view of the actual points. The arrows indicate the direction of gentle traction that the practitioner makes during contact.

Step 4

Action: Practitioner now releases contact for 5 seconds and waits (Fig. 7.96).

Note: This process of making successive contact for 10-15 seconds and releasing for 5 seconds now continues unbroken for another 5 or more minutes.

This simple "impulse strategy" at the upper trapezius origins is what will help to ultimately induce the PRM.

Throughout the first 2-3 minutes, the practitioner may feel that the vascular pulse slows to about the same rate as the rise and fall of

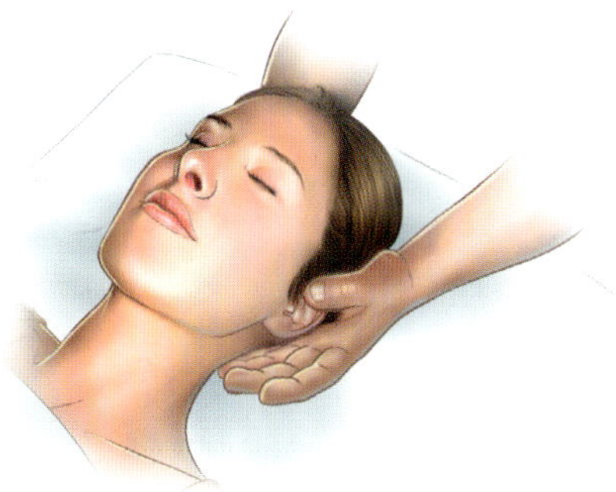

Figure 7.96 The image shows that once again, that although the practitioner's hands are in place, digital contact to the upper trapezius muscle origins has been released.

the patient's thoracic cavity of approximately 40 beats per minute.

This second pulse if referred to as a pulmonary respiratory pulse and will also continue become slower and slower throughout the next 2-3 minutes. Some practitioners feel it and other not. Regardless the technique works in any case.

Note: Successive repetitions of Steps 1-4 induce the PRM.

Step 5

Action: Once the practitioner notices that the pulse has become so slow that it stops or is otherwise very slow, the contact and release ceases, and the practitioner simply continues make soft contact to the upper trapezius muscle origins as in Step 1 (Fig. 7.97).

Note: At first, the practitioner may feel noting at all but then a single pulse may come without warning and then recede. A few seconds later, it will do the same. Providing the practitioner maintains contact, the pulse will continue to arrive and recede establishing a new rhythm "on average" of approximately 7-14 beats per minute. The rhythm can become as slow as two beats per minute up to 18 beats per minute.

This is the Primary Respiratory Rhythm and is the fundamental mechanism of the organism that helps to regulate cellular activity, and really sets the craniosacral rhythm of the body into optimal motion.

Once the practitioner feels this rhythm establishing itself, contact may be continued for another few minutes or longer if desired. The longer the contact the deeper the relaxation of the body.

Patients will frequently fall to sleep during this procedure, and it's a good idea that, once the practitioner has determined that it's time to stop, the patient is gently and softly informed that it will be time to open their eyes in a few minutes.

It's always wise to give the patient a few extra minutes to adjust to being "back in their body", as the procedure can cause a certain level of dissociation where the patient no longer feels their body lying on the table.

It's quite reasonable to expect that the whole Cranial procedure may take up to 10-15 minutes extra, and the practitioner really needs to plan for this additional investment of time.

However, the result will be a very satisfied patient who is even more likely to enjoy an even greater level of relaxation and sustainable results.

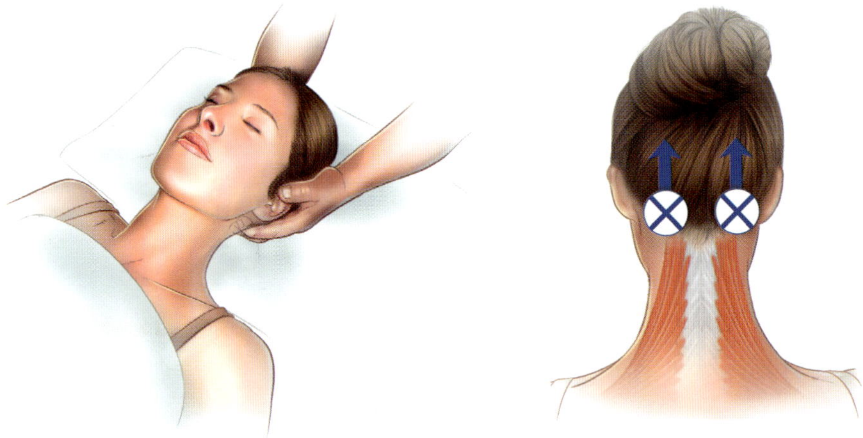

Figure 7.97 Once the ebb and flow of the PRM has been established, the practitioner simply continues to maintain contact for another few or more minutes. The image on the left once again shows the upper trapezius muscle origins being contacted, however this time contact is continuous. The image on the right once again shows a clearer view of the actual points to contact.

Once all prone and supine work has been completed, it's time for the patient to leave the table and become load-bearing through the dual activation of pressure receptors in the feet and sacroiliac receptors both being activated.

However, prior to the patient standing, they are invited unaided to come into a sitting position, with feet just touching the floor (assuming an electric treatment table is being used).

At this point checking to make certain that the cranium and body (Micro and Macro systems) will synthesize optimally, it's a good idea to spend a minute checking for range of motion differences and adjusting them if required.

This is entirely optional but always much appreciated by the patient.

Preceding this test however the levator scapulae muscles are quickly released again as follows.

Points 1a, 1b and 1c

Action: The practitioner prepares to apply a Pri-move to the left side levator scapulae muscle by stretching the skin over the muscle (this is exactly the same point as point 4 in DBB2). The patient is instructed to slowly turn their head to the left (Fig. 7.98).

Throughout the turning of the head, the practitioner crosses the levator scapulae muscle completing the Pri-move. The Pri-move is "retained" as the patient now turns their head back to the midline.

At this point the practitioner releases the retaining point (1a).

This same sequence is now repeated on the right side levator scapulae muscle (1b) (Fig. 7.99).

The practitioner now prepares to apply bilateral simultaneous Pri-moves to both levator scapulae muscles in an anterior direction. The patient is instructed to slowly flex their head

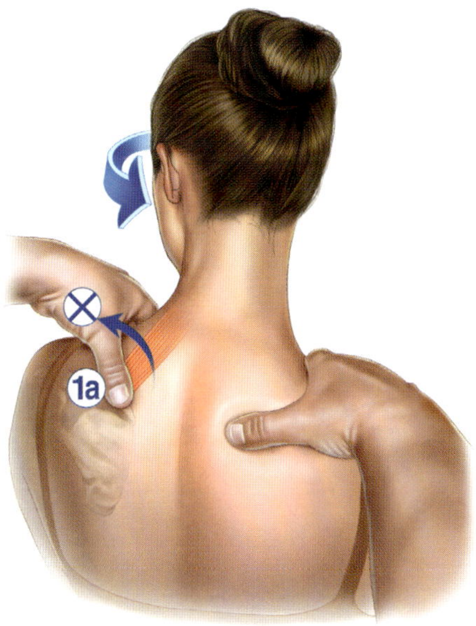

Figure 7.98 Image showing a Pri-move applied to the left side levator scapulae muscle, as the patient is turning the head to the left. The point is retained and the patient instructed to return their head to the midline.

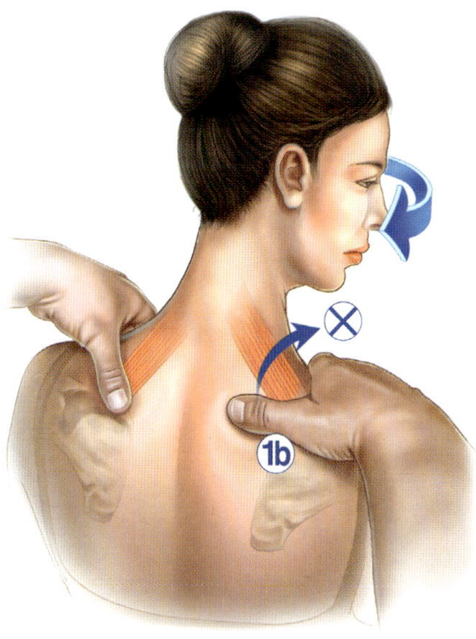

Figure 7.99 Image showing a Pri-move applied to the right side levator scapulae muscle, as the patient is turning the head to the right. The point is retained and the patient instructed to return their head to the midline.

anteriorly so that their chin contacts their sternum.

Throughout the process of moving anteriorly, the practitioner crosses both levator scapulae muscles completing the bilateral Pri-move. The Pri-move is "retained" as the patient extends their head posteriorly.

At this point the practitioner releases both retaining points (1c) (Fig. 7.100).

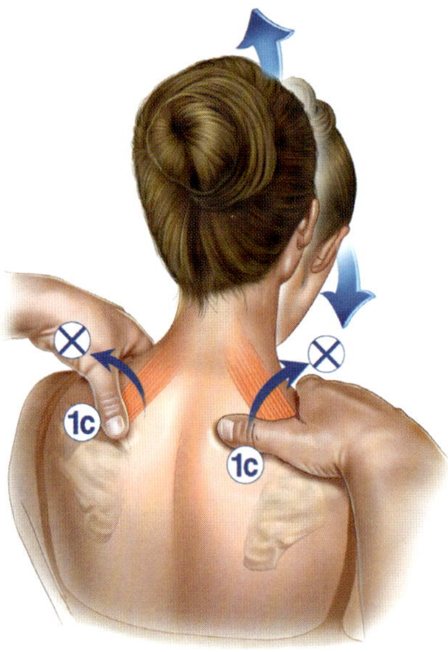

Figure 7.100 Image showing bilateral Pri-move applied to both levator scapulae muscles simultaneously, as the patient flexes the neck anteriorly towards the floor. The points are retained and the patient instructed to return their head to its normal resting position.

The patient is now invited to rotate their head towards the left shoulder and then the right, checking for any differential in range of motion or indeed any residual pain on one side or the other.

If restriction of motion or pain is felt on either side, Pri-moves 1, 2 and 7 from DBB3 may be reinserted to correct this situation (Fig. 7.101).

These points are performed exclusively on the restricted or painful side.

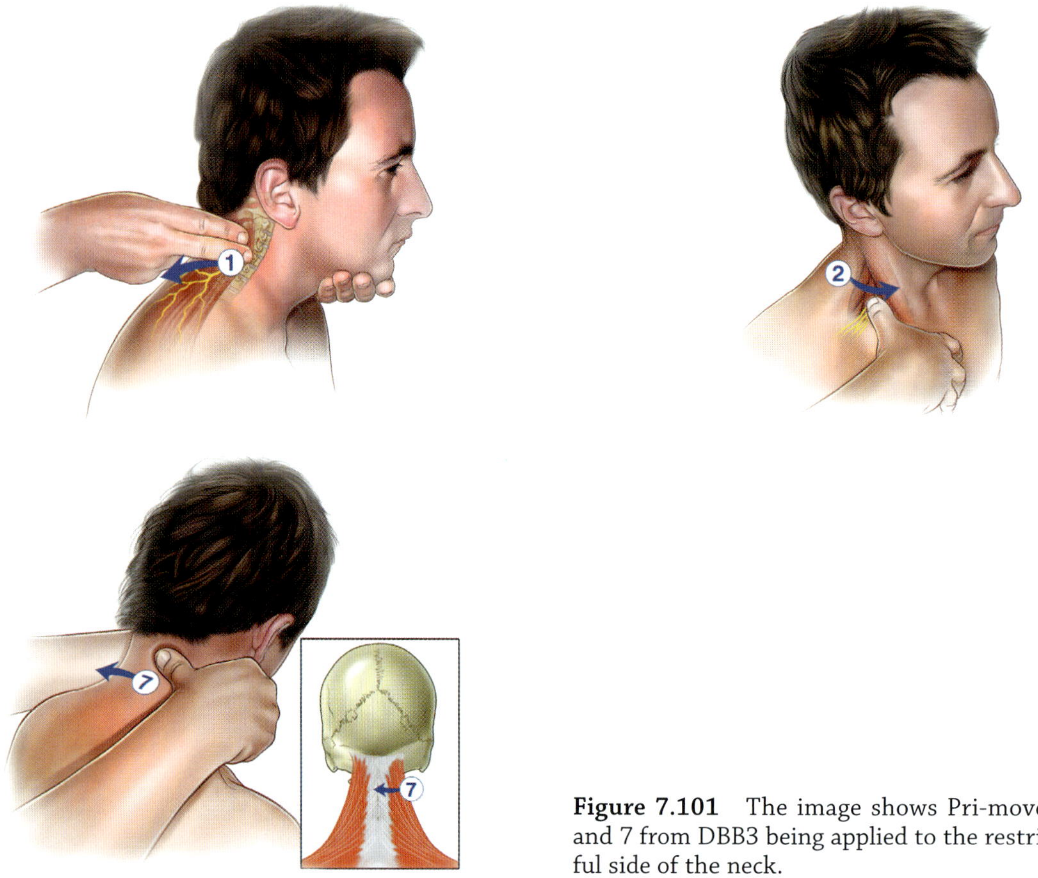

Figure 7.101 The image shows Pri-move points 1, 2 and 7 from DBB3 being applied to the restricted or painful side of the neck.

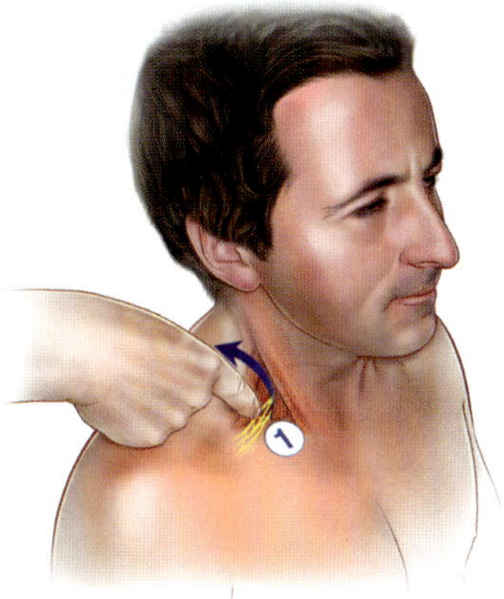

Figure 7.102 The image shows Pri-move point 2 from DBB3 being applied "in reverse" directly onto the brachial plexus, to the restricted or painful side of the neck.

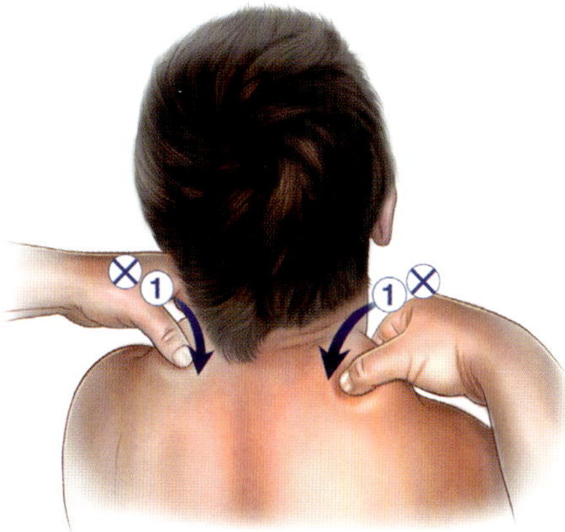

Figure 7.103 The image shows relatively rapid, bilateral Pri-moves being applied simultaneously, to the upper trapezius muscle borders in a posterior direction.

Should the pain or restriction still persist, a deep reverse Pri-move may be performed in the supraclavicular fossa, uniquely on the affected side. Essentially this is Pri-move 2 from DBB3 in reverse (Fig. 7.102).

Finally, if neither of the above strategies has resolved the condition, bilateral Pri-moves may be applied to the upper trapezius muscle as indicated (Fig. 7.103).

Note: Completing these final checks and releases should take no longer than 1-2 minutes.

CONCLUSION

Having now completed our final three Super core procedures for the pelvis, TMJ and cranium, plus of course the final cranium to body checks and adjustments, this brings us to the point where we are perfectly equipped to build a very thorough core – extremities – core session for a patient, should symptoms and indications demand.

Being able to work in such a highly integrated fashion, ensures that our NST work really has no limitations in terms of the various maladies and conditions that it may be applied to.

Importantly, the core – extremities – core approach enables us to achieve very rapid and thorough unlocking and integration, of the musculoskeletal system, thereby creating spinal integration even in the most chronic of cases.

As always, when building an integrated session that attends to all elements of the patient's presenting symptom pattern, we simply need to keep in mind that the procedures that we choose must firstly match the presenting symptoms of the patient, secondly match the indications we discover at the table, determined by positive tests (i.e., for coccyx, pelvis and TMJ) and/or thirdly be necessary prerequisites for a larger procedure (i.e., sacrum for coccyx, knee for pelvis, sacrum and shoulder for TMJ).

We have already seen how to combine DBB1, 2 and 3 to build one type of integrated session. And we have also learned how further detail a session by adding the sacrum, lung and some upper and lower extremities work to DBB1, 2 and 3.

So let's look at another hypothetical example of how to build an integrated session with the core – extremities – core approach, using the latest procedures that we have learned.

The session below is just a example of the flow of the session and includes all of the procedures covered indicating which procedures come first and where to give the pauses.

Note: the prerequisites provide the keys to determining the steps.

Although this is a hypothetical example, it is quite possible that it could nevertheless suit a patient's presenting condition.

PRONE SECTION

DBB1 ← *Pause for 5 minutes after point 5*
DBB2
Sacrum + iliolumbar ligament release
Hip procedure
Coccyx procedure
Hamstring procedure – prone part
End of prone procedures ← *Pause for 2 minutes*

SUPINE SECTION

Lung procedure
DBB 3 → Points 1-4
Knee procedure
Hamstring procedure – supine part
Ankle procedure
Foot procedure
DBB3 → Point 7
Shoulder procedure
Elbow & wrist procedure
Hand procedure
Reinsert points 6 and 7 from DBB3
End of extremities procedures ← *Pause for 2 minutes*
Pelvic procedure
TMJ procedure (assess → correct → reassess with psoas test → use MOJO if necessary)
End of super core procedures ← *Pause for 2 minutes*
Cranial procedure
Final "cranium to body" checks and adjustments – sitting position

Obviously, the example above is not going to be performed on every patient, and many will require much less work. However, if it needed to be performed, the time taken to complete such a session would be about 30-40 minutes including the pauses.

Some practitioners prefer to commence with DBB1, 2 and 3 only at the first session, and then see how the body responds. This is a valid way to work of course, but the risk is that there may be more reactions experienced than fewer as the body attempts to "grind" its way back to balance.

My person preference is to simply do what is required, but I always take a very commonsense and time saving approach by systematically installing all of the "prerequisite procedures" at every session. This saves a lot of time in having to go back and install them if any of the Super core procedures test positive.

This simply means that my session will include at the very least the following:

- DBB1 > DBB2 > Sacrum in the Prone position
- Lung > DBB3 > Knee > Shoulder in the Supine position

Further potential additions for the Prone position would be:

Hips, Coccyx or Hamstrings procedures.

Further potential additions for the Supine position would be:

Ankle, Foot, Elbow & Wrist, Hand procedures in the extremities and Pelvic, TMJ and Cranial procedures of the Super core.

In total, we have covered 17 parts or procedures and if you follow the above recommendation, 7 of those parts or procedures become the foundation for every session, while the remaining 10 procedures need to be added based on presenting symptoms, prerequisites or positive tests at the treatment table.

Note: Sitting position checks and releases can always included in every session.

Working in this way provides a very sound and reliable base strategy for all patients, and also simplifies the planning and further choices that need to be made.

In the NST system there are several other clever mini-protocols, alternative and time saving strategies that may be added or blended with the main work covered in this book, and this additional work will become the subject of future writings.

Ultimately attending live NST seminars and using the NST video trainings are excellent additional strategies for clarifying, deepening and expanding knowhow and honing NST clinical practice.

Clinical Management 8

STRUCTURING A TREATMENT PLAN

With every new NST patient, it is sound clinical practice from the outset, to book the consecutive sessions approximately a week apart, as this is the most typical number of sessions and optimal timing between the sessions, that over 85% of patients require to achieve total resolution of their presenting symptoms.

And while some patients will require just two sessions to reach total resolution others may need four or more sessions.

Obviously, every case is different and factors such as presenting symptoms, age, exercise behaviors, levels of hydration, diet, psychological status and levels of toxicity, all influence how quickly the patient responds and how effectively they hold their corrections.

Notwithstanding this, three sessions will ensure a successful outcome for most patients, who present with the typical symptoms that a general clinical practitioner would be familiar in dealing with (various spinal and pain conditions, to headaches, menstrual, visceral and respiratory conditions, injuries and more).

If three sessions are booked and the patient returns to for their third sessions and all symptoms have already abated, then there is no need to perform a third session. Of course, an option would always to do just DBB1, 2, and 3 in such a case.

However, neurological conditions do tend to require ongoing attention of approximately one session every one to three weeks, for the patient to remain symptom free or as symptom free as their particular condition permits.

In summary, the most straightforward way to plan is simply plan for three sessions, and then apply further sessions approximately one week apart until total resolution is reached, or until patient and practitioner agree that "this is as good as it's going to get", in the broader context of the patient's personal limitations, whatever they may be.

Once this point is reached, it will largely be the patient's lifestyle behaviors and experiences and their health limitations, that will determine when they might need a further session or two.

And every practitioner sees the subject of maintenance somewhat differently. I have many highly talented chiropractic and osteopathic colleagues around the world, who see it as their role to manage their patient's spine, and consequently have them return for regular sessions indefinitely.

This may obviously work for some, but it's not the way I recommend maintenance is performed with NST, as this level of frequency is just not necessary.

My suggestion to my patients is to simply return when they need to, but a session once every 2-3 months is a good maintenance plan. On average, my patients return for one or maybe two maintenance sessions every 2-6 months.

And many I do not see again for 12 or 18 months.

In terms of planning exactly what to do in the session, we have already covered this throughout Chapter 7 with various examples, but to reiterate to some extent, there are two fundamental approaches in planning what to do, in a "session to session" sense.

There's the "less to more" approach and the "more to less" approach and both work well.

i) "Less to more" simply means doing the bare minimum at the first session, such as

DBB1, 2 and 3, and then seeing what else needs to be added in subsequent sessions to address residual symptoms, which will typically mean adding more procedures.

The outcome of using this approach is that resolution is less likely after the first session, but becomes more and more likely with every subsequent session. Typically, however, more sessions will be required.

ii) "More to less" simply means doing everything required at the first session, to match the patient's symptom pattern, including coccyx, pelvis and TMJ if required. This approach will generally mean that the second sessions require a less complex approach, that becomes even less by the third session.

The outcome of using this approach is that resolution is much more likely after the first session, and sustainability of the patient's condition becomes more apparent sooner. Typically, fewer sessions will be required.

By comparison, i) is softly, slowly and steadily whereas ii) is quick, direct and definite.

My preference is to work in the second fashion as patient satisfaction is much better.

Once the patient leaves the clinic at the end of their first session, and indeed every subsequent session, it's important to provide them with some guidelines as to what to expect and how to manage themselves and their responses.

To achieve this, every patient is given an After Care sheet at the end of the session.

AFTER CARE

As good as our clinical work might have been, an uninformed patient can unintentionally "undo" things to some extent or even cause themselves a new injury if they do not follow the After Care recommendations set out below.

These simple recommendations have withstood the test of time and it is wise to give the patient a copy of them before leaving the clinic. This ensures that they have every chance of optimizing corrections and also avoid sabotaging the results.

The After Care recommendations are based around commonsense and intensive clinical experience with tens of thousands of patients, and are definitely important to follow.

NST AFTER CARE SHEET

Please strictly observe all recommendations for five days after any NST treatment.

1. Do not sit for any longer than 30 minutes at a time on the day of your visit. Lying down is fine.
2. Do as much walking as possible each day – at least 10-15 minutes twice daily.
3. Drink as much pure water as is comfortable – no less than 5 × 250 ml glasses per day. Avoid excessive usage of stimulating substances (coffee). Usage of painkillers and anti-inflammatory drugs are not contraindicated.
4. Move carefully – squat instead of bending when picking something up, do not forcefully cross the legs, be careful getting in and out of the car and bed – take your weight evenly on both feet when moving from sitting to standing.
5. Avoid all other forms of manipulation, e.g., massage, chiropractic, osteopathy, physiotherapy, acupuncture, kinesiology, etc.
6. Do not use excessive heat or cold on areas that have been treated. No ice baths or packs. No hot baths or packs. No saunas. Avoid using electric warming blankets in bed. Avoid using any form of magnetic mat.
7. Avoid strenuous exercise including gardening.
8. TMJ patients must avoid biting on hard foods-apples, carrots, nuts, confectionery, etc.
9. Avoid using orthotic appliances in shoes unless instructed otherwise.
10. Reactions ranging from hot and cold flushes, emotional releases, headaches and body aches may be experienced. These reactions

are a positive sign that the process of recuperation is working.

AFTER CARE EXPLAINED

The reasons behind these After Care recommendations are as logical and straightforward as the recommendations themselves. They are as follows:

1. Sitting and especially excessive sitting after the NST session, tends to prevent the sacrum from assuming its proper mobility and also prevents the mechanoreceptors in the sacroiliac joints from receiving the appropriate "load" that they need to fire, thereby keeping back, pelvic and leg muscles integrated.

The simple function of standing every 30 minutes loads the sacroiliac joints and helps to prevent a return to imbalance from occurring.

Office workers, taxi drivers, truck drivers or any patient whose occupation requires them to sit for long periods of time, are advised to purchase a specialized air-filled buttock cushion that ensures sacroiliac joint movement when sitting.

2. Walking has so many obvious benefits from muscular, nervous, lymphatic to circulatory, but the main reason for walking twice daily after NST, is to ensure that the "gait walking mechanism" is activated regularly, as this noticeably helps to settle the new neuromuscular pattern in.

Bike riding, jogging, and using trampolines do not count towards the patient's daily walking requirements.

3. Appropriate amounts of water significantly enhances lymphatic drainage, thereby reducing the toxic reactions to NST that can occur as muscles come back to balance. It is a natural function of muscles, organs and tissues to excrete bioaccumulation back into circulation, once they have been altered.

Proper hydration also facilitates better functioning of the nervous system.

A simple formula to calculate how much water a patient needs, is to double their body weight and divide by 100. So a person who weighs 75 kg is calculated as follows:

$75 \times 2 = 150 \rightarrow$ divide by $100 = 1.5$ liters per day.

This reflects a conservative but sensible amount, and can always be increased, but should not be reduced.

Water, herbal teas and fresh lemon drinks are regarded as appropriate liquids to drink. Soda drinks, fruit juices, coffee, milk and alcoholic, beverages, do not count towards the patient's daily water intake.

4. The function of maintaining equal load through the feet and sacroiliac joints, really assists in settling the musculoskeletal system into a balanced pattern. NST corrections typically take a few days to "set", which perhaps have more to do with the transient liquid to solid state of the changing fascia itself.

Quickly jumping out of the car and landing on one foot first, particularly after sitting for some time is not ideal after an NST session, as it can quite easily disturb sacroiliac function. There is much evidence to support taking the body weight evenly on both feet, and not just after an NST session but at all times. Information on the Alexander Technique provides ample insight on this subject.

5. Receiving other forms of manual therapy or spinal adjustments after and NST session, typically do one of two things. It may dilute the effectiveness of NST by interrupting the process of "autoregulation" or it may cause severe reactions.

Once the body is adjusted with NST it goes through a very particular "unraveling" process that is simply best left to work alone for at least three days.

6. Excessive, heat, cold or strong magnetic fields close to the body for prolonged periods,

tend to quickly stop the valuable "autoregulation" and may cause unwanted reactions as well.

7. Frequently after an NST session the patient feels like their body has "turned back the clock" and they feel as good or better than they did years before.

Deciding to go for a long run or do hard work in the garden, for example, particularly when the patient has not been able to do so for some time previously, is strongly discouraged as it will typically generate new issues to deal with and will likely block the body's attempt to complete its "unraveling" cycle.

8. When the patient presents with a TMJ condition, and particularly a chronic one, time has to be allowed for the TMJ tissues of the capsule and surrounding areas to resume some sense of normality again. This can mean allowing chronic inflammations to settle which will not happen overnight, but more so after a few days at least.

Applying strong force to the TMJ whilst the settling period is occurring, is not helpful and may quite easily render one or both TMJ into a state of imbalance again.

Conversely, MOJO usage is an excellent way to help optimize results after TMJ treatment.

9. Asking a patient to throw away their orthotic appliances that they have bonded with over months or years, can be challenging since another expert along the way has recommended that they use them.

Assuming that they were likely prescribed for functional correction, this would have been at a time when the patient had significant "tensegrity" imbalances, and perhaps pelvic rotation etc., that have now been corrected or are in the process of being corrected with NST.

Leaving the orthotic appliances in the shoes will only serve to reintroduce a state of imbalance.

Of course, if the patient has a structural leg length difference, then some form of mechanical device will be necessary whether that be adjustments to footwear or orthotic appliances.

10. Many patients will experience strong reactions particularly after their first NST session, when the largest amounts of bioaccumulation are being released and needing processing.

Arguably, the timing for this happening is not ideal given that a compensated musculoskeletal and visceral system is going to be less prepared for heavy detoxification.

However, it is both unavoidable and positive at the same time, since it is a clear confirmation that the body is "autoregulating" and coming back to balance.

If the reactions become intolerable, the patient may simply have a very hot soaking bath, which will stop the reactions but also any further benefits that would have been delivered with the ongoing "autoregulation".

Drinking copious amounts of water or herbal tea really helps to reduce the intensity of the reactions, and pain-killers are not contraindicated.

Providing patients follow the After Care Sheet judiciously, things settle nicely into place for the very vast majority and they will likely return for their second session a week later with reports that they had reactions for a few days, after which things settled nicely.

Their original presenting symptoms will typically be improved but not completely resolved.

This is a very desirable outcome, and will typically be followed by further improvement and stability of corrections after their second session.

However, whilst this is the case for the vast majority of patients, a small percentage may return to inform you that they have had no improvement.

This is unusual, and there are some practical steps to take and logical points to consider should it occur.

PROBLEM SOLVING

The main reasons why a patient may not respond to an NST session or not hold their corrections are as follows:

1. The patient is going back into a problematic situation and repeating the same behaviors that created or contributed to their condition in the first place.

There are endless examples of a patient doing this from:

- physical → too little movement or too much sitting
- hydration → drinking insufficient water
- nutritional → eating impoverished nutritionally deficient food
- chemical → engaging in chemical abuse like too much alcohol and/or drugs
- emotional → going back into a very stressful personal or employment situation.

2. The patient is not following the After Care recommendations in one of its many facets and sabotaging results.

3. The patient is in a state of advanced degeneration and the organism is close to exhaustion and simply cannot respond – cancer is a good example.

4. Some patients forget how badly they were in the beginning, and tend to think that they have not improved when there is ample evidence to suggest to opposite, albeit not yet fully resolved.

5. Perhaps the practitioner has missed adding some very important procedure, and the system as a whole is not "autoregulating". The main procedures that can create such an outcome are the four main system procedures:

- Coccyx
- Lung
- Pelvic
- TMJ

Each one of these four procedures has the capacity to block the SRM or SGS or both, if it has been overlooked when it needed to be done. Quite simply, the consequences can be that "autoregulation" cannot start and the symptoms do not change.

Although the importance of each of these procedures has been emphasized throughout Chapter 7 in the prone, supine and super core procedure sections, respectively, we will revisit them in Chapter 9 (System Procedures) and add further important details to re-emphasize their individual and collective importance.

System Procedures 9

INTRODUCTION

The System Procedures refer to four main NST procedures that are not only an integral part of the NST system, but also integral parts of the SRM, SGS and, consequently, the PRM.

In order of where they would be considered for inclusion, in the "flow" of any session, they are the Coccyx, Lung, Pelvic and TMJ procedures, and each one of them is significant in its own right and each one can directly affect the status of either the SRM or SGS or both.

In this way there is also a great degree of two-way interactivity between them, whereby imbalance in one can affect the other and viceversa.

The object of this chapter is to add further information to what has already been provided throughout Chapter 7, in relation to these System procedures, and to present it in a way that is relevant to clinical practice.

Indications, prerequisites and instructions have already been covered in Chapter 7 and will not be repeated here unless relevant to the content of the discussion.

Furthermore, in Chapter 3 (NST Operating Systems), much useful and relevant information has also been provided via the overviews regarding Spinal development, the SRM, SGS and PRM, and this should also be considered as part of the narrative and additional information provided in this chapter.

Coccyx Procedure – Additional Information

Often overlooked in many spinal and structural endeavors, the coccyx is tremendously important in NST as its influence, if unbalanced, can be multifactorial and manifest almost at any level of the body in mechanical, neurological and hormonal symptoms.

However, coccyx conditions are also sometimes confused with sacral conditions, and making the distinction between the two can be as simple as identifying pain, specifically to the side of the coccyx, as discussed in the Coccyx procedure test in Chapter 7, or indeed at the level of the sacrococcygeal junction.

Pain in the general area of the sacrum, piriformis and buttock muscles belongs to the sacrum and hips.

As part of one of the body's integral operating gears, the coccyx if inflammed, bent, angulated (or even worse, broken), is capable of causing not only local pain and urogenital symptoms, but also remote cranial symptoms.

Its pathways of connection to the rest of the body are many and any or all of them may be valid to consider when attempting to bring the coccyx back to balance (Fig. 9.1).

In energetic terms, the coccyx sits at the very bottom of the body's main energy cycle a feature that gives it the capacity to be able to effect the whole cycle (Fig. 9.2). And if the main energy cycle is compromised, in energetic concepts, the symptoms that can arise therefrom are limitless.

To draw a simple Einsteinian parallel, the "field" is the sole governing agency of the "particle" or Energy Governs Matter → $E = mc^2$ (Fig. 9.3).

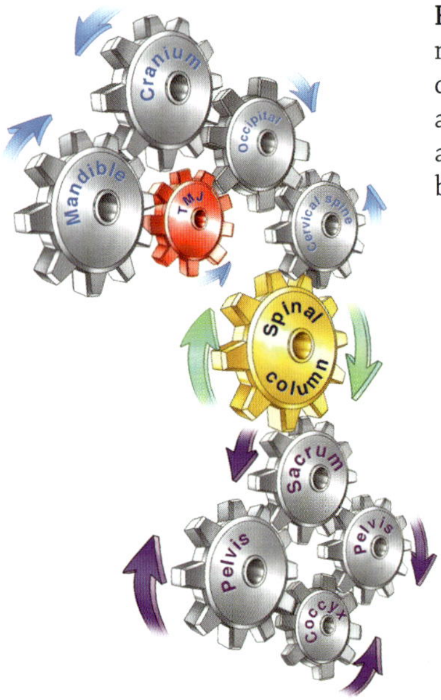

Figure 9.1 The image shows in simple mechanical terms that the reach of the coccyx is potentially local, remote and systematic. Ensuring that the TMJ and cranium are balanced, can greatly facilitate better balance of the coccyx.

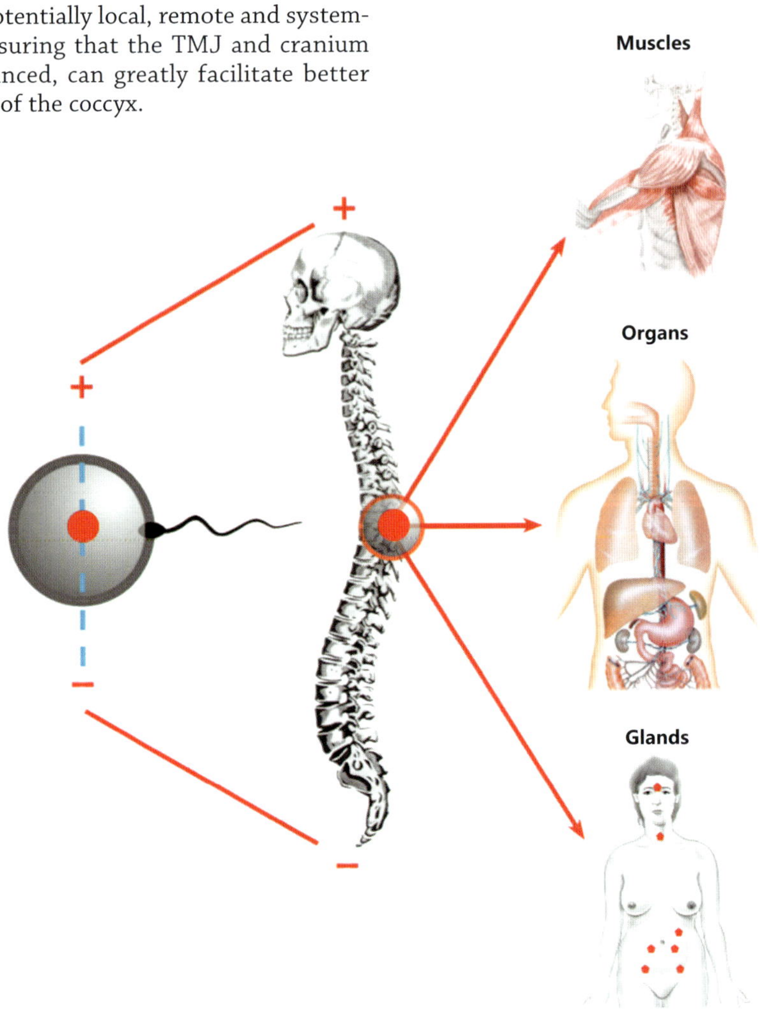

Figure 9.2 Image designed to communicate the important message that the coccyx not only sits at the bottom of the vertebral spinal column, but also the bottom of the body's energy cycle. As such its capacity to influence structures in its immediate proximity plus structures remote to itself, via various mechanisms, is highly probable. Consequently, correcting an unbalanced coccyx can result in favorable outcomes in the structural, neurological and hormonal systems of the body.

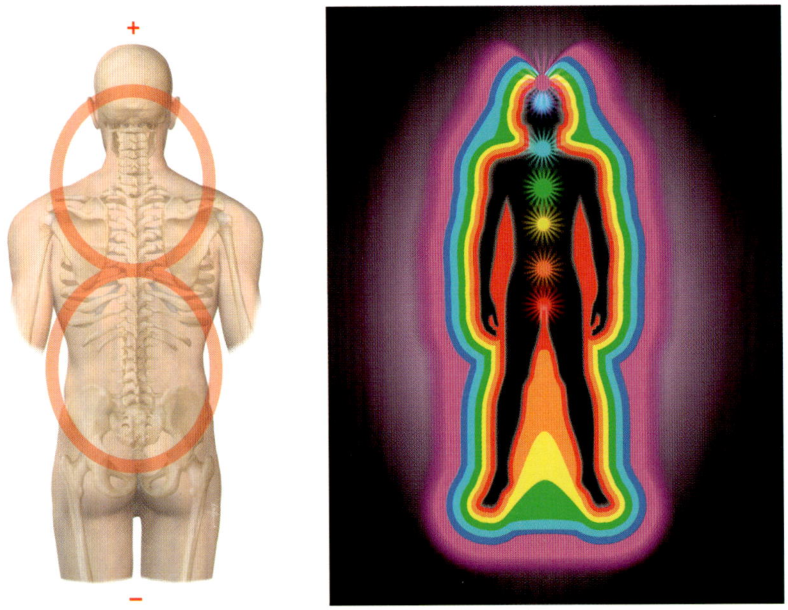

Figure 9.3 The left part of the image shows the rhythmic flows of the PRM or craniosacral system. The right part of the image supports the Quantum Physics findings, that the human organism receives energy, light and information from dimensions other than the third dimension - Energy Governs Matter → $E = mc^2$. Collectively, the images make the simple point, that with any health condition and subsequent adjustments for them to the body's various systems, that energy must and will be involved as well (Right image credit: Miro Kovacevic/Shutterstock).

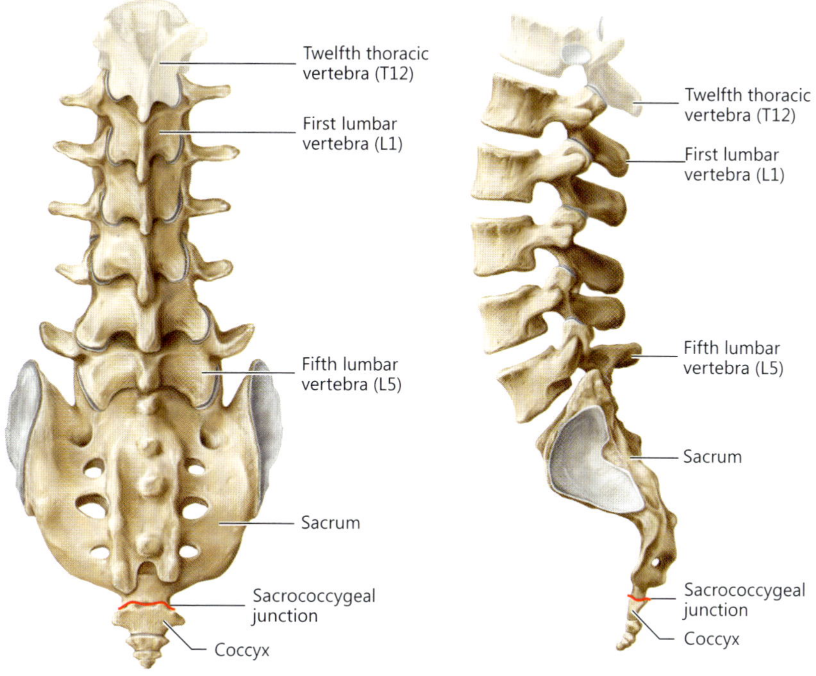

Figure 9.4 The image highlights the body of the coccyx and its connectivity to the sacral body at the "amphiarthrodial" sacrococcygeal junction.

However, before getting too far removed, let's look at some basics about the coccyx. First and foremost, the coccyx is a triangular fused bone with five small segments (Co1-Co5) and sits at the very bottom of the vertebral spinal column, where it articulates with the sacrum at the sacrococcygeal junction.

The sacrococcygeal junction is an amphiarthrodial joint, that connects the distal apex of the sacrum with the base of the coccyx, by strong cartilage and is capable of small flexing movements in most directions (Fig. 9.4).

Significantly, the coccyx is also connected to the sacrum via the filum terminale of the dura mater.

The filum terminale runs inside the dural tube from the conus medularis from whence it arises at the level of L2. It then descends, penetrating the dural mater at its main point of attachment at S2 of the sacrum, and finally inserts onto Co1 of the coccyx (Fig. 9.5).

One theory about the coocyx is that it acts as a take up mechanism, to keep appropriate dural tensions on the dural tube itself.

It is important to remember in this context that the dura mater is a 95% non-elastic covering of the spinal cord that has strong connections at S2 of the sacrum, C2 and C3 cervical vertebrae, the foramen magnum and then runs continuously inside the cranial vault.

The dura mater's length is a set length, whereas the vertebral column that it runs inside, can change its length. If there was not an adjusting mechanism between these two structures, there could be significant torsions on the dural tube with sweeping consequences for the nervous system and almost everything else therefore.

Over the last 100 years, in the fields of osteopathy, craniosacral and craniopathy, several researchers, including John Upledger, D.O., have elaborated on the effects and consequences that prolonged changes in dural tension have on the human nervous system and the systemic health of the individual as a whole.

When the dura is stretched, compressed, torsioned or distorted by the moving of bones attached to it, the spinal cord and brain alter their shape as well, which overtly expresses itself by changes in intensity, frequency and the amount of nerve flow to and from the brain. And it's not

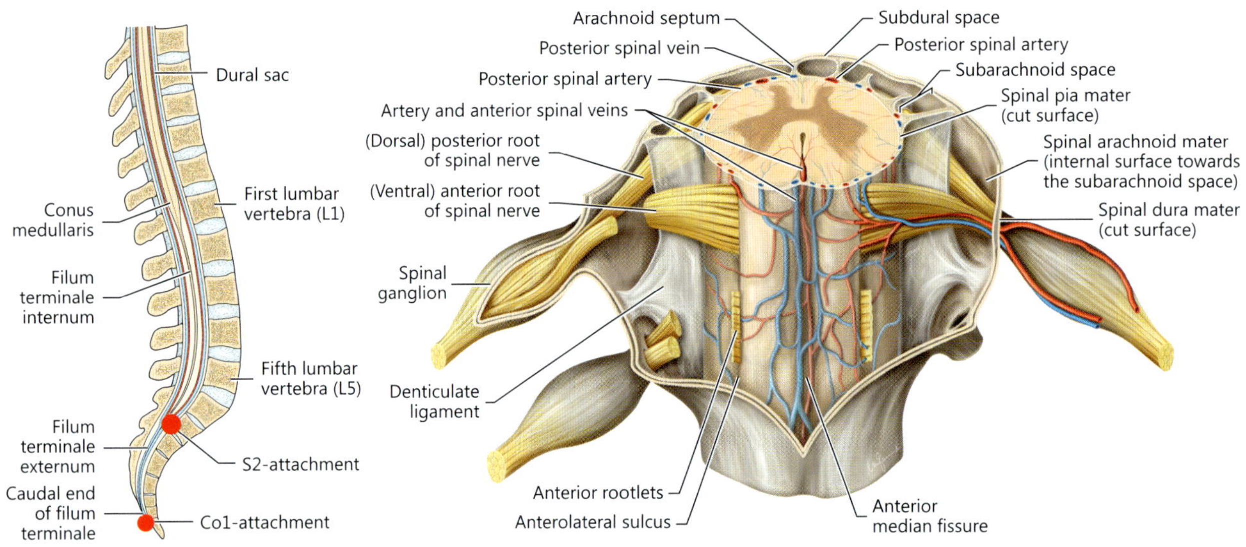

Figure 9.5 The image on the left highlights the continuous connectivity of the dura mater onto the coccyx via the filum terminale. However the filum terminale can also be seen to originate at L2 where it forms initially with the pia mater at the conus medullaris. It therefore starts its journey towards the coccyx from inside the dural sheath, anchoring and then leaving the sheath at S2 and inserting onto Co1 of the coccyx itself. The internal portion of the filum terminale stabilizes the entire spinal cord whereas the external portion forms the mechanical link to the coccyx. It's reasonable to conclude that a hooked or angulated coccyx may apply dural drag via the filum terminale, and even affect the conus medullaris. In both cases structural and neurological conditions may arise. The image on the right showcases the tough non-elastic nature of the dura mater itself, supporting the understanding that the dura mater is a valid mechanical link between the coccyx, sacrum at one end and the upper cervical vertebrae and cranial vault at the other end.

just the torsions alone, but the fact that the dural membrane system is a "pressurised" system containing cerebrospinal fluid that continually circulates through its cavities and cervices delivering vital oxygen and nutrition, while also removing waste products to and from the central nervous system and its supporting tissues.

We are closer to the truth of the matter when we view the dural membrane system as a "reciprocal-pressurised-tensional-membrane-system" in which a distortion in any one part will manifest elsewhere. And a distorted coccyx constantly distorts the system and most typically at the levels of the sacrum, cervical spine and cranium.

But apart from it articulating with the sacrum bone, the coccyx shares a mechanical partnership with the sphenoid bone of the cranium via the collective functions of the gait walking mechanism, SRM and SGS (Chapter 3) that not only affects the cranium as a whole (Fig. 9.6), but significantly, two of the eye muscles (superior oblique and levator palpebrae superioris) that originate from the sphenoid bone.

Hence, potential visual and balance disturbances and frontal headaches may arise.

Furthermore, in considering the sphenoid bone itself, we must not forget the all-important connection that both the lateral and medial pterygoid muscles share with it. Both pterygoid muscles are intimately involved in the process of mastication (chewing and biting), and thus belong to the SGS's important Micro system of muscles.

Significantly, the upper head of the lateral pterygoid muscle originates on the greater wing of the sphenoid bone and then inserts onto the articular disc and fibrous capsule of the TMJ itself.

This connection alone is incredibly significant for the whole body, as distortions at the level of the coccyx, can cause disturbance of the sphenoid bone's position and its movement, resulting in proprioceptive disturbance of the lateral pterygoid muscle affecting its inherent "tensegrity" (Fig. 9.7).

This disturbance can ultimately result in a predisposition for TMJ disc misplacement, occlusal faults and a myriad of other Micro system consequences that can arise from this. **Note**: Further discussed in the TMJ procedure section that follows later in this chapter.

It starts to become obvious then, that there is a potent two-way relationship at play between lower and upper parts of the body, whereby imbalances can be generated at the level of the coccyx that affect the TMJ or at the level of the TMJ that affect the coccyx.

Finally, as we turn our attention to the structures local to the coccyx, there are also considerations that are extremely valid and also have remote consequences via yet other pathways.

If for example chronic inflammation develops around the sacrococcygeal junction, as a result of an angulated or distorted coccyx through injury or too much sitting, or if a tumor develops on the anterior surface of the coccyx, there can be further dire consequences for the important ganglion impar.

The ganglion impar is an unpaired sympathetic structure located at the level of the sacrococcygeal junction and is the last and lowest ganglion of the paravertebral sympathetic chain. It innervates many of the structures located in this area of the body, including the lower third of the rectum, vagina, urethra, vulva, anus, coccyx and perineum (Fig. 9.8).

It also conveys pain signals back to the brain from these structures.

Furthermore, it can also strongly influence the visceral system's function via the ANS and enteric nervous system.

Disturbance of the ganglion impar can create therefore, a wide variety of symptoms in the structures it innervates and of the urogenital system generally (anything from sexual dysfunction in men and women, bladder conditions, incontinence, prostate conditions, constipation and more).

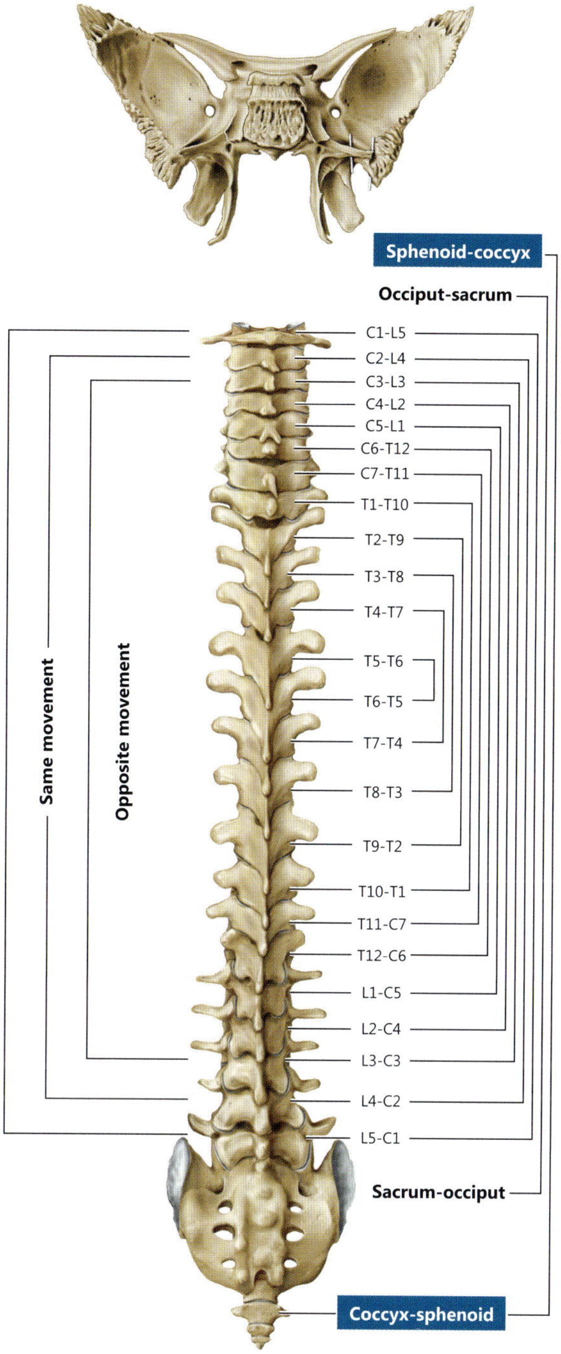

Figure 9.6 The Lovett reactor relationship is a set of natural compensatory movements that take place throughout the spinal column, pelvic girdle and cranium in response to the gait walking mechanism's operation. A subluxation or fault in one vertebral body will frequently affect its partner. Correcting the primary subluxation will typically correct both. However, correcting the secondary subluxation alone will generally not help. NST overcomes this issue by correcting the system as a whole.

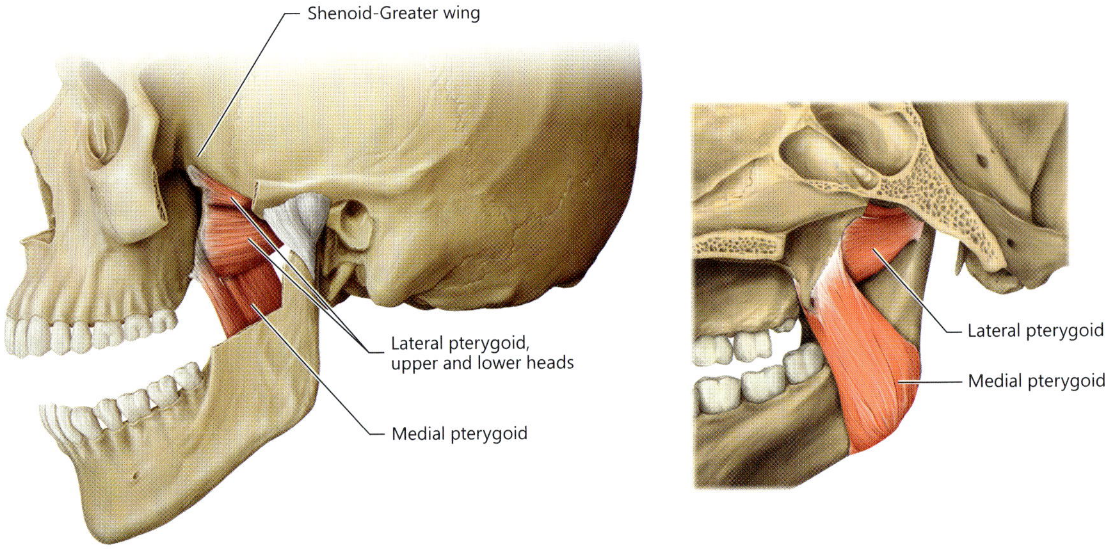

Figurc 9.7 Image highlighting the connection between the sphenoid bone and the TMJ. Through the Lovett reactor relationship a fault at the level of the coccyx will have consequences for its partner the sphenoid bone. In turn faults with the sphenoid bone, including suture faults, may affect the lateral pterygoid muscle, which in turn affects the TMJ by predisposing it to proprioceptive imbalance in the short term, and then presiding over its progressive demise in the long run. Nor should we discount the possibility that a faulty TMJ caused by clenching and grinding, might likewise, be able to interfere with the coccyx and the urogenital system.

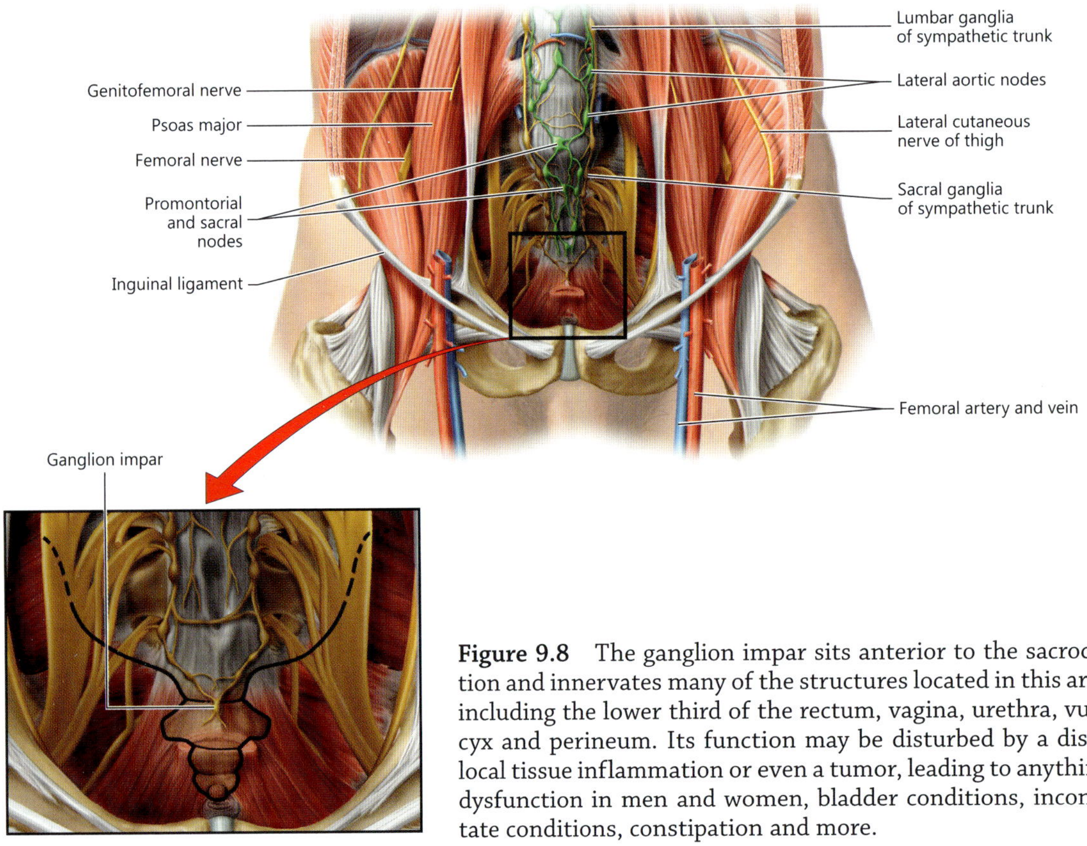

Figure 9.8 The ganglion impar sits anterior to the sacrococcygeal junction and innervates many of the structures located in this area of the body, including the lower third of the rectum, vagina, urethra, vulva, anus, coccyx and perineum. Its function may be disturbed by a distorted coccyx, local tissue inflammation or even a tumor, leading to anything from sexual dysfunction in men and women, bladder conditions, incontinence, prostate conditions, constipation and more.

Typical Coccyx Conditions

The main conditions of the coccyx that are typically at the source of coccyx symptoms are inflammation (Fig. 9.9), tumors (Fig. 9.10), distortions and dislocation (Fig. 9.11) and their causes are varied.

Typical contributing factors leading to coccyx conditions are accidents, childbirth and too much sitting.

I have treated many adults over the years who claim that their back and neck pain started after a fall on the coccyx as a youngster.

Nothing was detected via medical tests and they were told that it would "get better" with time. Sadly for so many the condition does not get better by itself, and intervention is required.

In Chapter 7, NST's general Coccyx procedure was presented, and it would be fair to note that this procedure, along with its prerequisites, will resolve a fair proportion of coccyx conditions, but not all.

However, following this procedure there are two additional coccyx strategies known as the advanced Coccyx procedure and a coccyx-cervical spine integrated release. These will be presented in later editions.

In some severe cases of a badly angulated coccyx conditions, intra-anal adjustments may be the best solution and should be carried out by a duly licensed physician skilled in doing so.

Note: Intra-anal or intravaginal corrections are not part of the NST system of adjustments.

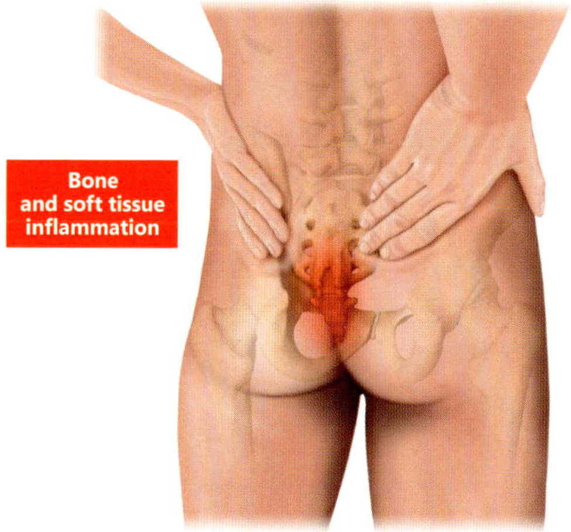

Figure 9.9 Image showing inflammation of the coccyx bone.

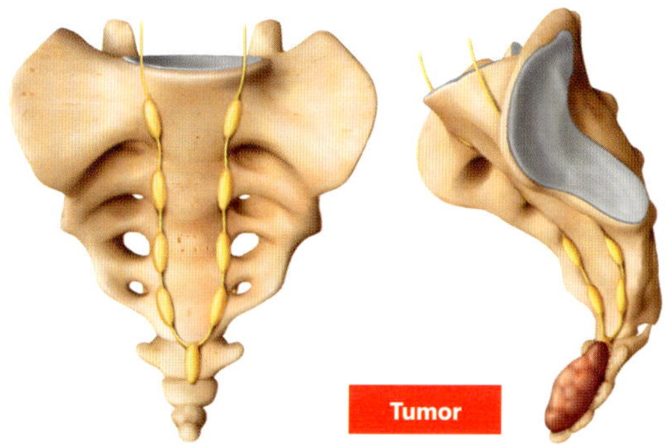

Figure 9.10 Image showing a tumor affecting the ganglion impar.

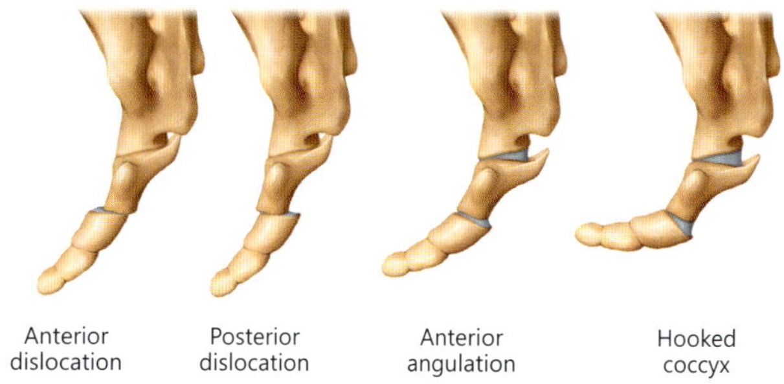

Figure 9.11 Image showing various typical structural distortions of the coccyx including, anterior angulation, hooked and dislocation.

CONCLUSION

Chronic coccyx and TMJ conditions in particular, are the hidden culprits in so many symptoms, illnesses and degenerative conditions, flourishing in their unsuspecting hosts bodies over many years, and invariably all courtesy of a perpetual imbalance cycle that was never detected or corrected when it first established itself (Fig. 9.12).

Fortunately, coccyx conditions are not as prevalent as some of the other more serious spinal and structural conditions found in general clinical practice, such as pelvic and TMJ conditions, but nevertheless they account for, or are involved in, about 15-20% cases.

However, although not as common as one might expect, the need for being able to identify and adjust the coccyx when necessary, is paramount in achieving optimal clinical success and sustainable corrections for the patient.

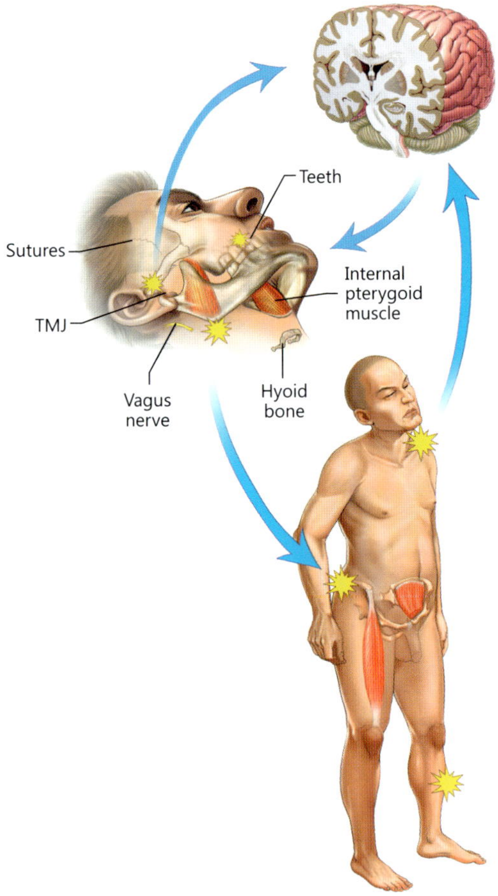

Figure 9.12 Image showing that an undetected coccyx fault, over time, may establish a perpetual imbalance cycle leading to a broad variety of chronic and degenerative conditions.

Lung procedure – Additional Information

The Lung procedure is so-called in NST because the lungs are the largest organ that are affected by this procedure, which in reality is dedicated to the release of the diaphragm muscle.

But the lungs are not the only organs to be dependent on or influenced by the proper function of the diaphragm muscle, as the muscle itself literally affects all organs that lay above it and all organs that lay below it. Specifically the organs are the lungs and heart in the thoracic cavity and the liver, gallbladder, stomach, pancreas, spleen, large and small intestines, kidneys and bladder in the abdominal cavity.

And when it comes to the organs that sit directly above it and lay directly below the diaphragm, we must keep in mind that it's not just the ongoing voluntary and involuntary movements of the diaphragm muscle that set the tone for the organs, but the story must also be considered the other way around, whereby the organs affect the muscle's operation.

A prolonged poor diet not only affects the operation of the nine "boiler-work" organs that reside in the abdominal cavity, but also places unnecessary load on the heart and lungs. Couple this with a prolonged lack of physical activity; the consequences for the heart and lungs in the thoracic cavity and consequently our health, can be dire.

A swollen and engorged liver, a constantly overloaded stomach, a pancreas struggling to produce sufficient insulin or constipated large intestine can quickly affect the diaphragm muscle's many "slip-like" fibers that emerge from its various points of attachment (xiphoid process, lower six costal cartilages and lumbar vertebrae) and insert into its large central aponeurotic tendon.

And indeed, when we consider that many of our patients who present with back and neck pain, are also sufferers from the above visceral conditions.

The diaphragm separates the thoracic cavity, containing the heart and lungs, from the abdominal cavity containing the visceral organs, and permits the all-important function of respiration to occur (Fig. 9.13).

Without a diaphragm muscle we cannot breathe, unless with the help of an external machine. Simply put, as the diaphragm contracts, the volume of the thoracic cavity increases and air is drawn into the lungs.

The muscle itself has two parts, consisting of a fibrous central tendon to which certain organs attach, and an external active muscular section that surrounds the central tendon.

The main muscular motor nerve input is via two phrenic nerves emerging from C3-C5 segments in the cervical spine. The central tendon is also supplied with two phrenic nerves for sensory nerve output. Further sensory nerve output from the external muscle fibers is supplied from T7-T10 segments of the thoracic spine.

The diaphragm muscle is penetrated by three significant structures, namely the descending aorta, inferior vena cava and the esophagus. Is it any wonder then that restrictions to its muscle fibers may exert inappropriate tensions on those structures, leading to further load on the heart and lungs plus digestive symptoms? (Fig. 9.14).

And of course, we must remember that the diaphragm and its inherent state of balance, optimal or otherwise, sets the tone for the rhythm of the secondary respiratory mechanism, and in many respects the whole body.

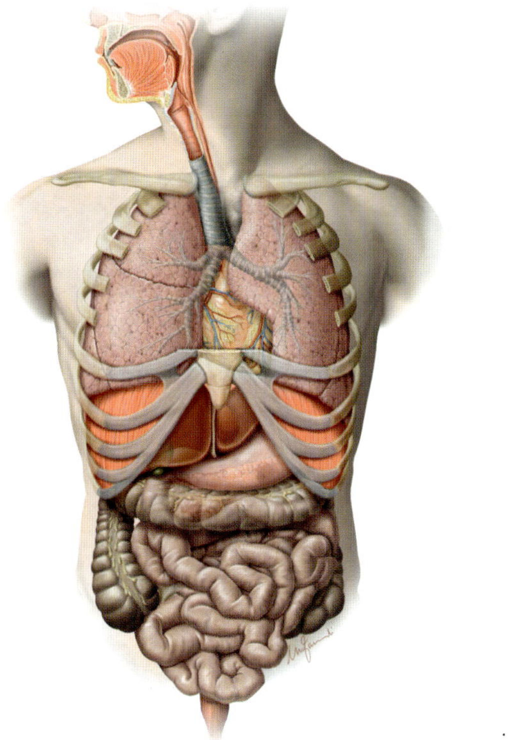

Figure 9.13 The diaphragm plays a crucial role not only in driving the rhythm of the body through the SRM, but also as a fulcrum between the thoracic and abdominal cavities. As activity increases in the thoracic cavity it decreases in the abdominal cavity, and vice versa. In this context the status of the diaphragm's intrinsic balance can facilitate or inhibit the complex procession of activities, that must take place on a daily basis, if indeed our boiler-works is to remain in top shape and produce the necessary energy to supply the muscles and other structures.

If we consider that the average adult, at rest, breathes about 1,000 times per hour, more if we run up and down stairs or do any other type of physical activity, and the diaphragm is involved with every one of those breaths.

Any activity that is performed 24,000 times a day is going to be registered and learned by the organism as being the status quo, and consequently whatever torsional (tensegrity) state the diaphragm is in, will be reflected into the pelvic floor muscles (lower diaphragm) via reciprocal pressures, which is further perpetuated into the neck and cranium (upper diaphragm) via particular tensions and drag.

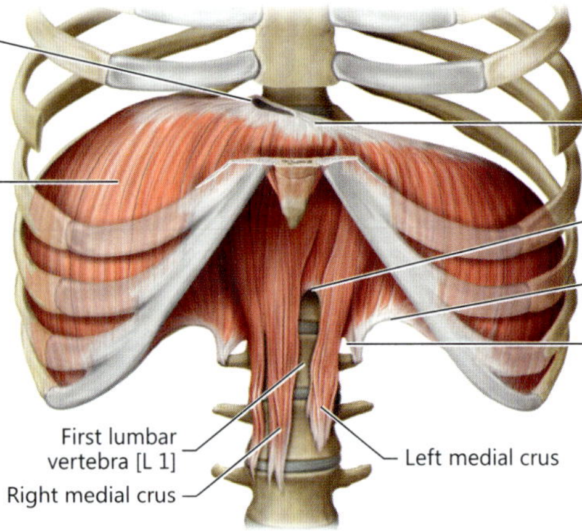

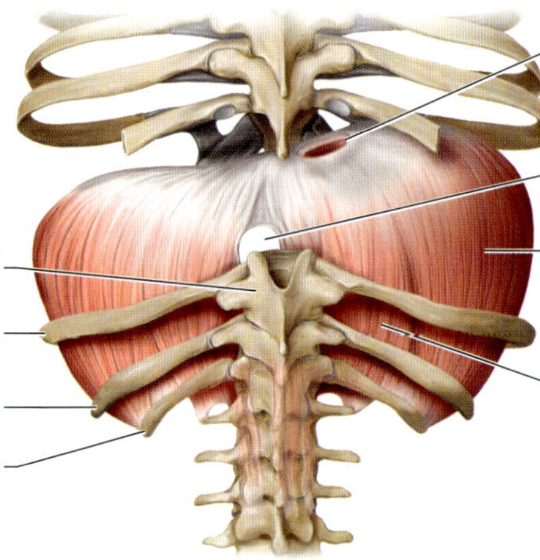

Figure 9.14 Anterior (**a**) and posterior (**b**) views of the diaphragm. Note the strong muscular attachments to the lumbar spine, the central tendon and the structures that pass through the muscle fibers. The diaphragm is also considered to be a skeletal muscle as it responds to nerve impulses and can be voluntarily controlled. It also uses actin, myosin and other proteins common to skeletal muscle.

Nor does the diaphragm muscle escape our emotional status or daily levels of stress. Persistent shallow breathing caused by stress, is closely associated with poor diaphragmatic action, meaning simply that the lungs do not take in as much oxygen, impacting on the level of oxygenation of the blood, the consequences for which can be multifactorial in themselves!

But in setting the muscular status, for the rest of the body in a Macro-sense, predispositions therefore, to further imbalances are established.

The evidence that this is indeed the case, is reinforced when we consider that it's not just the diaphragm muscle alone that is affected by the status of the organs, that have such a tactile relationship with it, or indeed by our breathing and emotional patterns, but all of the other muscles scattered around the body sharing inseparable viscerosomatic reflex relationships with those organs as well (Fig. 9.15).

The abundant neurolymphatic, neurovascular and neuromuscular reflexes are a testimony to this, and communicate intimately with their dedicated muscles acting as two-way circuit breakers for the congested organs they couple with.

A few examples of muscle-organ-reflex relationships:

- Heart → subscapularis
- Lungs → diaphragm
- Liver → rhomboid
- Gallbladder → anterior deltoid
- Stomach → pectoralis major, clavicular head
- Pancreas → latissimus dorsi
- Large intestine → tensor fascia latae
- Small intestine → quadriceps femoris
- Kidney → psoas
- Bladder → tibialis anterior
- Reproductive organs → gluteus medius

And all of these muscle associations may have a direct or indirect impact on the status of the cervical spine and pelvic girdle, affecting dura mater and the function of the SRM and SGS.

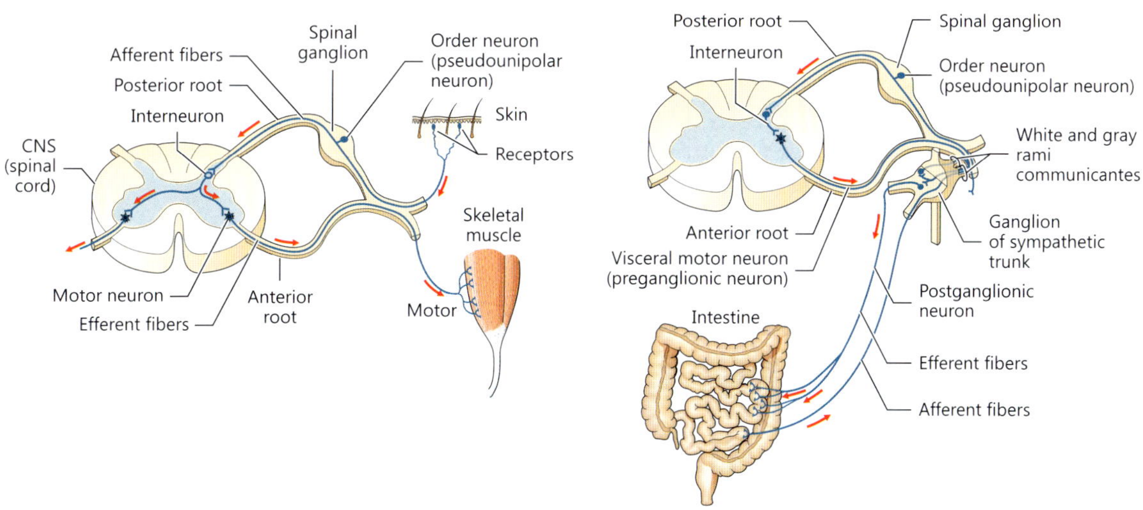

Figure 9.15 Image illustrating the intimate relationships shared between muscles and organs, mediated through the various neurolymphatic, neurovascular, neuromuscular and viscerosomatic reflex systems that control them.

And if the story was not complex enough already, it does not stop with muscles and reflexes alone. When we talk about the visceral abdominal cavity, its contents and their function, we are also obliged to consider the potential involvement of the mesh like enteric nervous system, embedded in the lining of the gastrointestinal system from the esophagus to the anus. Its 500 million neurons out number the neurons in the neurological spinal cord by five to one and by comparison amount one two-hundredth of the neurons contained in the brain itself.

Having its own self-contained reflex activity, it can and does function independently to the spinal cord and brain, however its activity is intimately linked with the ANS's sympathetic and parasympathetic activities, the vagus nerve in particular being a major player.

And as we will see in our final section on the TMJ, the function of the vagus nerve can be affected by TMJ syndrome, just as much as it can by a compromised visceral system.

Indeed, the enteric nervous system and the gut itself are often referred to our "second brain" not only for their unique nervous activity but also because of the fact that 90% of the

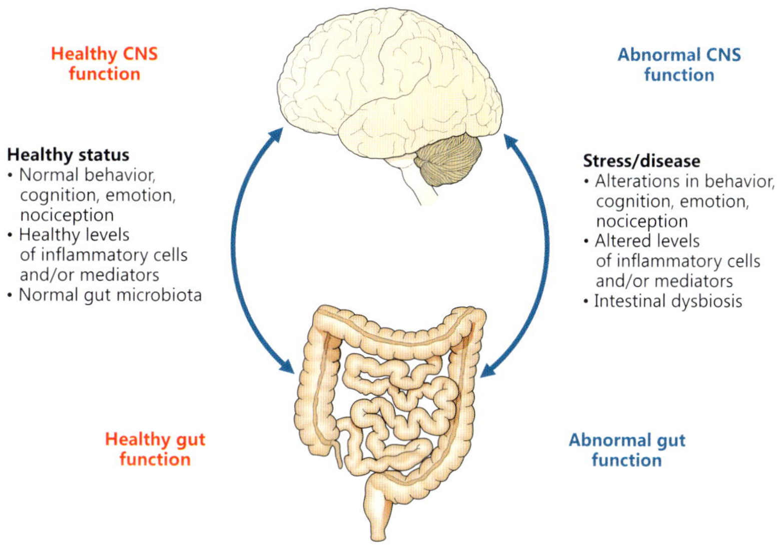

Figure 9.16 The enteric nervous system and gut are often referred to as our "second brain" as we now know that 90% of the body's mood, sleep and appetite hormone, serotonin, is produced in the gut. And the 100 trillion microorganisms that inhabit our gut are responsible for ultimately determining the quality of digestion, blood, tissue and therefore physiology itself. Is it our brain that controls our gut or our gut that controls our brain?

body's serotonin is created in the gut. When we consider the brain's needs for serotonin to help regulate, mood, sleep and appetite we start to expand our thinking even further.

Given that the 100 trillion microorganisms that inhabit our gut are responsible for ultimately determining the quality of digestion, blood, tissue, and therefore physiology itself, is it our brain that controls our gut or our gut that controls our brain? (Fig. 9.16).

And are the choices we make and behaviors we engage in on a daily basis, to do with our diet, detoxification, physical culture, stress management and breathing patterns all somehow interwoven with the way our diaphragm muscle works, and indeed how our whole system operates?

CONCLUSION

Our patients so urgently seek pain relief for the various ailments they present with, but often what they need just as urgently, is simple fundamental education about how to better manage the amazing human organism that they find themselves in charge of.

When Dr. Andrew Still, the father of osteopathic medicine, said: "Through you, we live, and through you we die", in reference to the diaphragm, was he referring to pulmonary respiration alone, or was the simplicity and wisdom his comment contains, intended to highlight a much more important relationship between the health of the and function of the diaphragm and how life itself is lived?

Pelvic procedure – additional information

The center of gravity of the body is located at S2 of the sacrum, which is curiously also the point of attachment of the dura mater to the sacrum, and geographically speaking half way from the bottom of the feet up and the top of the head down.

The sacrum sits in between the innominate bones of the pelvis, together creating the pelvic girdle.

The abdominal and back muscles that insert and attach to it from above are balanced by the leg and hip muscles that insert and attach to it from below.

That it moves, flexes, extends and twists as we walk and move about in various ways, is a testimony not only to the muscles that are attached to it, but the pelvic girdle's capacity to act as a dynamic mechanism, that can influence the status of the muscles above and below it as much as they can affect it.

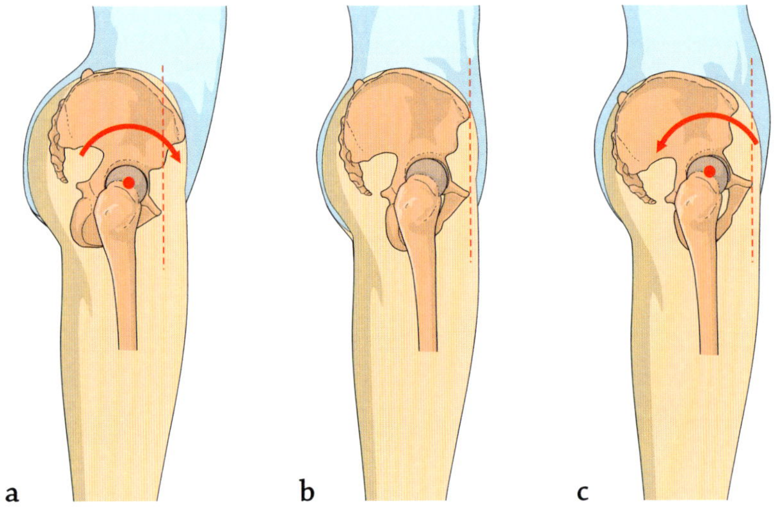

Figure 9.17 The pelvic girdle's position is at the mercy of so many intersecting forces from within, above and below. The diaphragm, abdominal, back and pelvic floor muscles can all influence its position. Leg muscles are no exception and the sacrum itself can exert its own unique influence. The image shows the pelvic girdle in three typical positions – (**a**) anterior pelvic tilt, (**b**) neutral and (**c**) posterior pelvic tilt. The aim of NST is to achieve neutral position and for this reason the pelvic girdle is assessed at every session.

But if things are amiss with the pelvic girdle generally, the result is typically an anterior or posterior tilt or rotation pattern, the consequences of which can be sacral, lower back, hip and groin pain locally and then knee, shoulder and neck pain more remotely (Fig. 9.17).

Subscribing to the simple rule that what lays above and below an imbalance are likely contributing factors, the reverse must also be true, in that what's in the middle, affects what is below and above it.

Like so many parts or systems in the human organism it is an interdependent and "symbiotic" relationship that the pelvic girdle shares directly or indirectly with almost all other moving parts of the body.

The pelvic girdle is intimately involved in the muscular activities of the "gait walking mechanism", and as a consequence, the compensatory spinal and cranial muscle activities that are obliged to take place as well.

We have already learned that the pelvic girdle is affected by the functioning of the diaphragm muscle, and can itself affect the function of the cranium via the SRM and SGS.

Furthermore, our modus operandi in using NST is to always do at least DBB1, 2, 3 while adding Sacrum and Lung procedures gives just that bit of additional surety, in knowing that the SRM will come back to balance.

But there are times when the pelvic girdle as an entity needs specific additional release, to be able to fully and accurately participate in the process of walking and moving about, and the function of the SRM itself (Fig. 9.18).

And this is behind the reason to evaluate the pelvis at every session (as described in Chapter 7 by using the FABER test) after the extremities work has been completed in the supine position.

Indeed, if there are residual pelvic faults left undetected at the session's end, the patient may find themselves coming back for further appointments sooner rather than later, as an unbalanced pelvic girdle can effect almost anything in the body via its systematic involvement with, and influence over, both the SRM and SGS.

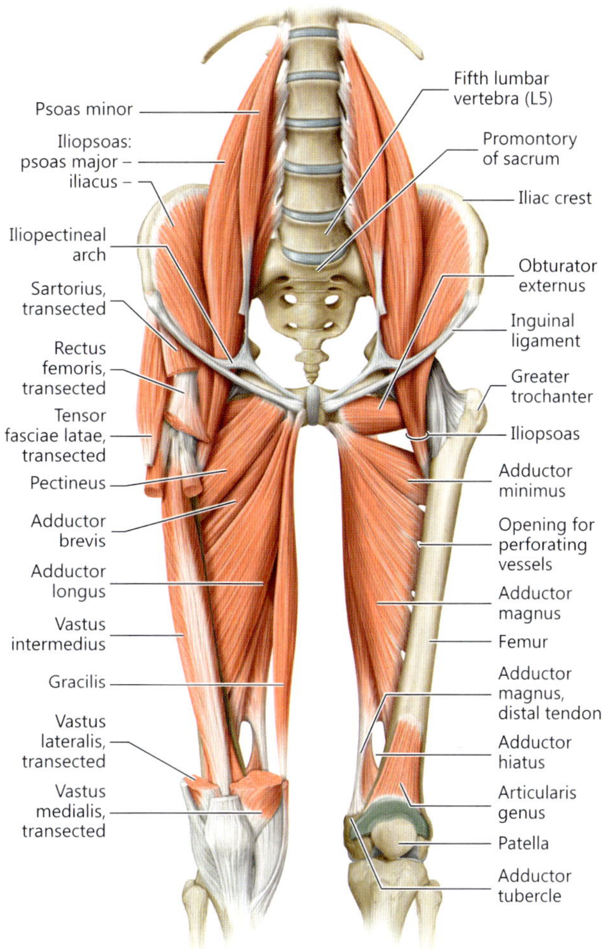

Figure 9.18 The image shows the muscles and structures involved in the NST pelvic procedure. Note the origins and insertions of the gracilis, adductors, sartorious and iliacus muscles, and the inguinal ligament itself. Muscles that warrant further consideration yet not directly stimulated in the Pelvic procedure are psoas and pectineus muscles. The abdominals although dealt with in the Lung procedure should also be considered.

We often talk about and treat the sacrum, pelvis and coccyx as if they were separate entities, but in reality they all belong to the one interactive complex of bones, muscles, ligaments, tendons and fasciae.

The coccyx can affect the sacrum and the sacrum the pelvic bones, just as much as the pelvic bones affect the sacrum, and in turn, the coccyx.

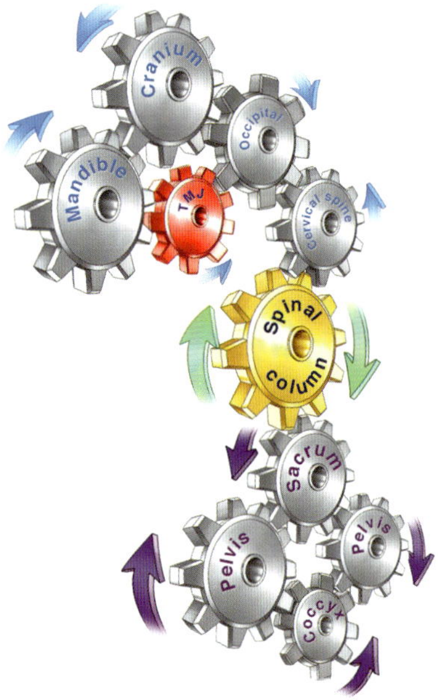

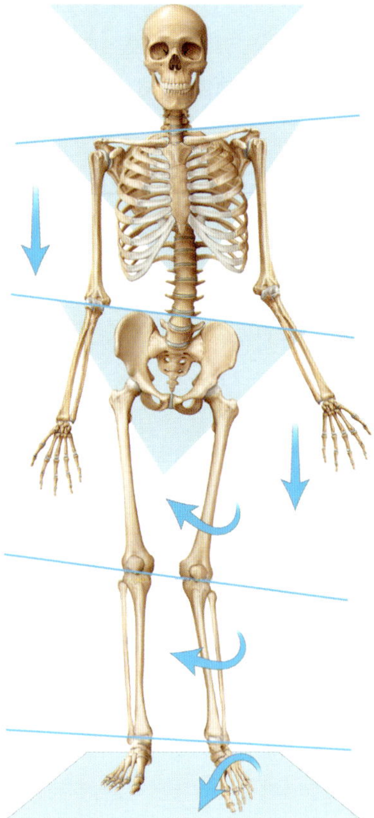

Figure 9.19 The image on the left shows that spinal and cranial structures are dynamically poised and balanced atop the pelvic girdle – all gears must move in natural compensatory directions to maintain pelvic and systematic balance. The image on the right highlights the skeletal and postural consequences that may arise from an unbalanced pelvic girdle.

Like a heavy superstructure poised on top of the lower extremities, yet a foundation for the spinal column and cranium, that are balanced on top of it, the free flowing interactivity and interdependence that the pelvic girdle is designed for, is paramount to preserve, if we hope and expect to maintain the dynamic balance within the body, and thereby assist our patients in creating sustainability of corrections (Fig. 9.19).

In my own clinical evaluation of many thousands of patients, the Pelvic procedure is far more frequently indicated than the Coccyx, with approximately 70-80% of patients testing positive for pelvic imbalance.

Apart from performing the FABER test at every session, some of the other clues that the pelvis may be out balance are:

- Differences in the range of movement in the leg when rotated laterally - point 4 of DBB1.
- Leg length differences in the prone or supine positions.
- Visible eversion of one foot or the other in the supine position.
- Pelvic rotation.
- Groin pain especially when moving from standing to sitting or sitting to standing.
- Pubic symphysis pain.

Some of the most common reasons why the pelvis has inherent imbalances are:

- Too much sitting.
- Not enough walking.
- Prolonged usage of inappropriate footwear (stilettos).
- Unnecessary or poor fitting orthotic appliances.
- Not preparing adequately or properly before sport activities (jogging, tennis, football).
- Pregnancy and childbirth.
- Endometriosis.
- Digestive conditions.

CONCLUSION

Correcting the pelvic girdle when necessary as part of NST treatment will deliver extremely pleasing results, not only in rapid pain reduction but also in excellent sustainability of corrections, via better dynamic balance within the SRM and SGS.

TMJ Procedure – Additional Information

Always performed as the very last of the procedures in any integrated NST session, the TMJ procedure is perhaps the most astounding of all when it comes to the amount and variety of symptoms that become resolvable by its proper assessment, correction and stabilization (Fig. 9.20).

And being left till last, means that its effects will have a positive and powerful integrative effect on all other corrections achieved adding real stability to the session.

Conversely, it must be remembered that the amount and variety of symptoms that an unbalanced TMJ and hence SGS can cause is almost limitless.

In Chapter 7 (Supine Position Procedures – Super core), we covered the complete assessment, correction and stabilization procedure,

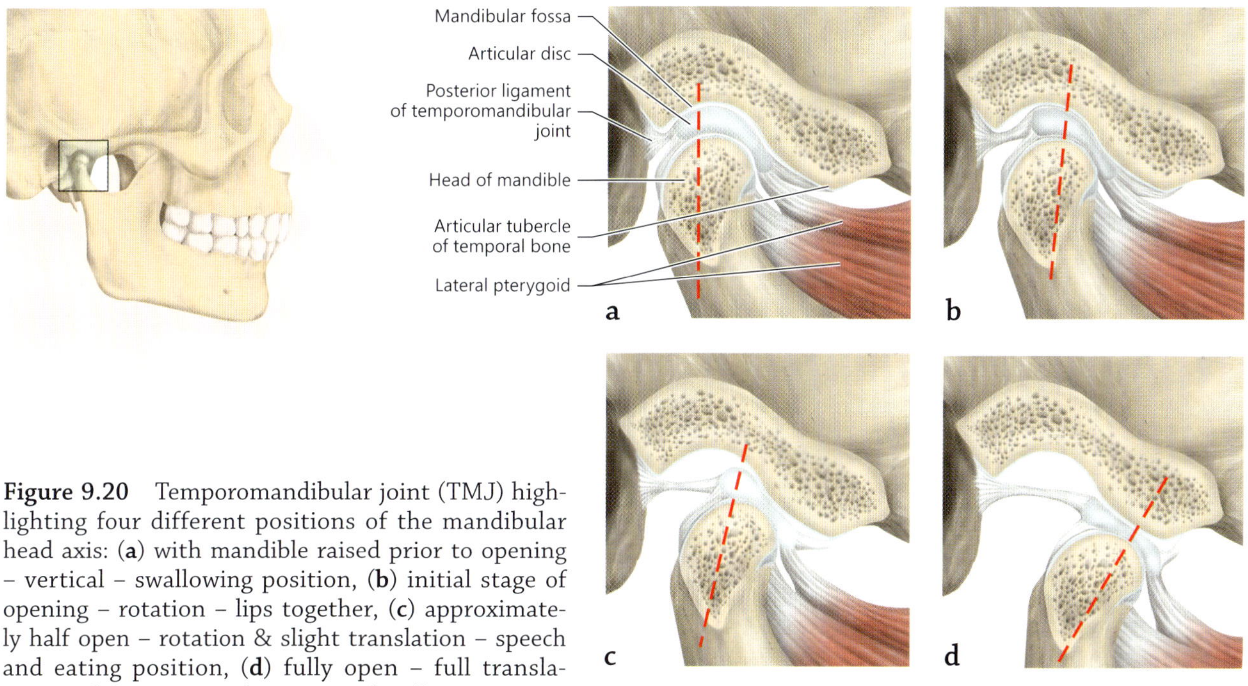

Figure 9.20 Temporomandibular joint (TMJ) highlighting four different positions of the mandibular head axis: (**a**) with mandible raised prior to opening – vertical – swallowing position, (**b**) initial stage of opening – rotation – lips together, (**c**) approximately half open – rotation & slight translation – speech and eating position, (**d**) fully open – full translation & depression – cheering and yelling position. Apart from the bony structures of the mandibular condyle and temporal fossa, the TMJ consists of a mobile soft tissue capsular joint that contains an intracapsular meniscus, that sits between an upper and lower synovial cavity complete with synovium. There is also a rich blood supply servicing the posterior portion of the meniscus rendering it capable of regeneration. The lateral pterygoid muscle is attached to the anterior portion of the capsule, and is responsible for ensuring that the capsule and its meniscus remain cushioned between the bony surfaces throughout slight opening (rotation) or fully opening (translation and depression) and the reverse when closing. As the mouth closes the responsibility for maintaining the appropriate position of the meniscus, largely falls to the elastic retracting ligament that is firmly attached to the posterior aspect of the TMJ capsule. In other words, throughout closing the lateral pterygoid muscle is inhibited, and the natural elasticity of the retracting ligament performs the task of ensuring the appropriate position of the meniscus.

containing much valuable TMJ information throughout, while in Chapter 3 (NST Operating Systems) we looked at the Stomatognathic System (SGS) and noted how the TMJ was one of its components, and that if unbalanced or degenerated could cause the whole body to remain in a state of perpetual imbalance.

We also covered the Micro-Macro system relationships that exist in the SGS and detailed its many components.

Quick review:

The temporomandibular joints are so-called because of the articulation of the mandible in the temporal fossa, of the temporal bone, of the cranium – hence temporomandibular.

The joints belong to the closed Micro system

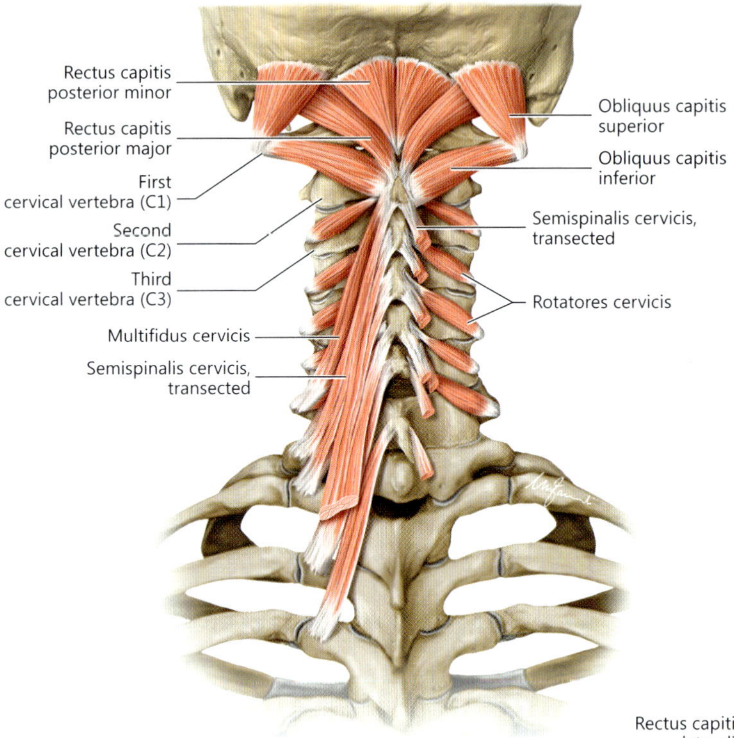

Figure 9.21 Image showing the posterior suboccipital muscles, potentially implicated in delivering tensegrity faults, from and unbalanced Micro system, into the upper cervical vertebral bodies. In turn, distortions in the upper cervical vertebral bodies affect the dura mater, sacrum and ultimately the SGS. Note in particular the rectus capitis posterior major and minor and obliquus capitis superior and inferior muscles.

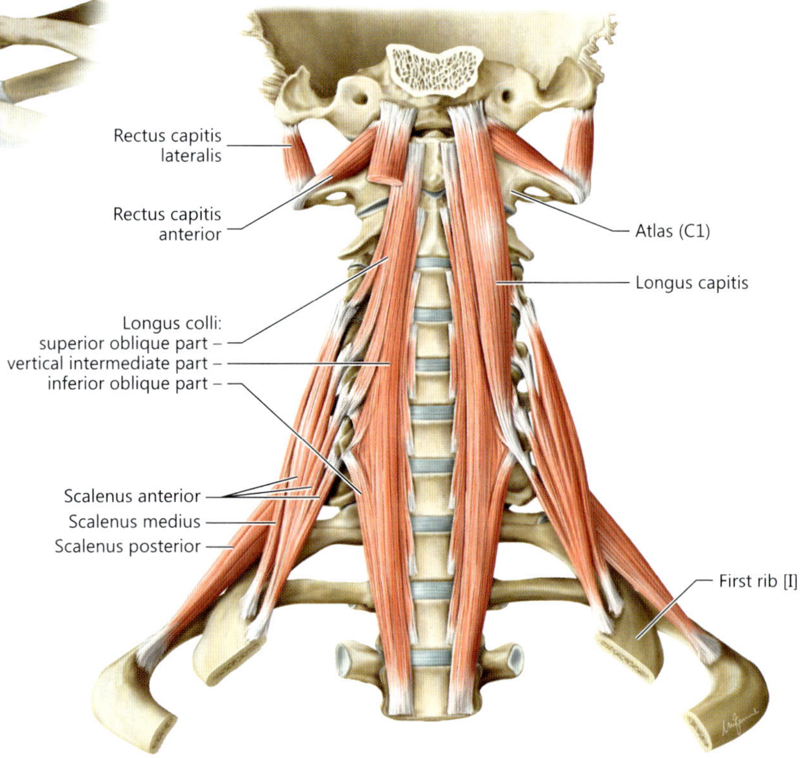

Figure 9.22 Image showing the anterior suboccipital muscle – longus capitis – that could potentially be implicated in delivering tensegrity faults, from and unbalanced Micro system, into the upper cervical vertebral bodies. In turn, distortions in the upper cervical vertebral bodies affect the dura mater, sacrum and ultimately the SGS.

of structures that sit above the shoulders, and are just one of the components of the Micro system. Other components have previously been identified in more detail but include bones, muscles, ligaments, nerves, teeth and TMJ.

All components must function synchronistically as we chew, bite, swallow and speak for the Micro system in and of itself to stay balanced.

Should any component of the Micro system be out of balance, the whole system is affected, resulting in suboccipital muscles namely rectus capitis posterior major and minor, obliquus capitis superior and inferior (all posterior neck muscles) and capitis longus muscles (anterior neck muscle) distorting C2 and C3 upper cervical vertebrae. This, in turn, creates "dural drag" from the upper cervical vertebrae down to the sacrum via the dura mater, thereby disturbing the pelvic girdle and its musculature (Figs. 9.21 and 9.22).

At this point, the Micro system has disturbed the Macro system, and now the whole body is involved potentially creating a perpetual imbalance cycle that is maintained by ever more poor ongoing afferent input, to the somatosensory cortex of the brain and equally poor efferent motor output to the Micro and Macro system musculature (Fig. 9.23).

In this circumstance, the body has no way out, and has entered onto a trajectory that is progressively degenerative in nature, with many dire consequences, manifesting in a variety of symptoms from A-Z along the way.

To help explain the above, if we think of the

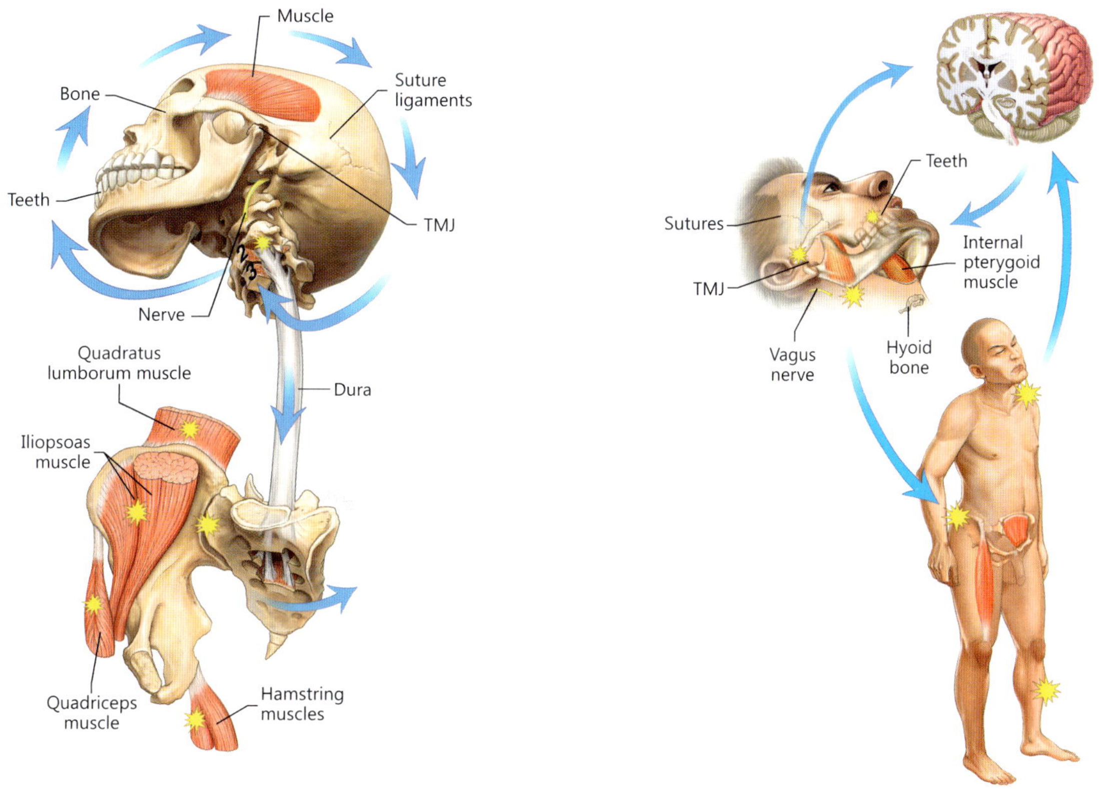

Figure 9.23 The image on the left is illustrating that all components of the cranium (Micro system) need to be integrated for the spine and rest of the body (Macro system) to be integrated. If not the consequences quickly become systematic. The image on the right is illustrating that when Micro-Macro system integration is lost, the body enters a perpetual imbalance cycle that is frequently evident in chronic and degenerative conditions. The brain depends on balanced input to produce balanced output, and if input is compromised through chronicity and degeneration, output will be corrupted as well. The body literally becomes locked in a perpetual self-sabotaging cycle that is progressive in nature.

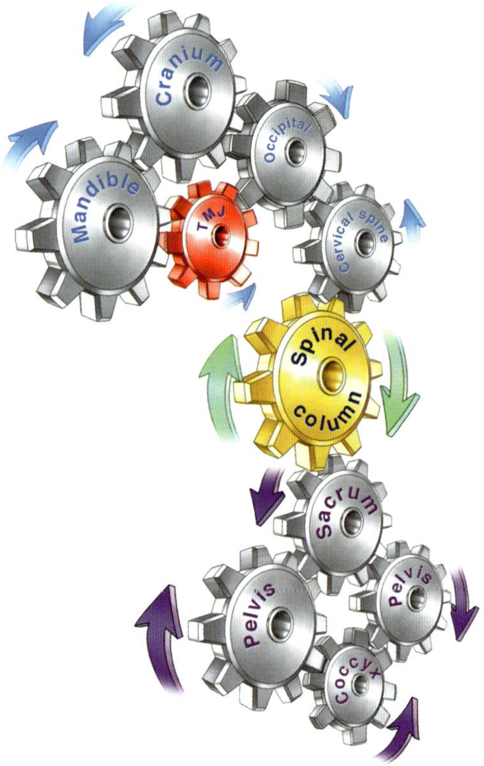

Figure 9.24 Note the cranial section in the system of interlocking gears. Imbalances in the mandible, cranial gears and especially the occiput gear share an intimate micro relationship with the TMJ gear. If the TMJ is unbalanced, various muscles and structures within the Micro system will follow, and the resultant consequence will be that unbalanced forces will be transmitted to the cervical spine gear. Once in the cervical spine gear the whole body in obliged to compensate, or over time, degenerate. The interlocking system of gears should be regarded as a metaphor for what happens as a result of an unbalanced TMJ, and is clearly an over simplification as to what can actually occur at structural, neurological and hormonal levels.

TMJ and its relationship to the rest of the body in a purely mechanical sense, like a system of gears, as illustrated in Figure 9.24, we can see that the TMJ gear is articulating with the mandible, cranial and occipital gears in an interlocking system of four gears.

The occipital gear is articulating with the cervical spine gear, indicating that if there any imbalances at all in the TMJ – mandible – cranium – occipital system (the Micro system), the resultant forces will be "dumped" into the cervical spine.

From here, the cervical spine gear now articulates with the spinal column, which is continuous with the integrated gear system of the pelvic girdle, consisting of the sacrum, pelvis and coccyx gears.

The image is designed to highlight the complete interactivity that the body has and that imbalances can be generated from any gear or part of the body.

All gears mentioned represent significant components of the NST system that correspond to the Dynamic Body Balance and important procedures.

Importantly, the discussion regarding the TMJ and SGS centers around the Micro system only, for the simple reason that the Macro system aspect of the pelvic girdle, will already have been attended to in any integrated NST session, in which all necessary prerequisites have been properly carried out (DBB1, 2, 3, Sacrum and Shoulder).

The fundamental principle that we always need to keep in mind with any NST adjustment, and there is no difference when working with the Micro system is "tensegrity".

Specifically, our NST TMJ procedure has been designed to correct the complex "tensegrity" that exists in the muscle systems from the shoulders up to and including the cranium. Collectively, these are the general muscles of the cervical spine, hyoid muscles, tongue muscles intrinsic and extrinsic, muscles of mastication and deglutition, facial muscles, eye muscles and cranial muscles.

When these muscle systems are all balanced and well integrated as they are designed to be, the positioning of the cervical spine is balanced and there is no disturbance to the cervical spine and in particular the upper cervical vertebrae C2 and C3.

If there is a fault (disc misplacement or deterioration) at the level of one or two TMJ, the chewing muscles (masseter, pterygoid and temporalis muscles) pull too tight throughout the repetitive action of chewing and, as a consequence, the introduction of inappropriate

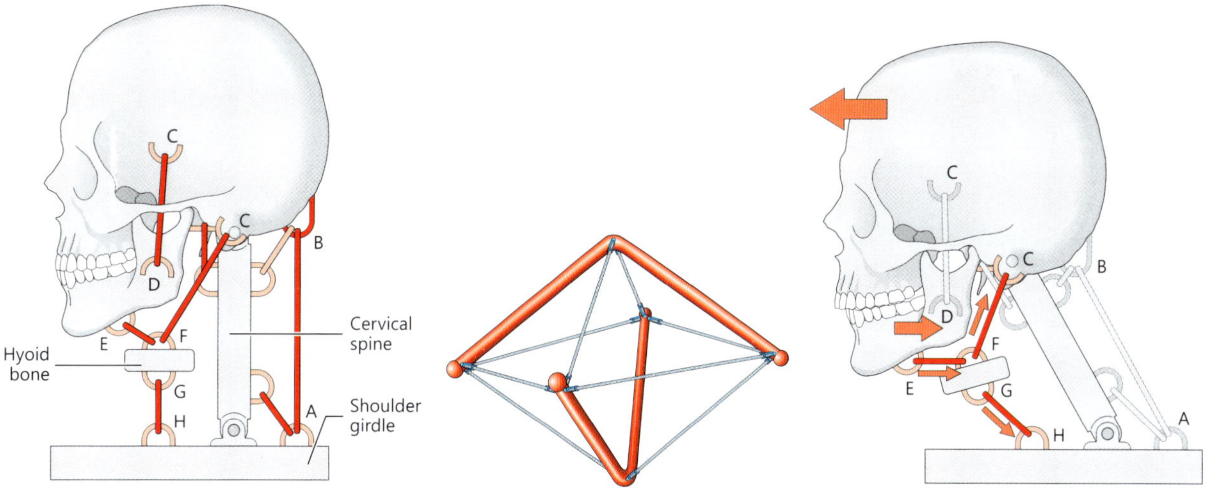

Figure 9.25 The image on the left shows the cervical spine delicately poised between the head and shoulder girdle. The band of muscles A-B represents the general head on neck musculature that are generally dealt with in NST – DBB3. The collective bands from C-D-E-F-G-H represent the Micro system of muscles (hyoid, facial, cranial, chewing, biting, swallowing, tongue and eye). If the tensegrity of the two opposing systems is balanced, then the head-neck-shoulder girdle relationship will be structurally sound, and consequently everything below the shoulders (Macro system) will be balanced. The image in the middle shows a typical tensegrity model discussed in the introduction of this book, and simply highlights that tensegrity is the key principle at play when considering the assessment and treatment of the Micro system. The image on the right shows the consequences for the cervical spine when appropriate tensegrity is lost in the Micro and Macro systems of muscles. Of course from this point we have to assume the consequences will be pain and dysfunction.

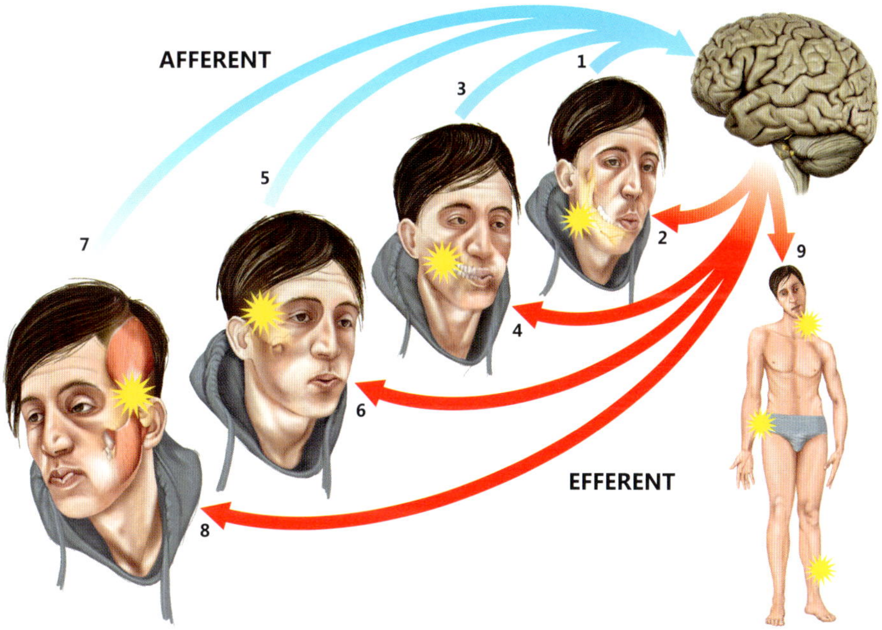

Figure 9.26 The image shows that SGS disturbances typically start at a very superficial level – such as a muscle imbalance, which in turn may have an inhibitory effect on other muscles in the Micro system – arrows 1 and 2. The bite may be affected leading to malocclusion, with further compromised afferent and efferent relationships – arrows 3 and 4. Over time periodontal ligament receptors may fire inappropriately and chewing muscles may be compromised – arrows 5 and 6. Confusion within the SGS becomes so complex, that degeneration of the TMJ and chronic inflammation become unavoidable – arrows 7 and 8. Equilibrium proprioceptors are now compromised rendering the body incapable of holding appropriate neuromuscular status and chronic disorganization sets in. The organism is now predisposed to pain and eventually degeneration.

tensional cables has been introduced into the complex system of cables that is the SGS Micro system of muscles.

As soon as we disturb one cable, more will follow. If we disturb a whole group, such as the chewing muscles, others follow suit, and it is very common therefore to discover that many hyoid muscles will have lost their "tensegrity" as will neck muscles (Fig. 9.25).

Bit by bit, if left uncorrected further mechanical and soft tissue faults build into the complex of imbalances. Cranial sutures may jamb, cranial nerves may receive too much pressure from tight and inflammed muscles and fascia that surround them.

Teeth may wear (poor occlusion) providing an unstable base against which the act of swallowing that we must do approximately 800-1,000 times per day, must occur.

In summary, the condition becomes progressively degenerative in nature until the closed Micro system affects the Macro system, and the body is riddled with neuromuscular compensations and predisposition for more and more of the same to develop (Fig. 9.26).

It is clearly not a positive picture to paint, but nevertheless a realistic one, and one that can be comprehended, identified and corrected with NST.

Following are typical examples of how the TMJ and SGS can affect the body as a whole.

The three basic categories of faults that can be generated are as follows:

1. Mechanical
2. Neurological
3. Hormonal

MECHANICAL FAULTS

The fundamental principle with mechanical faults is that patterns of muscular imbalance pull the bony skeletal system out of place, causing pressure on nerves and intervertebral discs, resulting in stagnation of the vascular, visceral, endocrine, energy and fluid systems of the body, creating further consequential muscular imbalance with more chronic and degenerative outcomes.

This is a classical tension – pain – tension cycle and is perpetual in nature leading to ever increasing levels of neuromuscular imbalance and more pain and physiological dysfunction.

And typically, when we disturb one or two spinal vertebral bodies, other become affected and the consequences become far more complex than just a single bone applying pressure to a single nerve.

But in doing so we must factor in the consequences that muscle pressure on surrounding nerves has as well.

Nerves need appropriate amounts of pressure to fire both electrically and hydraulically, and when muscles become too tight or too laxed, nerves fail to transmit effectively with yet further consequences.

This principle can be applied to any muscle pair anywhere in the body and the consequences are always the same, with unbalanced tensions leading to either excessive bone or muscle pressure, or both, on nerves creating compromised muscle function elsewhere, leading to circulatory problems, inflammation, and pain (Fig. 9.27).

Conclusion

The goal is to correct the "tensegrity" ensuring that appropriate balanced tensions allow the skeletal system and therefore nervous system to function normally (Fig. 9.27).

It's worth keeping in mind that, whenever wasteful muscular contractions are removed, the organism conserves energy and physiology functions optimally.

Chapter 4 (Further Operating Principles), goes into more detail on this subject and should be read in combination with this section.

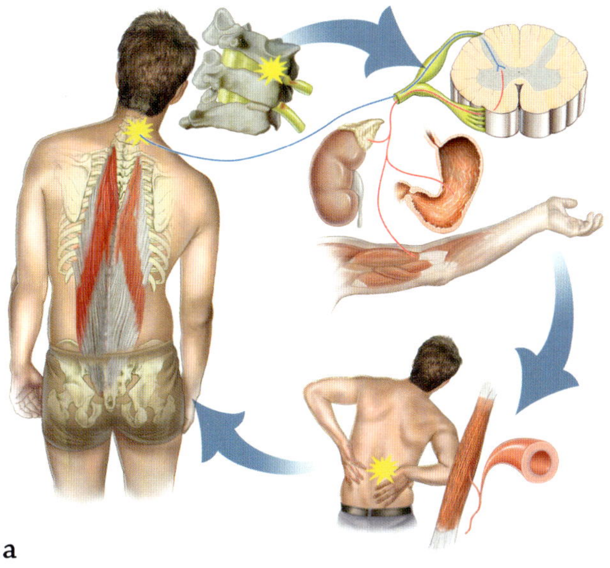

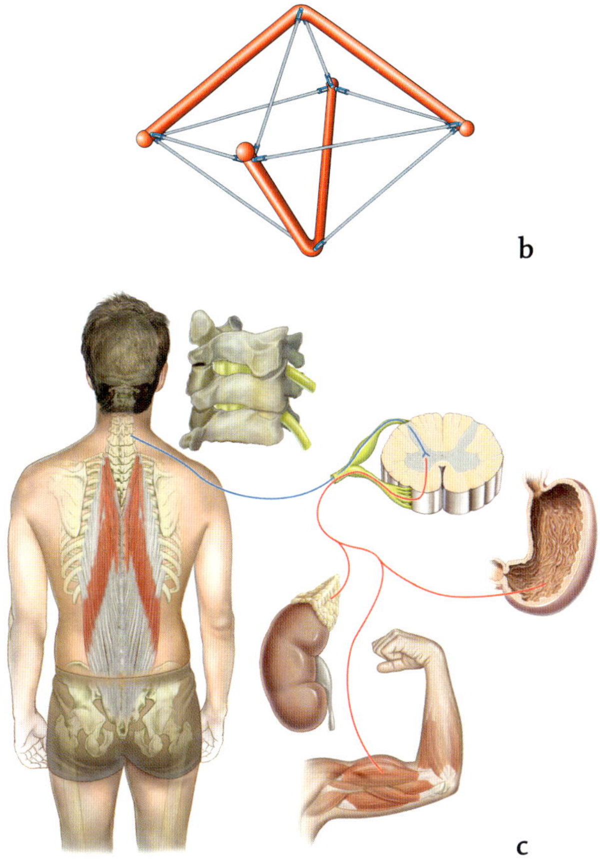

Figure 9.27 The image (**a**) shows that mechanical faults generated by poor tensegrity result in pain and more tension. The image (**b**) is a reminder that the fundamental principle of tensegrity is paramount in the assessment and treatment of health conditions. The image (**c**) shows that good tensegrity leads to good physiology and robust health.

NEUROLOGICAL FAULTS

Apart from the obvious nervous involvement in the previous example, where peripheral nerves are mainly involved, we must also consider another very important part of the nervous system.

When it comes to the TMJ and its surrounding structures, landmarks and foramina, we are obliged to consider the impact that the inflammation of the tissues surrounding the TMJ may have on cranial nerves in particular.

Typically inflammation is created by the negative forces of clenching, bruxing and subsequent disc misplacement and deterioration that consequently occur.

The sheer number of symptoms that can be generated by such inflammation and TMJ syndrome generally, are both multifactorial and limitless.

Scattered throughout the small area between the medial-posterior aspect of the mandibular fossa of the TMJ, the lateral aspect of the occipital condyles of the cranium (very close to the general area where the occipital, temporal and sphenoid bone cranial sutures meet), are important foramina, through which some extremely important cranial nerves pass on their way to the equally important structures that they innervate.

There are also foramina that sit either just posterior to, and anteromedial to, the mandibular fossa and TMJ, and also one canal, that are all of interest to us as well (Fig. 9.28).

The foramina that are mainly involved with the potential negative effects of TMJ dysfunction and their surrounding tissue tensions and inflammations, are as follows:

- The jugular foramen that sits between the mandibular fossa and the occipital condyle, and is formed by both the occipital and temporal bones.

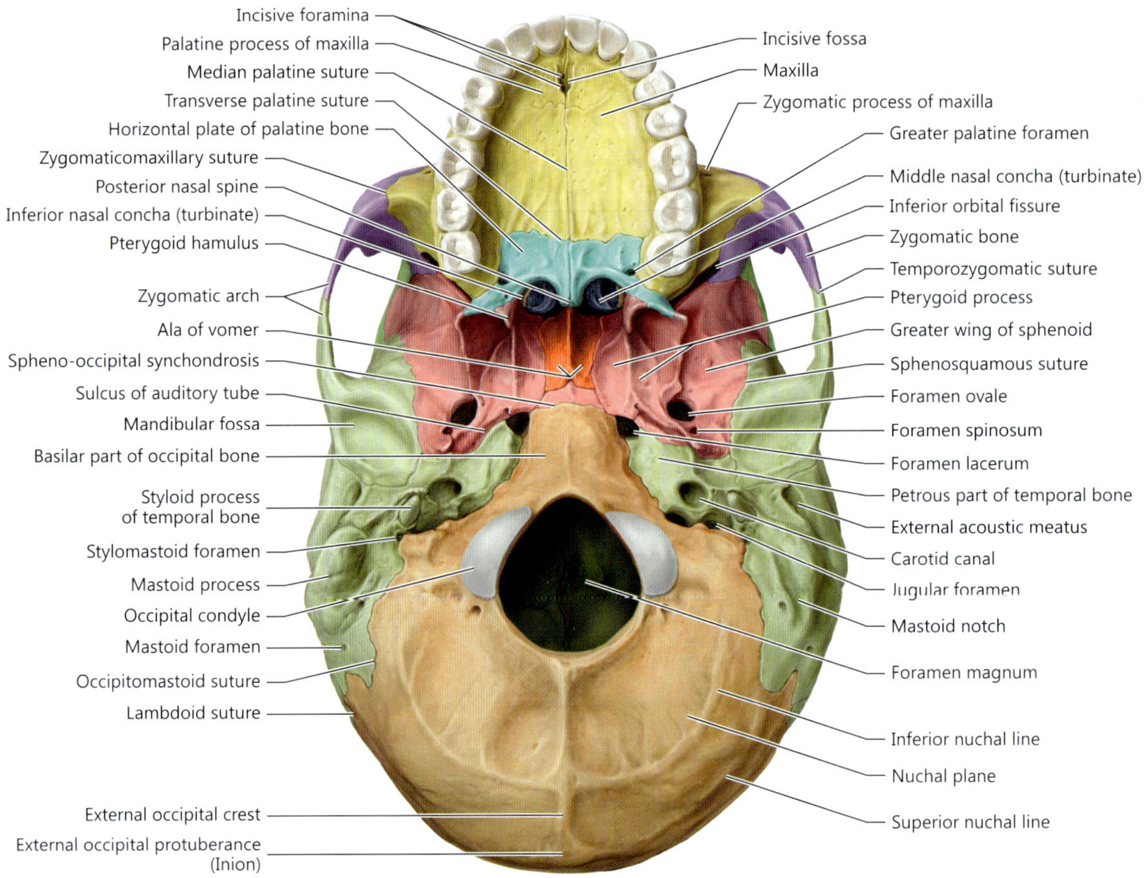

Figure 9.28 This inverted view of the cranium helps to appreciate more clearly, the close proximity that the jugular foramen, stylomastoid foramen, foramen ovale and hypoglossal canal have to the mandibular fossa of the TMJ. A dysfunctional TMJ will create tissue and sometimes bone inflammation potentially affecting the cranial nerves that pass through the foramina and canal adjacent to them. Potentially the function of cranial nerves 5, 7, 9, 10, 11 and 12 may be implicated.

- The stylomastoid foramen that sits posterior to the mandibular fossa in the temporal bone.
- The foramen ovale that sits anteromedial to the mandibular fossa, in the sphenoid bone.
- The canal that is of interest to us is the hypoglossal canal.

The important nerves that pass through the foramina and canal area as follows:

- Jugular foramen → Glossopharyngeal, Vagus and Accessory – 9th, 10th, 11th Cranial nerves.
- Foramen ovale → Trigeminal – 5th Cranial nerve (mandibular division).
- Hypoglossal canal → Hypoglossal – 12th Cranial nerve.
- Stylomastoid foramen → Facial – 7th Cranial nerve (Fig. 9.29).

Functions of the Cranial Nerves and Consequences

Glossopharyngeal → sensory nerve → carries sensory information from the pharynx (initial portion of throat) and some portion of tongue and palate.

Potential symptoms: Swallowing, taste, saliva production, speech conditions.

Comment: Restricting the glossopharyngeal nerve's function, is an insidious imbalance because one of the functions of the Micro system's muscles is to perform swallowing.

This points to the negative spiraling effects that typically occur in the SGS when further poor sensory input leads to poor motor output,

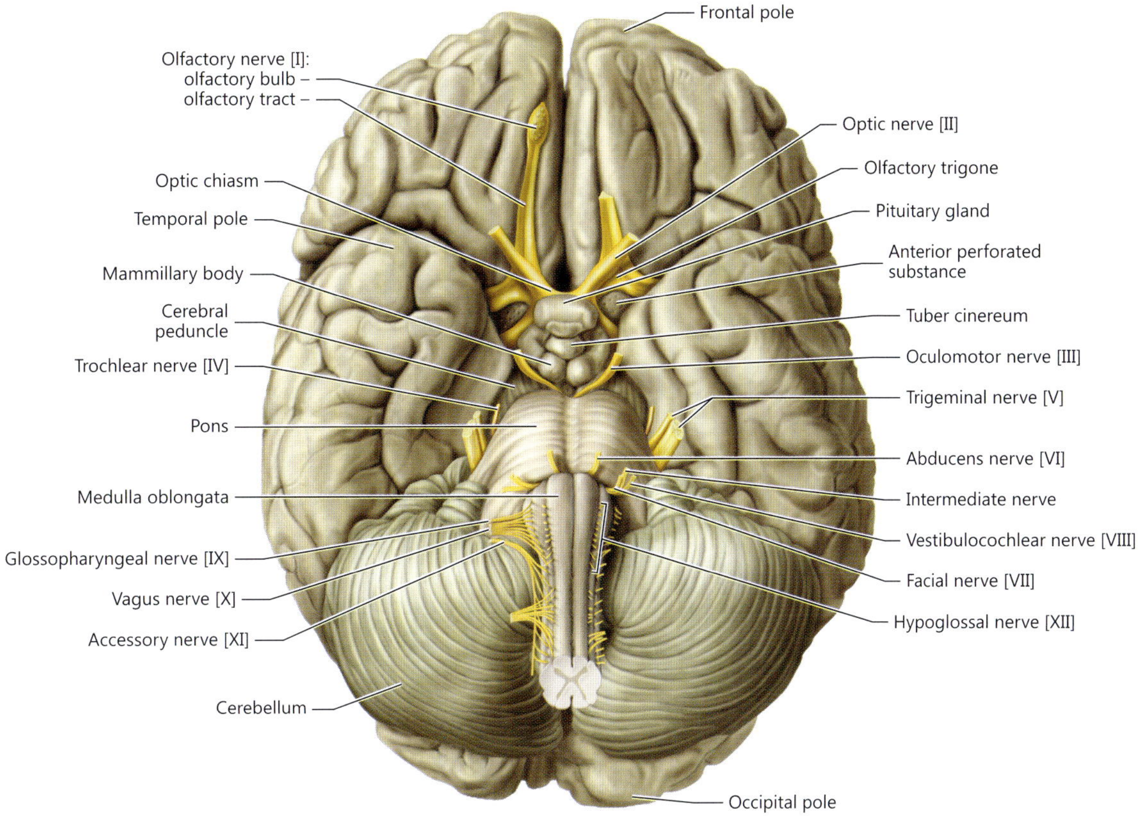

Figure 9.29 Image showing the twelve paired cranial nerves exiting the brain and brainstem. TMJ dysfunction may in particular affect the function of cranial nerves 5, 7, 9, 10, 11 and 12.

and further poor sensory input, and so the spiral into degeneration goes.

In simple terms, the Micro system blocks its own nerve supply and becomes progressively dysfunctional.

Vagus → sensory, motor and autonomic nerve → Sensory functions in the lungs, heart, stomach, liver, spleen, kidneys, intestines, ears, tongue, palate, epiglottis and dura mater in the posterior cranial fossa (housing the cerebellum, medulla oblongata and the pons).

Motor functions in the diaphragm, heart, stomach, pharynx, larynx.

The vagus nerve also shares specialized connections with the first two spinal nerves, the phrenic nerve, accessory nerve, facial nerve, glossopharyngeal nerve, hypoglossal nerve and large sympathetic nerve of the ANS.

Potential symptoms: Almost anything and everything. See all TMJ Procedure indications in Chapter 7.

Comment: The vagus nerve is arguably the most important of all the nerves that can be affected by TMJ dysfunction. It is the predominant neural effector of the parasympathetic nervous system that comprises 75% of all parasympathetic nerve fibers.

If the parasympathetic nerve supply is compromised, the multitude of symptoms that can arise are limitless, as its involvement with the function of the ANS is both intimate and profound.

Furthermore, by compromising the parasympathetic supply to the ANS, a context is established for the sympathetic division of the ANS to become too predominant, leading to amongst other things, an over excitation of the adrenal cortex and an excessive release of is many corrosive hormones such as adrenalin and cortisol.

Specifically, inflammatory signals in peripheral tissues activate afferent signals in the vagus nerve, which are relayed to the hypothalamus and stimulate the release of ACTH.

The vagus nerve may also be involved in an immunological regulatory capacity.

Accessory → Motor nerve → Motor supply to the sternocleidomastoid and trapezius muscles.

Potential symptoms: Neck and shoulder conditions, upper back conditions and headaches. May also interfere with the general "tensegrity" of the Micro system's musculature, predisposing it to TMJ dysfunction.

Comment: The accessory nerve's innervation of the sternocleidomastoid and trapezius muscles, underscores why it is so important to consider adding both the TMJ and Cranial procedures to NST work, as direct interventions for neck and should pain conditions, that have perhaps not responded to DBB1, 2, 3 and the Shoulder procedure alone.

Trigeminal → Sensory and motor nerve → It is divided in three branches that are ophthalmic, maxillary and mandibular branches. The branch most affected with TMJ conditions is the mandibular branch.

Sensory functions: Facial skin in the lower portion of the face, bottom row of teeth, anterior two thirds of the tongue.

Motor functions: Chewing muscles including masseter, medial and lateral pterygoids and the temporalis.

The mandibular branch is also involved with other muscles, namely mylohyoid and digastic anterior belly both of which elevate the hyoid bone during swallowing, and tensor veli palatini that elevates the soft palate to prevent regurgitation, and tensor tympani that stabilizes the malleus bone in the middle ear to dampen sounds.

Potential symptoms: Chewing, biting and swallowing conditions, clenching and bruxing conditions, reflux, facial muscle pain, spasms and neuralgia conditions, tooth pain, taste and speech conditions, and tinnitus. Creates predisposition to TMJ syndrome.

Comment: Restricting the trigeminal nerve's function, is an insidious imbalance because of the many functions of the Micro system's muscles such as chewing, biting and swallowing that are compromised.

This points to the negative spiraling effects that typically occur in the SGS, when further poor sensory input leads to poor motor output, and further poor sensory input, and so the spiral into degeneration goes.

In simple terms, the Micro system blocks its own nerve supply and becomes progressively dysfunctional.

Hypoglossal → motor nerve → controls muscles of the tongue.

Potential symptoms: Speech and swallowing conditions.

Comment: Not unlike the glossopharyngeal nerve in some respects, restricting the hypoglossal nerve's function is an insidious imbalance because two of the functions of the Micro system's muscles are to perform speech and swallowing.

This points to the negative spiraling effects that typically occur in the SGS when further poor sensory input leads to poor motor output, and further poor sensory input, and so the spiral into degeneration goes.

In simple terms, the Micro system blocks its own nerve supply and becomes progressively dysfunctional.

Facial → sensory, motor nerve, parasympathetic → Motor supply responsible for various facial muscle actions related to facial expression, posterior belly of the digastric "hyoid" muscle and the stapedius muscle of the ear.

Sensory supply for providing information about touch to the face, and special taste sensation to the anterior two thirds of the tongue.

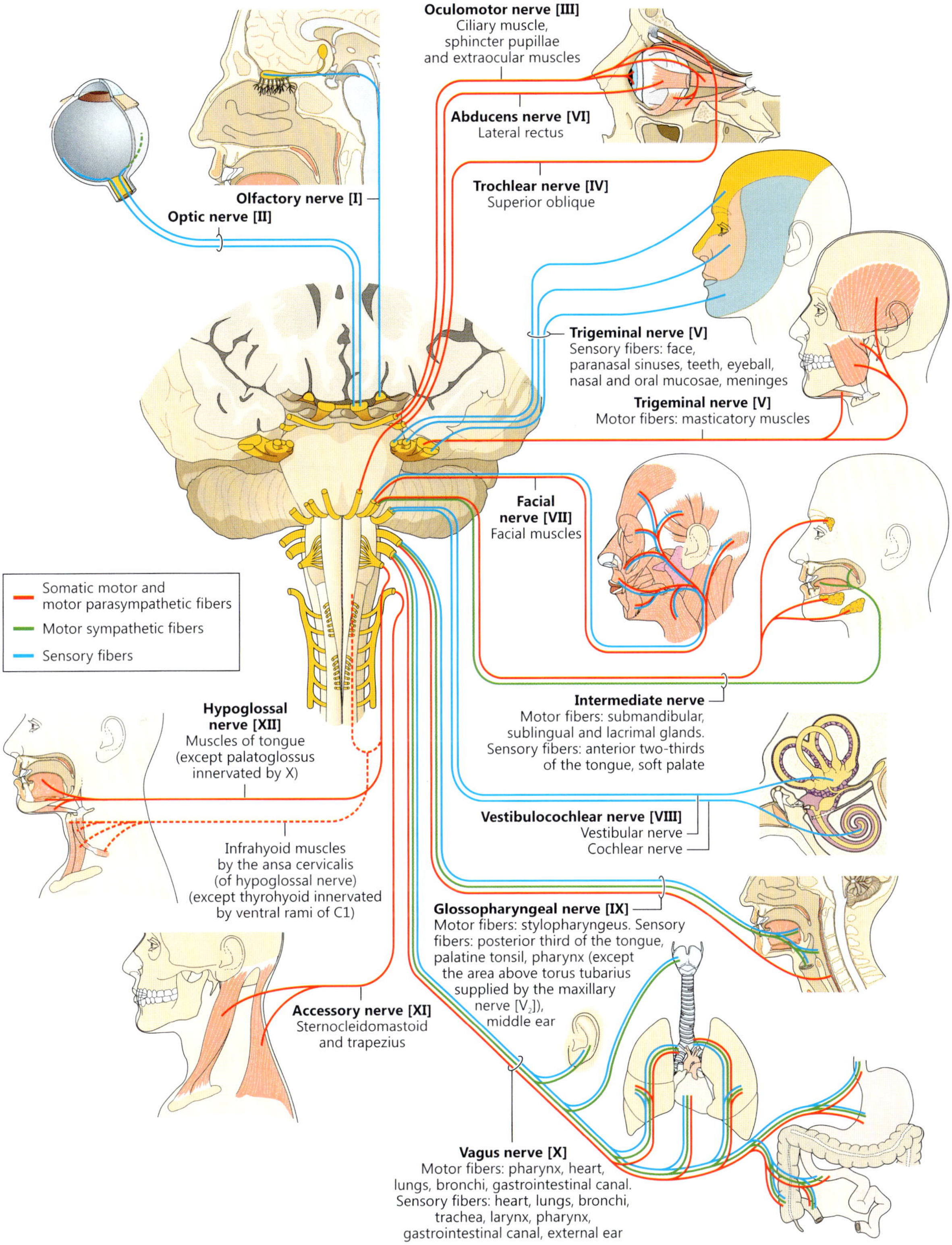

Figure 9.30 The image of the twelve paired cranial nerves and the typical structures they innervate, whilst instructive, could be regarded as a convenient simplification of the actual consequences that may arise when even a single cranial nerve is impinged or interfered with. The complex inter-branching that occurs between the cranial nerves, the overlapping of functions and even compensatory mechanisms that come into play when called upon, should also be considered in the broader context of the effects of the TMJ on neurology.

Parasympathetic supply to many of the glands of the head and neck, including the submandibular and sublingual salivary glands, nasal, palatine and pharyngeal mucous glands and lacrimal glands.

Potential symptoms: Bell's palsy, facial muscle pain and spasms, sagging of facial muscles, tooth pain, tinnitus, hyperacusis, may interfere with the general "tensegrity" of the Micro system's musculature predisposing it to TMJ dysfunction.

Comment: The facial muscles are an important set of Micro system muscles, whose proper balance are significant to the general "tensegrity" of the Micro system itself. In terms of correcting the TMJ and creating sustainability of corrections the facial muscles may be strengthened by exercising the orbicularis oris muscle with an intra oral appliance such as the NST MOJO (Chapter 7 – TMJ Procedure – Stabilization).

Conclusion

When we consider that any one of the six cranial nerves mentioned can lead to a broad variety of symptoms, we are are obliged to regard this part of the body and our clinical treatment thereof with a great deal of significance.

Of particular significance is the vagus for its individual ability to generate almost anything and everything from pain to degenerative diseases.

But in some ways the foregoing information regarding these six nerves, as complex as it sounds, is really an over simplification of the true situation masked for convenience, because the very real subject of cranial nerve "inter-branching" that exists between all cranial nerves must be considered as well.

It's quite feasible therefore to consider, that symptoms to do with the remaining cranial nerves may be generated via the imbalances in the six covered herein. Vision, hearing and balance conditions are typical symptoms that may arise for example (Fig. 9.30).

Nevertheless, as important as the subject of cranial nerve involvement is in TMJ care, there is still one final manner whereby the TMJ and SGS may affect the organism. Specifically, this is via disturbance to the proper output of the pituitary hormones and the all-important, Hypothalamus-Pituitary-Adrenal axis.

HORMONAL FAULTS

To appreciate just how the endocrine system may have anything to do with structure, the spine and muscles, and hence the TMJ and SGS, we need to turn our attention once again to the function of the SRM, covered in detail in Chapter 3 (NST Operating Systems).

Through millions of years of hard fought evolution of the human species, nature has wasted nothing, and at the same time learned to be breathtakingly ingenious in its design, integration and precisely engineered interrelationships with all systems of the body.

Consequently, we see the evidence that many parts of the body, be they muscular, nervous or hormonal play multiple roles ensuring the organism functions and functions optimally according to the directions of its master program – survival.

Indelibly encrypted into the organisms brain and structures, no other emotion is more powerful than survival, and this master emotion exerts its influence though all regulatory systems of the body, ensuring that appropriate checks and balances occur to optimize physiology and homeostasis, for the ultimate cause of preservation of the organism for as long as possible.

The organism literally adapts and adapts until it can no longer do so, and as exhaustion sets in, survival is obliged to stand aside and allow the organism to disintegrate and return to its fundamental elements.

But until that happens life is taking place, and one of the cleverest of all regulating structures that the body has at its disposal, to keep things ticking along, is its pea-sized pituitary gland that sits in its own specially designed

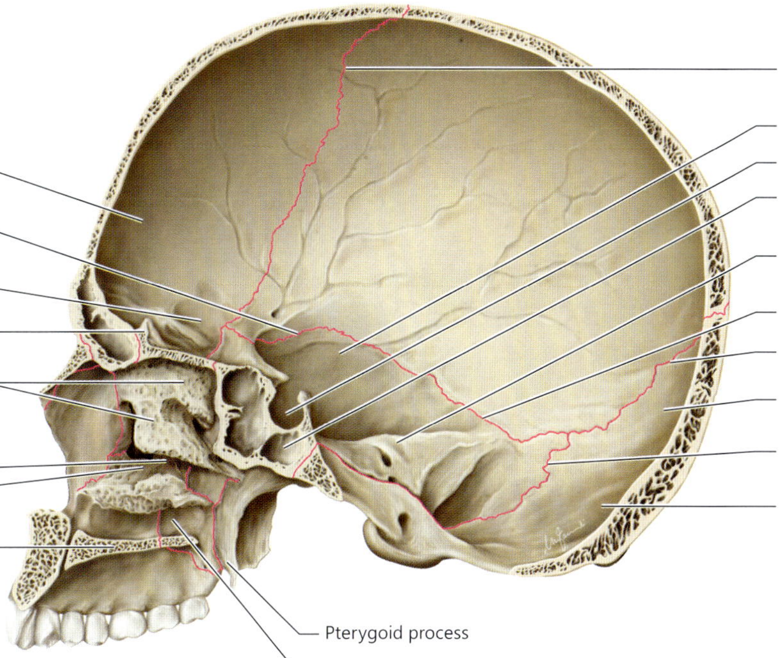

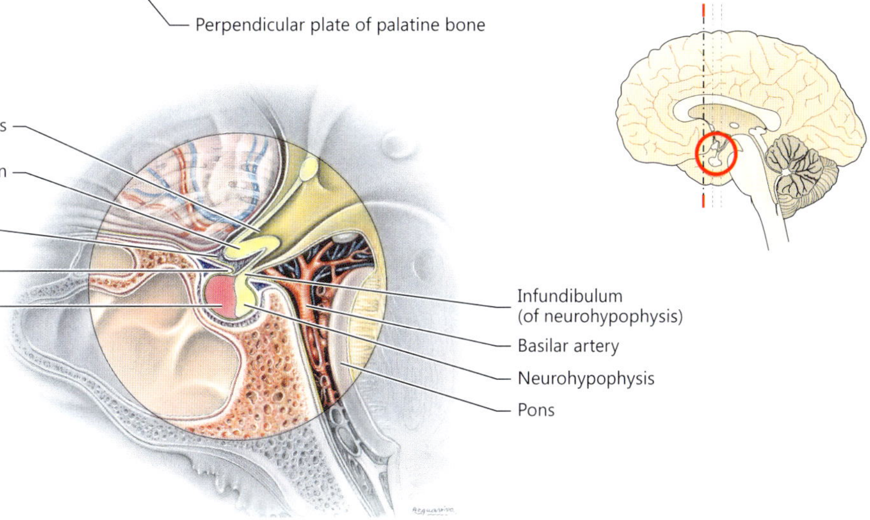

Figure 9.31 The sella turcica is located in the sphenoid bone, just above the junction of the occiput and the sphenoid bones (at the sphenobasilar junction), the cranium's first point of flexion in response to respiration. The rhythmic flexion and extension of the cranium induced by the SRM is crucial in coercing the pituitary gland to release its hormones, in perfect timing with the demands of the autonomic nervous system – ANS.

seat – the sella turcica, strategically formed in the sphenoid bone (Fig. 9.31).

As nature would have it, the sella turcica is located in the sphenoid bone, just above the junction of the occiput and the sphenoid bones, at the sphenobasilar junction, which is the cranium's first point of flexion in response to respiration.

When ongoing inhalation and exhalation take place, the sphenobasilar junction flexes and extends, essentially giving the pituitary gland a free ride, almost in a rhythmic rocking motion.

The ride is made that much smoother by the fact that the pituitary is bathed in cerebrospinal fluid, whose swirling currents, along with

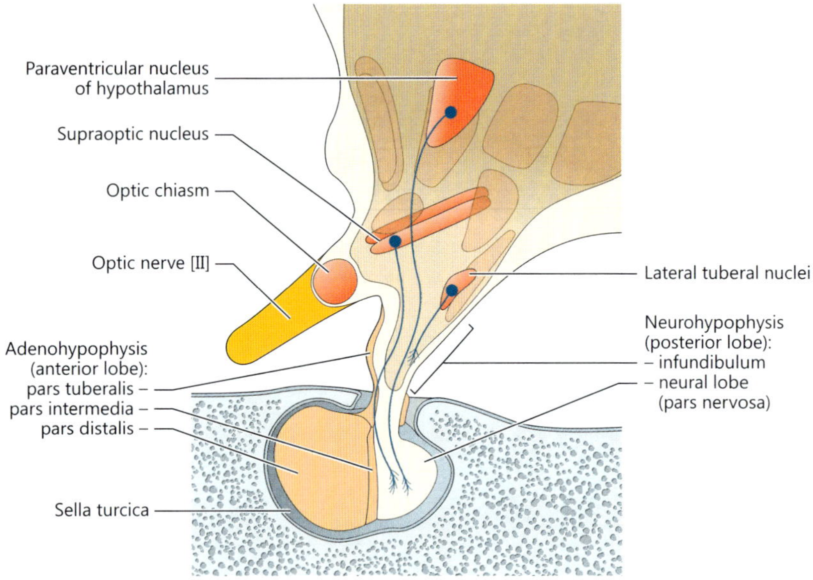

Figure 9.32 The image illustrates the position of the pituitary gland in the sella turcica, and also its close proximity to and therefore relationship with, the hypothalamus whose commands it is beholden to. Of course the limbic system, and its intimate relationship with the hypothalamus, must be considered to complete the simple understanding that the pituitary gland does not operate in isolation.

the rocking motion, coerce it to release its hormones, in timing with respiration, and as needs dictate, based on the chemical directions it receives from the hypothalamus that sits above it, and to which the pituitary is connected by way of a short tube called the infundibidulum (Fig. 9.32).

When cranial respiratory motion is compromised by faults in the diaphragm, pelvic girdle and cranium, including the TMJ, the pituitary gland hormones cannot be released in an optimal or organized sense, as other protective survival mechanisms are activated and prioritized to preserve the organism at all costs.

The pituitary itself has an anterior lobe and a posterior lobe and both release hormones as follows below.

Anterior pituitary

- Thyroid-stimulating hormone (TSH)
- Adrenocorticotropic hormone (ACTH)
- Human growth hormone (HGH)
- Luteinizing hormone (LH)
- Follicle-stimulating hormone (FSH)
- Prolactin (PRL)
- Melanocyte-stimulating hormone (MSH)

Posterior pituitary

- Antidiuretic hormone (ADH)
- Oxytocin (Oxt)

Collectively the hormones perform a variety of very specific tasks in the body and work intimately with the hypothalamus and adrenal glands to regulate our responses to stress, immunity, digestion, energy, sexual responsiveness, mood and emotions.

Conversely, the types of symptoms generated by lack or over secretion of these hormones, is directly related to the functions they are designed to regulate. An inability to conceive is one example. Struggling with weight control another.

Furthermore, the extremely important association that the Hypothalamus, Pituitary gland and Adrenal glands share, is referred to as the HPA Axis, and these powerful neuroendocrine relationships, ultimately couple with the ANS to regulate our physiology, keep homeostasis in check and essentially keep us alive (Fig. 9.33).

That this ingenious regulating system can be compromised by a malfunctioning SRM or SGS simply further highlights the need to ensure that at every session, the TMJ are properly, assessed, corrected and stabilized if necessary.

Targets and function of the pituitary hormones

	TARGET	*FUNCTION*
		HORMONE ANTERIOR LOBE
TSH (Thyroid-stimulating hormone or Thyrotropin)	Thyroid	Stimulates the thyroid gland to secrete its hormone called thyroxine. Regulates body's metabolic rate, heart and digestive functions, muscle control, brain development and maintenance of bones
ACTH (Adrenocorticotropic hormone or Corticotropin)	Adrenal glands	Stimulates the adrenal gland to produce a hormone called cortisol. Converts protein storage to glucose in time of stress. Anti-inflammatory action in injury. Overstimulation leads to blood-sugar problems
HGH (Human growth hormone)	All body cells	Regulates growth, physical development, effects body shape, regulates body fluids, muscle and bone growth, sugar and fat metabolism
LH (Luteinizing hormone)	Ovaries	Triggers ovulation and regulates reproduction function. Can assist testosterone production. Works synergistically with FSH
FSH (Follicle-stimulating hormone)	Testes	Stimulates testes to produce testosterone and sperm. Stimulates the growth of ovarian follicles in women. Works synergistically with LH
PRL (Prolactin)	Breasts	Stimulates the mammary glands of the breasts to produce milk during pregnancy and breastfeeding. Assists male's LH in sperm development
MSH (Melanocyte-stimulating hormone or Melanotropin)	Skin	Stimulates the production and release of melanin for skin darkening. Contributes to sexual arousal
		HORMONE POSTERIOR LOBE
ADH (Antidiuretic hormone)	Kidneys	Controls the blood fluid and mineral levels in the body by affecting water retention in kidneys. Also known as Vasopressin (AVP)
OXT (Oxytocin)	Uterus and breasts	Provokes contractions of uterus in labor and childbirth and stimulates subsequent release of breast milk

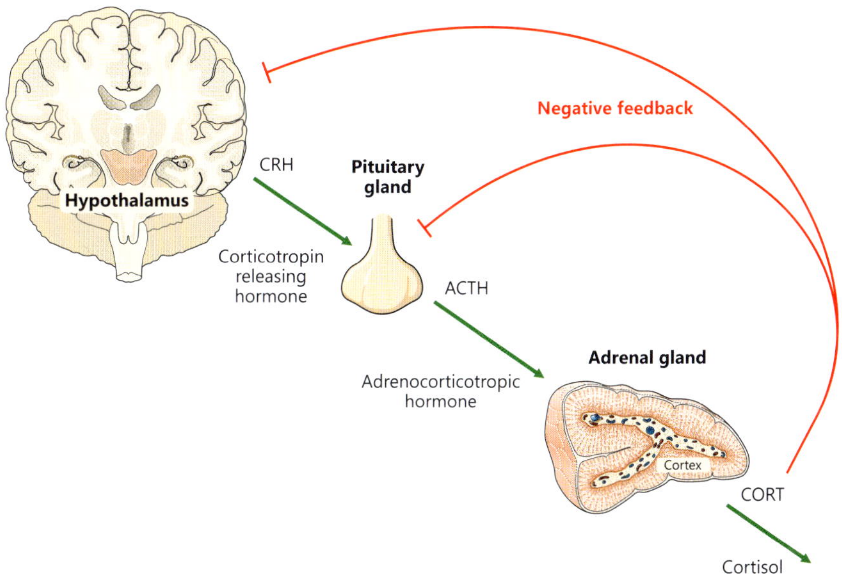

Figure 9.33 Image highlighting the HPA axis which is a powerful neuroendocrine relationship between the Hypothalamus, Pituitary gland and Adrenal glands that serves to regulate our ANS, and thereby maintains homeostasis in the organisms ongoing quest to hold onto life, and indeed flourish.

CONCLUSION

When we consider the totality of outcomes, symptoms and health conditions that mechanical, neurological and hormonal imbalances may provoke, we are indeed reminded of the incredibly significant role that proper TMJ work has in all clinical endeavors, be they NST or otherwise.

In many years of clinical practice dealing with a broad variety of chronic degenerative diseases and conditions, I have found it to be extremely rare "not to find" a TMJ involvement in each and every such condition.

This begs the question: "was TMJ dysfunction the precursor or causative factor for the chronic condition, or was it a consequence of the condition, or perhaps to some extent both?"

Whatever the case, the more chronic the presenting symptom or condition, the greater the likelihood that TMJ dysfunction will be involved, and in most cases the level of chronicity of the condition is mirrored by the level of chronicity in the TMJ.

As perplexing and confounding as it can be, for patients to have gotten themselves into a "perpetual imbalance cycle" with apparently no way out; by the practitioner judiciously following the guidelines of proper assessment, correction and stabilization of the TMJ, combined with their designated prerequisites, excellent clinical results can be achieved.

In most cases within just a few NST sessions, the patient can find themselves on a pain-fee path with new hope that leads to better lifestyle choices going forward.

But there is no doubt that therapy, no matter how effective it is, can only take us so far, and better lifestyle choices in diet, movement and oxygenation in particular, are the most powerful form of medicine that patients can subscribe to, not only to hold the corrections, but indeed to gravitate to a whole new level of health.

Mechanisms of Health and Disease - Life Expectancy 10

"We do not deteriorate because we grow old but we grow old because we deteriorate".

INTRODUCTION

The sun shines warmly on a homeless beggar living in filth and squalor, as it does a king living luxuriously in his palace. It makes no distinctions and nor do the Laws of Nature that govern our health.

They are simply immutable laws, and the smarter we learn to live by them and not against them, the easier our path becomes and the better our health seems to flourish, helping us to live to our genetic potential.

I can choose to drink pure water as part of my daily regime and there will be a consequence as a result of this choice. I can choose to drink pure vodka as part of my daily regime and similarly there will be other consequences.

If we want to be very neutral we can say that neither are good or bad, they are just choices that generate their own particular consequence or outcome.

So functions the mechanism of Nature's Laws!

Of course there are a variety of other such choices. I can choose to eat processed foods or whole foods, I can choose to incorporate adequate healthy movement into my daily lifestyle or I can choose not to.

Maybe I'm a truck driver, taxi driver or office worker and I don't have the chance to walk.

Nothing wrong with that of course, but according to the laws that we are obliged to live by, there will be consequences in the sense that the body will manage what it has been given to manage the best way it can. And lack of movement has significant consequences for our health.

My personal observations and conclusions reached in treating several thousands of individuals, over twenty years using NST alone, and longer using other methods, is that the variety of different maladies from back and neck pain to autoimmune issues, menstrual disorders, digestive disorders, headaches and more, are created unintentionally by the individuals themselves.

Fundamentally, they create their own health issues, by having adopted poor lifestyle choices and maintaining them over many years.

And hence the opening quote.

"We do not deteriorate because we grow old but we grow old because we deteriorate".

Literally it's poor lifestyle choices maintained over many years that cause deterioration, and not simply living more years.

Death is guaranteed, but when and how it arrives (barring accidents, murder and war) is largely determined, I believe, by the way we live our lifestyles.

That our DNA is capable of getting us to 120 years of age, sadly belies the figures we see on most gravestones around the world, which typically have just two digits.

As an example, in my country Australia, the average age adults will die in rounded figures, is at 82 years. In the USA it's 79 years, China 76 years and India 68 years.

That's a whopping one third of our lives gone missing – just chopped off the ledger!

There is nothing "toxic" per se about old age itself, except that it appears to be when most people get sick and die, leading to the belief that we are destined for gloom and doom once we turn the corner after age 65. This is when most people start developing more chronic illnesses and notice a big drop off in energy and capabilities.

I hear it from my patients all the time. "I can't climb the stairs any more without huffing and puffing – I guess I'm just getting old" or "I used to be able to open a jar of marmalade but my hands and wrists have lost their strength – I guess I'm just getting old" or "my husband can't do the gardening any longer so we have to get someone in to help – I guess he's just getting old".

This sorry and energy depleting refrain is devoid any optimism and engorged with resignation. And I dare say at a psychological level the organism is being "trained" into the inevitability of it all.

And why not, everybody else around us is experiencing the same thing, so it must be true. There is no doubt that "herd mentality" can have its downside, and this is a good case in point!

In observing my own patients and countless others over many years, I came to the clear conclusion long ago, that simply accumulating years, in and of itself does not have to mean that chronic illness will be more likely, providing throughout the accumulation of those years we are conducting our lifestyle in a way that is close to nature.

This simply means that we need to design a lifestyle plan that is going to deliver health and not sickness.

DIET, MOVEMENT AND OXYGENATION

And the fundamental pillars of the plan need to be built around the three most important requirements of all living organism – diet, movement and oxygenation.

Diet simply means the type, amount and quality of the food we put into our bodies for processing.

Eating the right foods in the right balance of alkaline and acid, healthy carbohydrates, fats and proteins combined with "systematic under-eating" and "intermittent fasting" can produce marvelous outcomes in generating health and vitality.

But most people's diets are abominable, and it's not for lack of money. For whatever reason modern day man has come to the conclusion that eating whatever is on the supermarket shelves is good and will keep them healthy, but this could not be further from the truth.

Movement, simply means doing an amount of daily motion or exercise that is tailored to your needs, given your current state of health. If you have not been exercising for some time doing a little bit at first is fine providing there's an eye on the future in terms of how much better it can get. And some level of cardiovascular elevation needs to accompany whatever type of exercise.

Walking is the simplest of all exercises and in many respects the "king" of all exercises for the many health benefits it delivers.

Oxygenation is just so vital to completing the trilogy of fundamental activities that can quickly lead to good health.

We live at the bottom of an ocean of oxygen not by chance, but because this is where humans can flourish the best, and take advantage of this most precious gas "oxygen" that is free and in abundance.

Fish live in water and we live on land because this is where both species function best.

We all know that putting a fish on land or a human underwater does not work.

Oxygen fires so many systems in the body and its proper intake in copious amounts is vital to health and longevity. Sadly, breathing deeply for modern day man seems to be a lost function.

Nevertheless, this book is not about diet, movement or oxygenation, so my comments about the three subjects will remain brief.

However, my simple point is, that having the right diet, exercise regime and oxygenation habits takes just a little planning and working out at first, and there are many good guidelines these day's to help out.

But keeping this simple formula working in our lives, ultimately builds good blood, and from good blood comes good tissue, and from good tissue comes good physiology, and from good physiology comes good health and longevity.

Something to think about: every second the body produces 2.5 million new red blood cells, every minute 150 million new blood cells are formed and throughout approximately every 90 days, our complete 5-6 liters of blood will be completely renewed.

It does not have to get more complicated than that.

For years I have encouraged many of my patients to commit to a 90 day program with adjustments to diet, exercise and breathing habits, and for those who have run with it, the results have been life changing.

Sadly however, getting the diet, movement and oxygenation formula out of balance, typically results in bioaccumulation (toxicity) building in body tissues, nerves getting irritated, muscles pulling tight, and circulation becoming impeded.

The organs struggle to function optimally further inhibiting other muscles reflexively, and the organism starts to manifest "symptoms" in a vain attempt to express its inability to interact with its environment in a meaningful way.

Chronic neuromuscular compensations throughout the body is one way of knowing for sure that something is not going well in a person's lifestyle. Be it that diet is out of balance, daily movement habits are inadequate and poor respiration habits are the norm.

Nervous, muscular, immune and circulatory systems of the body suffer the most profoundly.

Having such neuromuscular compensations is akin to driving your car with the handbrake on. Of course it is possible to drive your car with the handbrake on, but in doing so you consume much more fuel, cause wear and tear and eventually cause damage (Fig. 10.1).

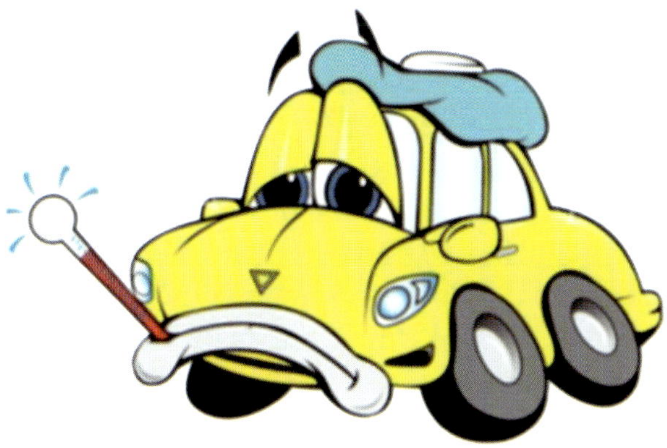

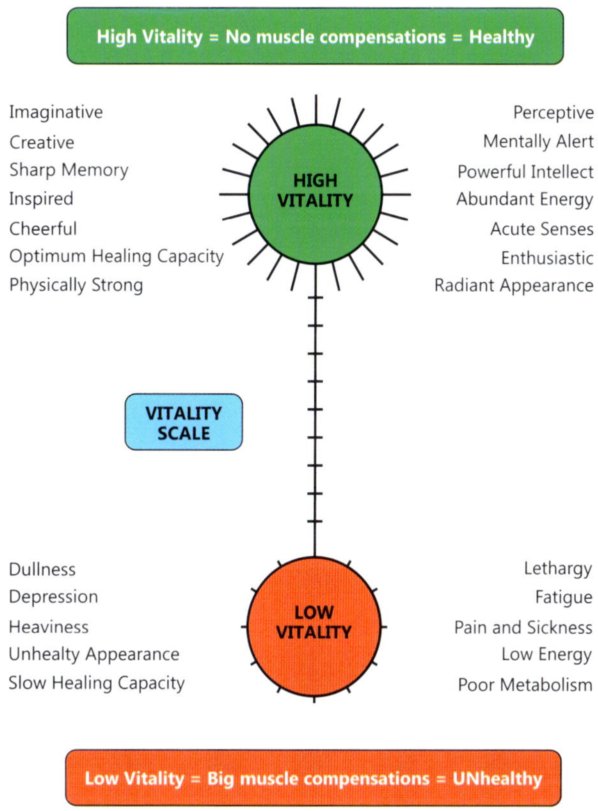

Figure 10.1 The image of the sick and exhausted car simply makes the point that you can drive a car with the handbrake engaged and it will move – but in doing so will consume much more energy than it would without the handbrake on. Leaving the handbrake on too long will result in damage. The parallel for the human body is that muscular compensations are the handbrake and the consequences are the same as for the car. The image of the high and low vitality scale simply shows the particular characteristics that belong to individuals who have high and low vitality. It also makes the point that low vitality is consistent with high neuromuscular compensation within the body. And high vitality is consistent with low or no neuromuscular compensation in the body.

Of course there is always medical intervention and the number of anti-inflammatory medications, pain-killers, antibiotics and other wonder drugs available is increasing by the month.

Again these substances are not evil in and of themselves, but are they the best choice, and is there another or better way to live life without them?

Voltaire, the French philosopher in the 17th century, observed the tendency of his fellow man to misunderstand the Laws of Nature while rushing into life without thinking too much about consequences, and had the following to say on the subject:

"In the first half of our lives we sacrifice our health, to accumulate wealth and in the second half of our lives we sacrifice our wealth to buy back our health".

Voltaire (1694-1778)

The current Dalai Lama when asked what surprised him most about humanity echoed similar sentiments and added a bit more:

"Man...because he sacrifices his health in order to make money.

Then he sacrifices money to recuperate his health.

And then he is so anxious about the future that he does not enjoy the present.

The result being that he does not live in the present or the future.

He lives as if he is never going to die, and then dies having never really lived".

The last part of the Dalai Lama's quote has had significant relevance for me as a health practitioner, because I have literally had to remind hundreds of patients over the years that they are going to die, if they do not abort their current life's trajectory that they are on.

It's something I have referred to for many years now as the "death conversation" and I often have it in one form or another at the very first session. It is in no way disrespectfully delivered, rather a sobering conversation that links the symptoms they present with to the state that their bodies are currently in, and the lifestyle they are currently living. And of course what other options they have at their disposal to plan for the future.

We can talk about Life span but there is also Health span.

Life span is how long we live. Health span is how long we live without illnesses, low energy and frailty.

Many medications can chemically preserve life but there is no quality left.

So, I start by reminding my patient that the process that we are all living is a temporary one, and we can make it more temporary or less temporary by our lifestyle choices. Of course less temporary means that we live longer!

And I use it to bluntly bring awareness into the therapeutic setting, by respectfully reminding the patient that should they continue to embark on the same path they are currently on, that illness and death will come sooner rather than later.

Luckily it has awoken countless individuals over the years, who have adopted better health plans for their life.

In 1991 I was working in a wealthy part of Melbourne, Australia called Caulfield. Caulfield is the suburb in Melbourne that has the highest number of Jewish residents at almost 100%.

If there is one thing that many Jewish people have in common, it is their ability to make money, and I worked with some exceedingly wealthy people.

Wealthy in the sense that they had millions or billions of dollars in property, cash, gold and assets. But when it came to being healthy many of them were "broke" and plagued with one type of chronic illness or another.

I was frequently offered more money for a more "premium" service that would "fix" them quicker or better. But the sad reality for many was, that they had run their health bank account so low that they were literally bankrupt or close to it.

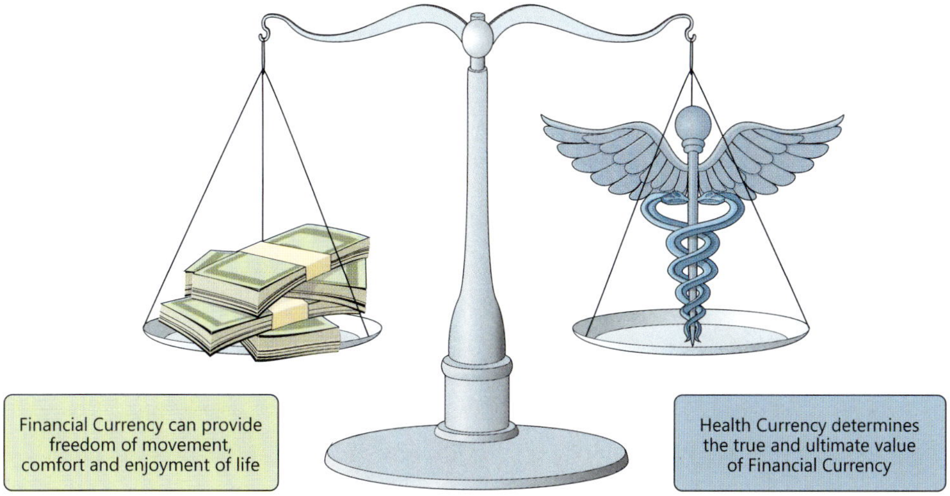

Figure 10.2 We can have all the money in the world, but it will count for little if we do not have the health to use and enjoy what it can bring. Our physical life is temporary and will expire eventually, but how long it lasts can be strongly influenced by how successfully we have accumulated health currency. It is a personal and unavoidable challenge for every individual to get the balance right!

I was personally saddened on many occasions to have to report that there was nothing else I could do to reverse the situation they were in. Degeneration had gone to far.

Many of the experiences that I had in those days, galvanized my thinking to the very sobering reality, that the value of any property, cash, gold or assets is determined by our ability to use it, and our ability to use it is determined by our health.

So I came up with this simple image to help convey the point and it spoke in terms that they could understand (Fig. 10.2).

For those that it was not too late for, I'm glad to say that they made more informed and productive choices from that point on, and started to put some currency back into their health bank accounts.

But it's also at this point that I make the very clear distinction for patients that, even though they may be pain free after two sessions, this does not automatically mean that they are now as healthy as they can be. It just means that the pain has gone and the system is in a better state of balance.

TRIAD OF HEALTH

"The doctor of the future will give no medicine, but instead will interest his patients in the care of the human frame, in diet, and causes and prevention of disease".

Thomas Edison, 1903

To help add meaning and understanding as to why being pain free is not a guarantee of health, I frequently use the Triad of Health model, to provide my patients with a concept or framework, to see themselves objectively through.

And by objectively, I mean, so that they can see how they have most probably created their symptoms and also how to create a new path ahead toward sustainable health.

The Triad of Health is used in many forms of clinical therapy and is particularly common in the world of Applied Kinesiology.

It embraces the concept of "whole person" therapy and shines a light on fundamental areas that a clinician needs to focus her/his work on, to bring about an optimal outcome for the patient.

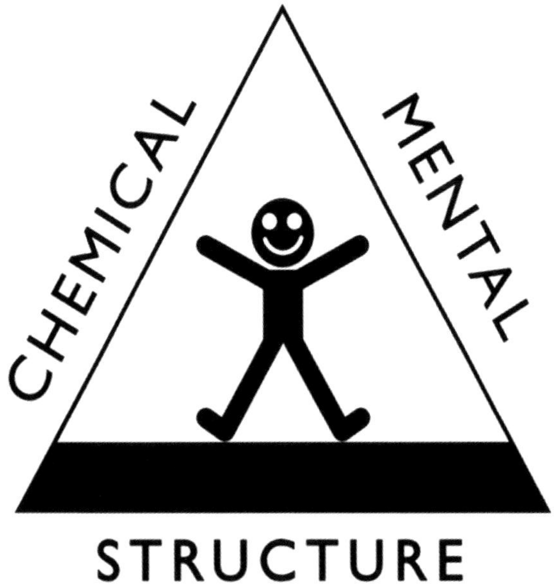

Figure 10.3 Image showing the basic aspects of the Triad of Health. It makes the point, that we can attain sustainable health if we keep three important aspects in balance.

It makes the very clear point that if we want to be balanced and healthy, that we need to attend to and maintain equilibrium between, three important aspects of our bodies. These aspects are structure, chemical and mental.

Structure refers to the spine, skeleton and neuromuscular system and encompasses physical culture.

Chemical refers to toxicity and nutrition, in the tissues and blood and encompasses our nutritional intake, including general diet and specific nutrition such as vitamins, minerals, amino acids, fatty acids, etc.

Mental refers to stress, emotional well-being and the brain, and encompasses everything to do with how we think feel and behave. It includes such things as negative or unresolved emotions (worry, stress, panic, grief and endless other emotions) plus how we manage relaxation and recreation (Fig. 10.3).

The concept is simple and logical to follow and adheres to the basic principle that if any aspect of the Triad of Health is out of balance, the individual will struggle to attain and maintain optimal health and pain and symptoms will manifest.

Furthermore, all aspects are totally interactive, and can therefore support or compromise one another (Fig. 10.4).

Structure can compromise or support both mental and chemical.

Chemical can compromise or support both structure and mental.

Mental can compromise or support both structure and chemical.

So, patients quickly come to understand that although they may have previously not considered it, the other aspects of their life (such as diet and emotions that are arguably, not in balance) may have been contributing to their pain or health condition all along, without them really knowing it.

It's a powerful wake-up call for many, that has several positive outcomes, as individuals suddenly have an answer, and also a plan to work to, that is both logical and capable of delivering tangible results. Frequently, I have found that the effect it has on my patients, is to make them feel relieved, clear, empowered and in control again.

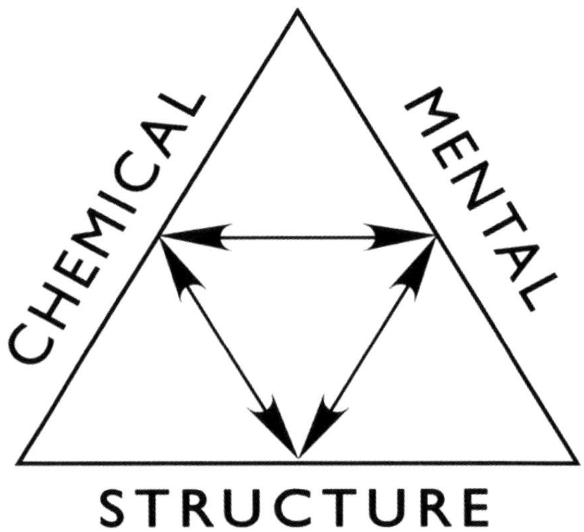

Figure 10.4 The image highlights that all three aspects of the Triad of Health can both compromise or support each other. And all three need to be considered, when either removing symptoms or creating sustainable health.

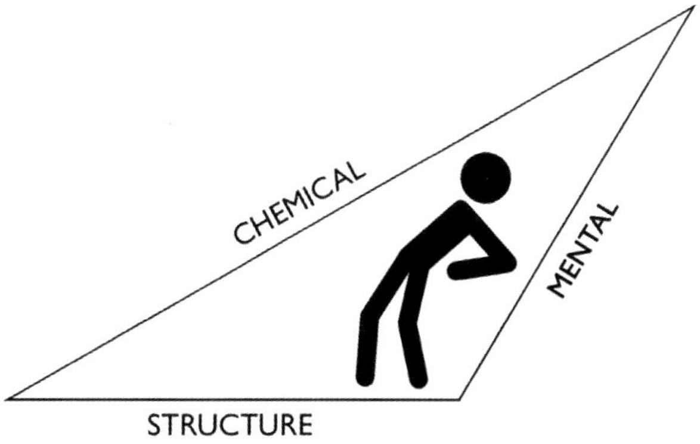

Figure 10.5 Image showing that the source of back pain may be a chemical excess (toxicity) or deficiency (nutrition).

We can think of the Triad of Health working in the following manner.

Using a basic example – we all understand that if a spinal lumbar vertebral body is pushing on a nerve, that back pain will result.

We can conveniently assume that the vertebral body has just rotated by itself (too much sitting perhaps) and that's why it's in the wrong position, irritating the nerve and causing pain.

But what if the patient's nutritional status is so poor, that the muscles supporting the troublesome vertebral body, cannot contract and extend properly, and become too tight or too loose? Or what if there are levels of toxicity in the patient's tissues, that are irritating the same muscles or even the nerve(s) supplying those muscles, and become too tight or too loose?

Excessive sitting may have been the obvious cause, but was the patient already pre-disposed to this happening via nerve and muscle imbalance firstly?

Could chemicals in excess or deficiency, be the cause of back pain? – Absolutely!

I have had countless patients over the years tell me, that ever since they started their specific nutrition program in combination with NST sessions, that their back pain is not returning like it used to (Fig. 10.5).

And we can ponder similarly, about the mental side of the Triad of Health. Is our patient under so much stress at work or home that they are constantly in a state of worry, stress or panic, and could this me irritating a nerve or muscle.

Remember, the same nervous system that performs the raising of an arm, the bending of a leg or the flexing and extending of back muscles, also controls our emotions. There is no disconnection whatsoever, between the central, peripheral, autonomic and enteric nervous systems.

Similarly, over work and lack of rest can play havoc with muscles, causing them to demand higher and higher levels of metabolic support, against an unrelenting barrage of stress, and consequently they become tight or over facilitated.

Could emotions in excess or deficiency, be the cause of back pain? – Absolutely!

Once again, I have had countless patients over the years tell me, that ever since we did the emotional corrections at the end of the NST session, that their back pain is not returning like it used to (Fig. 10.6).

Of course, the Triad of Health concept can then be flipped, to help explain to patients, that if they want to maintain a healthy body, that they will need to do the positive things that keep it balanced – exercise, diet and emotional strategies.

And of course, the principle holds true in the positive. If we exercise, our levels of toxicity are

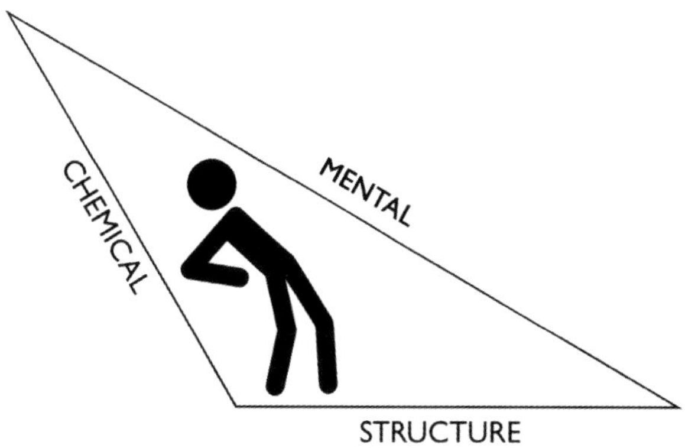

Figure 10.6 Image showing that the source of back pain may be stress or unresolved emotions.

reduced and our nutritional uptake is greatly enhanced.

If we exercise, our energy levels, mood, sleep and productivity are all so much better.

If we have a great diet, and our gut health is optimal (think healthy gut flora and serotonin – dopamine production) then once again our energy levels soar, and our mood and sleep improve and we become more productive.

If we do some intermittent or longer fasting, toxicity reduces and the same beneficial outcomes result.

If we attend to our emotional well-being by focusing on the personal things that work for us, be they relaxation, recreation seeking help when necessary, then the same very positive benefits become apparent.

Clearly attending to all three aspects of the Triad of Health is the optimal approach.

In summary, the Triad of Health is used as blueprint for helping individuals to firstly remove pain, dysfunctional physiological conditions and emotional conditions, and then secondly, to maintain those corrections by building sustainable health via a practical ongoing plan that attends to physical culture, diet and emotional well-being.

I have found working in this way, to be a highly successful approach, in helping individuals shift from a dependency on repetitive clinical intervention, to a state where they can regain and maintain their health, without the need for regular visits NST sessions to correct pain and symptoms, that they continue to re-create.

These additional clinical strategies that can be built around the Triad of Health are very different to NST bodywork, but nevertheless are very much an integral part of NST as well.

They belong to the section of NST I affectionally call "beyond the spine" which refers to a system of principles and techniques, that are taught via an NST training known as, Deep Cures.

Using NST bodywork alone will produce extremely satisfying results for around 85% of patients. Adding the additional strategies not covered in this book will increase that number to about 95%.

GENERAL ADAPTATION SYNDROME

In the previous section on the Triad of Health, we have looked at general concepts around testing and correcting patients in a whole person manner, and by doing so we can significantly help them stave off the typical ravages of old age and premature death, that typically afflict the millions of people who have no knowledge or access to these.

But what happens to the organism when it is left to its own devices to deal with one stressor or another – be it physical, nutritional or emotional?

In this section on the General Adaptation Syndrome, we will get to see more precisely, just how the organism responds to unrelenting stressors, and the ongoing and eventual consequences of this.

The General Adaptation Syndrome or GAS, developed by Dr. Hans Selye in 1936 in Canada, is a well-known model for observing and interpreting the effects of stress on living organisms.

The model has three distinct phases (Fig. 10.7):

- The Alarm Reaction – first exposure to the stressor.
- The Stage of Resistance – the organisms defense to and containment of the stressor.
- The Stage of Exhaustion – the organisms inability to resist further due to exhaustion of all physiological resources.

The three stages were characterized as follows:

- Alarm Reaction – Symptoms - Acute phase of illness.
- Stage of Resistance – Apparently normal – not yet sick but not healthy – low energy.
- Stage of Exhaustion – Chronic illness - Death.

Selye quite randomly discovered the GAS while he was working in his laboratory at the

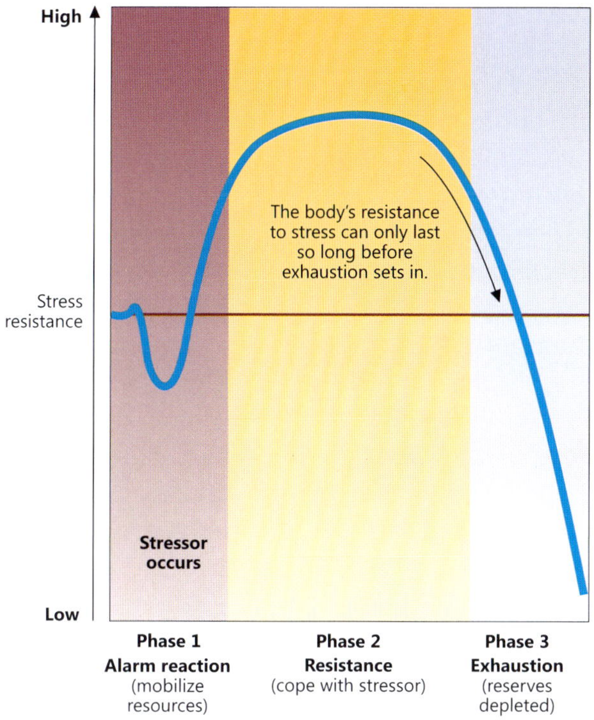

Figure 10.7 The General Adaptation Syndrome – GAS, popularized by Dr. Hans Selye in 1936 is as relevant today as it was then. Observing the alarm, resistance and exhaustion responses of the organism, provides us with a practical and logical template, through which we can see life, health, adaptation, sickness and death, in a more pragmatic manner.

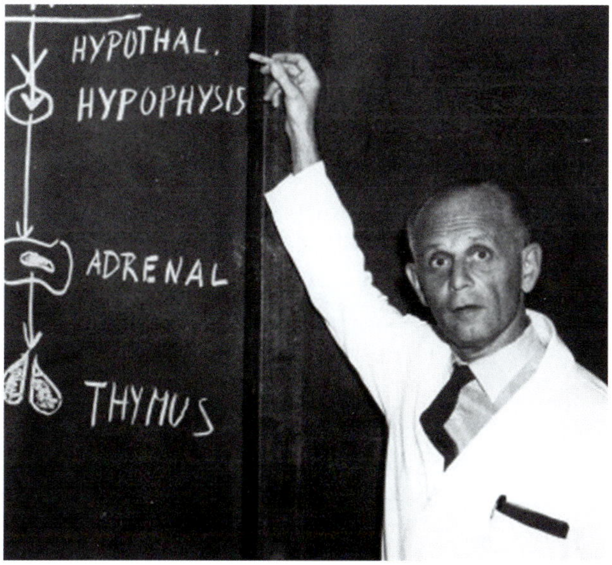

Figure 10.8 Photograph of Dr. Hans Selye explaining the mechanisms behind his GAS theory. Note the referencing of the hypothalamic-pituitary-adrenal axis on the chalkboard.

McGill University in Montreal, Quebec in Canada (Fig. 10.8).

He had been conducting tests into the effects of ovarian hormones on the glandular system of rats. He discovered that injections of the ovarian hormone stimulated the outer tissue of the adrenal glands of the rats, causing deterioration of the thymus glands and producing ulcers and other symptoms.

Selye wrote many books and papers on the subject of stress, perhaps his most renowned book was The Stress of Life.

I have heard and read many accounts of Selye's work and about some of his experiments and a popular one is as follows.

Apparently, Selye exposed rats to various types of other "stressful" experiments as well and placing them in a refrigerated space was one such experiment.

On being placed into the refrigerated space, at first the rats huddled in a corner and over time developed the symptoms of common cold with watery nose and eyes, sweating, heart rate increase, etc. – Alarm Reaction.

However, to Selye's surprise; leaving the rats in the cold space did not kill them, and after some days, they started moving around, eating food and seemingly behaving normally. Over time their coats thickened and they had apparently adapted to their environment. But there was also evidence of increased glucose, fat and protein concentration in blood, attesting to the overworking adrenal cortex in converting protein to energy – Stage of Resistance.

After several further days without warning the rats returned to huddling in the corner and the initial symptoms returned, but this time they became worse, due to lack of any meaningful immune response. Chronic conditions such as cardiovascular disease, diabetes, intestinal bleeding all preceded death – Stage of Exhaustion.

In subsequent experiments, at various stages, Selye would remove certain rats from the refrigerated space, kill and dissect them, analyzing their contents chemically and biochemically.

What he discovered is that the Hypothalamus-Pituitary-Adrenal – HPA axis, discussed in the previous chapter, was the coping mechanism the animals were utilizing to survive, and the results were quite outstanding, in the sense that the adrenals, thymus, intestines and liver were clearly involved in the defense, inflammatory and degenerative processes.

Even in the Alarm Phase, symptoms that became apparent often resembled Addison's Disease - adrenal insufficiency, with the subsequent slow onset of symptoms such as weakness, abdominal pain and weight loss.

I believe that many of the patients who come to see us with chronic aches and pain, blood pressure conditions, diabetes, digestive conditions, autoimmune conditions, kidney and liver conditions, reproductive conditions, etc., are more than likely in the Stage of Resistance already.

Living in the Stage of Resistance is physiologically and energetically speaking an "expensive" place to live because costs are high. The organism is alive but at what cost?

Surely if researchers are right and our DNA is capable of permitting the human organism to live 120 years, have we not found a reason as to how and why we are not achieving that, because we are simply using more than our allotted "day's worth of energy" to survive in every single day?

For example, if at the age of 40 years, less than ideal lifestyle practices (poor diet, poor detox habits, poor movement habits, poor breathing habits) lead to excessive levels of bioaccumulation (toxin) in the body's tissues, inflammation of tissues in muscles and joints and general aches and pains, it's highly likely that the body's protective systems are already at work.

This can mean that our heart and adrenals are performing an amount of work in every day, that they could normally spread out over two or three days. The net cost is that we deplete our physiologic reserves. The math becomes easy to perform.

If after 40 years of age, we have 80 years of life potential remaining from a DNA perspective, and we use two days worth of that energy in every passing day, we are not going to reach 120 years. It will be more like 80 years.

This is a simple example but it highlights just how important it is to keep our lifestyle on the right trajectory.

CONCLUSION

As wonderful as NST is, and as miraculous as the results can be, it is not a guarantee of radiant health.

I sometimes have to convince my patients that simply being pain free does not mean they are suddenly optimally healthy. And doing NST to them every day of their lives will not make them healthy either.

In other words, the absence of pain is not a confirmation of health, but a starting point from which better health may be garnered or attained.

However, if the absence of pain does anything well, it's that it quickly engenders hope.

To see a patient who has felt trapped by their health condition, suddenly be free of its burdensome pain and tyranny, quickly breeds new found hope and energy follows.

The relationship between hope and energy is astounding. As hope fades with all of its negative entrails, so too does energy. As hope returns with all limitless optimism, so too does energy.

"Grasp the opportunity" I tell my patients, and make some meaningful life changes while you are feeling good. Humans often have a tendency to go into "cruise mode" when they are no longer in pain, and then start looking for the next hedonistic experience and forget that there's still a lot of work to do. This can amount to a missed opportunity in the end.

Using the Triad of Health is a great blueprint to follow, and having simple pillars around which to build it can help. Remember to give it 90 days so that the full benefits of healthier blood are starting to manifest.

Some general steps to follow, that always produce great results are:

- Detoxification of the body – intermittent fasting or longer fasting.
- Change the diet to a more alkaline one based around 70/% fruit and vegetables and 30% healthy carbohydrates, fats and proteins. Add specific nutrition as well – vitamins, minerals, amino acids, fatty acids, etc.
- Daily exercise, suited to your current state of health, and if possible, for at least 30 minutes. If not daily then no less than 5 times a week. Make sure that the exercise produces cardiovascular elevation.
- Incorporate adequate relaxation and recreation into your lifestyle, so that you frequently have the feeling of being refreshed.
- Limit the usage of pharmaceutical medications. Use only when absolutely necessary.
- Use surgical intervention only if there is no other way. If you are going to use surgery, make sure that you are as healthy as possible beforehand, as this will ensure optimal recuperation.

Of course, in combination with the above steps, remember to seek professional help from a structural, nutritional or emotional therapist to regain any lost integration, if necessary.

Humans are not robots, and we therefore are never ever really fully integrated. In fact, we go in and out of integration all the time.

Nevertheless, long periods of integration are the goal, as these relate to good physiology, good health and longevity.

Short periods of dis-integration are normal and even desirable at times, as they function as a reset.

Long periods of dis-integration are not ideal, and are typically associated with poor physiology, poor health and premature death.

Ultimately, the process of life is temporary for all of us, but it can become "more temporary" or "less temporary" depending on how we manage our lifestyles.

To last the journey, we alone, simply must take control of our health!

Bibliography

Anastasi G, Gaudio E, Tacchetti C (Eds.), Mtui E (Editor English Edition). Human Anatomy – Atlas. Milan, Italy: Edi.Ermes, 2019.

Black D. Inner Wisdom. Springville, UT, USA: Tapestry Press, 1990.

Bragg PC. The Miracle of Fasting. Santa Barbara, CA, USA: Health Science, 1979.

Cramer GD, Darby SA. Basic and Clinical Anatomy of the Spine, Spinal Cord and ANS. 2nd ed. Oxford, UK: Elsevier Mosby, 1995-2005.

DeJarnette MB. The Philosophy, Art and Science of Sacro Occipital Technic. 3rd ed. Nebraska City, NE, USA: Major Bertrand DeJarnette, 1967.

Gallo F, Vincenzi H. Energy Tapping. Oakland, CA, USA: New Harbinger Productions, Inc., 2000.

Gerber R. Vibrational Medicine. Santa Fe, NM, USA: Bear & Company, 1988.

Johnson D. Discovering the Art of Effective Counselling. Bendigo, Victoria, Australia: Ampersand, 2003.

Juhan D. Job's Body. Barrytown, NY, USA: Station Hill Press, Inc., 1987.

Keown D. The Spark in the Machine – How the Science of Acupuncture Explains the Mysteries of Western Medicine. London, UK and PA, USA: Singing Dragon – an imprint of Jessica Kingsley Publishers, 2014.

Krebs C, Brown J. A Revolutionary Way Of Thinking. Melbourne, Australia: Hill of Content Publishing Company Pty. Ltd., 1998.

Maciocia G. The Foundations of Chinese Medicine. UK: Churchill Livingstone, 1989-1991.

Magoun HI. Osteopathy in the Cranial Field. 3rd ed. Kirksville, MO, USA: The Journal Printing Company, 1976.

Myers TW. Anatomy Trains. Australia, Canada, United Kingdom, USA: Churchill Livingstone, 2001.

Netter FH. The CIBA Collection of Medical Illustrations, Volume 1: Nervous System, Part 1, Anatomy and Physiology. Summit, NJ, USA: CIBA, 1983.

Niel-Asher S. The Concise Book of Trigger Points. 3rd ed. Nutbourne, UK: Lotus Publishing and Berkeley, CA, USA: North Atlantic Books, 2008.

O'Hanlon B, Weiner-Davis M. In Search of Solutions: A new direction in psychotherapy. New York, NY, USA: W.W. Norton & Company, 2003.

Panksepp J. Affective Neuroscience: The Foundations of Human and Animal Emotions. New York, NY, USA: Oxford University Press, 1998.

Pert C. Molecules of Emotion. New York, NY, USA: Simon & Schuster, 1997.

Reed-Gach M, Marco C. Acu-Yoga. Tokyo, Japan and New York, NY, USA: Japan Publications, Inc., 1991.

Richter P, Hebgen E. Trigger points and Muscle Chains in Osteopathy. Stuttgart, Germany: Georg Thieme Verlag, 2009.

Rosenberg S. Accessing the Healing Power of the Vagus Nerve. Berkeley, CA, USA: North Atlantic Books, 2016.

Selye H. The Stress of Life. New York, NY, USA: McGraw - Hill Book Company, 1984.

Sinclair I. You can overcome Asthma. Ryde, NSW, Australia: Ian Sinclair, 1993.

Upledger JE, Vredevoogd JD. Craniosacral Therapy. Seattle, WA, USA: Eastland Press, 1983.

Upledger JE. Craniosacral Therapy II: Beyond the Dura. Seattle, WA, USA: Eastland Press, 1987-1995.

Walther DS. Applied Kinesiology: Synopsis. Pueblo, CO, USA: Systems DC, 1988-2000.

Walther DS. Applied Kinesiology, Volume 2: The Stomatognathic System. Pueblo, CO, USA: Systems DC, 1983.

Williams W, Dyson B. Gray's Anatomy. 37th ed. Edinburgh, UK: Churchill Livingstone, Longman Group UK Limited, 1989.